**THIRD EDITION**

# COMMUNICATION AND COMMUNICATION DISORDERS

## A Clinical Introduction

**ELENA PLANTE**
*The University of Arizona*

**PÉLAGIE M. BEESON**
*The University of Arizona*

Boston   New York   San Francisco
Mexico City   Montreal   Toronto   London   Madrid   Munich   Paris
Hong Kong   Singapore   Tokyo   Cape Town   Sydney

**Executive Editor and Publisher:** *Stephen D. Dragin*
**Editorial Assistant:** *Katie Heimsoth*
**Marketing Manager:** *Kris Ellis-Levy*
**Production Editor:** *Gregory Erb*
**Editorial Production Service:** *Walsh & Associates, Inc.*
**Composition Buyer:** *Linda Cox*
**Manufacturing Buyer:** *Linda Morris*
**Electronic Composition:** *Publishers' Design and Production Services, Inc.*
**Cover Designer:** *Kristina Mose-Libon*
**Photo Researcher:** *Annie Pickert*

For related titles and support materials, visit our online catalog at www.ablongman.com.

Between the time website information is gathered and then published, it is not unusual for some sites to have closed. Also, the transcription of URLs can result in typographical errors. The publisher would appreciate notification where these errors occur so that they may be corrected in subsequent editions.

*Library of Congress Cataloging-in-Publication Data*

Plante, Elena
  Communication and communication disorders : a clinical introduction /
Elena M. Plante, Pélagie M. Beeson. — 3rd ed.
    p. ; cm.
  Includes bibliographical references and indexes.
  ISBN-13: 978-0-205-53209-4 (alk. paper)
  ISBN-10: 0-205-53209-8 (alk. paper)
  1. Communicative disorders. 2. Communicative disorders in children.  I.
Beeson, Pelagie M. II. Title.
  [DNLM: 1. Communication Disorders. 2. Communication. 3. Speech-Language
Pathology.   WL 340.2 P713c   2008]

  RC423.P59 2008
  616.85'5—dc22

                                                          2007019129

Printed in the United States of America

10  9  8  7  6          RRD-VA      11

Photo credits appear on page 368, which constitutes an extension of the copyright page.

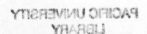

*To our patients, who continued to teach us.*

*To our colleagues, who share our enjoyment of the science and service of our profession.*

*To our students, for whom this book is written.*

# CONTENTS

# PREFACE

When we wrote the first edition of this textbook, our intention was to speak to the undergraduate student encountering speech, language, and hearing sciences for the first time. We strove to present concepts in a simplified, yet interesting manner. As we taught from the textbook and received feedback from others who used the book, we found that we hit the mark in many respects. In our second, and now third, edition, we directed our efforts to improve the book by further simplifying difficult concepts, removing excess detail, and strengthening the clarity of writing. We updated the content for this edition to make it consistent with the science and evidence-based practice of the professions, and also included a number of new figures to further illustrate the concepts. We have retained a clinical emphasis by introducing communication disorders with case examples, which have proved effective in bringing the reality of the disorders and the professions to life. We added to the lists of books from the popular literature that include personal accounts of individuals with communication disorders as the reading of this literature has been a valuable and enjoyable activity for our students.

As we worked to revise this text, we were again impressed by the breadth and depth of our field. We continue to be fascinated by the science within and outside our field and within and outside our respective specialties. We feel fortunate to have the privilege to work with such impressive and delightful colleagues in the process. We thank Drs. Julie Barkmeier-Kraemer, Anne Marie Tharpe, Linda Norrix, Fran Harris, and Ted Glattke for their excellent chapters and gracious responses to our editorial efforts to unify the tone of the book. We also appreciate the generous contributions of other faculty in our department, including Brad Story and Barbara Cone-Wesson, who help to keep our knowledge current. We appreciate the time and input of reviewers Patricia Mercaitis (University of Massachusetts, Amherst) and Benjamin Munson (University of Minnesota). Finally, we are indebted to Susan Carnahan, who provided significant editorial assistance for this revision, and we thank Celeste Connelly, HyeSuk Cho, and Jennifer Parrott for their support as well. We are pleased with the outcome of the combined efforts in this editorial process, and look forward to teaching from this new edition. We hope that others will find it useful as well.

Elena Plante, PhD, CCC-SLP

Elena Plante completed bachelor's and master's degrees in speech-language pathology at Loyola College in Maryland. Before returning for a doctorate at The University of Arizona, she worked as a speech-language pathologist in the public schools. Since completing her doctorate and postdoctoral studies, she has been on the faculty in the Department of Speech, Language, and Hearing Sciences at The University of Arizona, where she is currently the department head. Her research has focused on the behavioral and biological correlates of developmental language disorders using magnetic resonance imaging (MRI). Subsequent investigations have used electrophysiology and functional magnetic resonance imaging to examine the brain correlates of language processing. In addition, she has produced a series of studies that focus on identification of developmental language disorders in both children and adults through diagnostic testing. She has received support for her research from grants from the National Institutes of Health. Dr. Plante is a Fellow of the American Speech-Language-Hearing Association. She is on the editorial board of the *Journal of Communication Disorders* and has reviewed for several of ASHA's professional journals. She speaks regularly at national and international conferences on the topic of developmental language disorders.

Pélagie M. Beeson, PhD, CCC-SLP

Pélagie (Pagie) Maritz Beeson received her bachelor's and master's degrees in speech-language pathology from the University of Kansas. She began her clinical career at a community speech and language center in Fairbanks, Alaska, where she provided service to a diverse clinical population. She later completed her doctoral work at The University of Arizona, where she also served as the coordinator of the American Indian Professional Training Program in Speech-Language Pathology and Audiology. Currently, Dr. Beeson is Associate Professor in the Department of Speech, Language, and Hearing Sciences at The University of Arizona. Her research and clinical work have been devoted to neurogenic communication disorders in adults, with a particular emphasis on the nature and treatment of aphasia, alexia, and agraphia, as well as the cognitive mechanisms and neural substrates of written language. She is board certified in Adult Neurogenic Communication Disorders by the Academy of Neurologic Communication Disorders and Sciences. Dr. Beeson is a Fellow of the American Speech-Language-Hearing Association and previously served as coordinator of the ASHA Special Interest Division 2:

Neurophysiology and Neurogenic Speech and Language Disorders. She frequently speaks at national and international conferences on the topic of acquired language impairments in adults.

### Julie Barkmeier-Kraemer, PhD

Julie Barkmeier-Kraemer has extensive experience with assessment and treatment of voice and swallowing problems. She worked in the Department of Otolaryngology–Head and Neck Surgery at the University of Iowa Hospitals and Clinics for seven years, where she initiated assessment and treatment services for patients with dysphagia. In addition, she coordinated and participated in the assessment and treatment of individuals with voice problems in the University of Iowa Voice Clinic. After completing her doctoral studies in speech pathology at the University of Iowa in 1994, Dr. Barkmeier-Kraemer worked as a research scientist in the Voice and Speech Section of the National Institute on Deafness and Other Communication Disorders (NIDCD). Her research at the NIDCD focused on modulation of laryngeal reflexes during swallowing as well as studying long-term effects of botulinum toxin treatment on adductor-type spasmodic dysphonia. Her clinical work while at the NIDCD focused on assessment and treatment of neurogenic voice disorder. Dr. Barkmeier-Kraemer is presently a member of the faculty in the Department of Speech, Language, and Hearing Sciences at The University of Arizona.

### Theodore J. Glattke, PhD

Theodore Glattke is a professor in the Department of Speech, Language, and Hearing Sciences and the Department of Surgery at The University of Arizona. He is the former editor of the *Journal of Speech and Hearing Research* and the *Journal of Communication Disorders*. He provides clinical services in the areas of diagnostic audiology and electronystagmography and conducts research in noninvasive physiological measures of the auditory system. Dr. Glattke is a recipient of the Honors of the American Speech-Language-Hearing Association, as well as the American Academy of Audiology's Distinguished Achievement Award.

### Frances P. Harris, PhD

Fran Harris is a practicing audiologist and an adjunct faculty member in the Department of Speech, Langauge, and Hearing Sciences at The University of Arizona. Among her areas of specialization is rehabilitation of hearing loss in adults. She has also conducted research on the characteristics of otoacoustic emissions in adults with and without impaired hearing. She has over twenty years of experience as a clinical audiologist, primarily in an outpatient medical facility and in a state institution for individuals with developmental disabilities. She has published numerous scientific articles, primarily on otoacoustic emissions, and has presented her work nationally and internationally.

## Linda Norrix, PhD

Linda Norrix is a clinically certified audiologist who has experience assessing and treating individuals with hearing disorders. She worked at McFarland Clinic in Ames, Iowa, for two and a half years, where she performed audiologic testing and provided rehabilitation services that included counseling and the fitting of hearing aids. After completing her doctoral studies at The University of Arizona in 1995, she worked as a research scientist in the Center for Neurogenic Communication Disorders at The University of Arizona. Her research involved examining the perception and integration of auditory and visual speech. During her doctoral and postdoctoral studies she has continued to assess and treat individuals with hearing disorders at several medical facilities in Tucson. Dr. Norrix is currently a clinical faculty member in the Department of Speech, Language, and Hearing Sciences at The University of Arizona.

## Anne Marie Tharpe, PhD

Anne Marie Tharpe is a professor of audiology in the Department of Hearing and Speech Sciences of the Vanderbilt Wilkerson Center for Otolaryngology and Communication Sciences. Dr. Tharpe has been involved in the provision of clinical audiology services to the pediatric population for over twenty years. In addition to clinical service, her activities include research, writing, and teaching. Her clinical and research work has focused on assessment and management of children with hearing loss, normal auditory development in infants, and practitioner education. She has published numerous scientific articles and pediatric audiology chapters and has coauthored a text on amplification in children.

# CHAPTER ONE

# INTRODUCTION TO THE PROFESSIONS OF AUDIOLOGY AND SPEECH-LANGUAGE PATHOLOGY

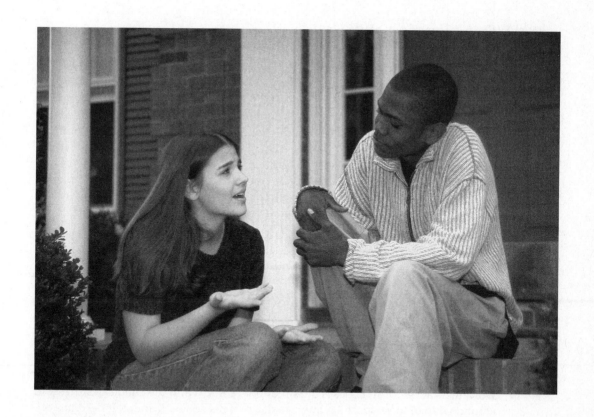

■ ■ ■ ■ ■

## PREVIEW

Communication is so pervasive in daily life that we often take it for granted until something goes awry. In this chapter, we introduce the field of communication disorders, starting with an examination of normal communication in its various modalities. Then we profile six individuals with disorders of speech, language, or hearing. These cases represent the estimated 10 percent of the population for whom communication is impaired. We can begin to understand the bases of these disorders by determining where normal communication breaks down and what components are affected. Later chapters examine these components in detail. For individuals with communication impairments, the services of a speech-language pathologist or audiologist may improve the quality of daily life. We will meet some professionals in communication disorders and sciences who shared their perspectives regarding the rewards and challenges of this broad, dynamic field.

## NORMAL COMMUNICATION

Human communication embodies a rich tapestry of information conveyed through vocalizations, gesture, and emotional expression. **Communication** includes all means by which information is transmitted between a sender and a receiver. By this definition, we know that animals communicate through posture, movement, facial gestures, scent, and sound production. Humans are unique among animals in that we have a highly developed system of symbolic communication that we call language. Language may be spoken, written, or signed. Although all forms of language are used to communicate ideas, not all forms of communication involve language. A look at some real-life examples of normal communication illustrates that language and communication can take many forms.

> A father carried his 18-month-old son in his arms as he walked through a public park. His son leaned over and excitedly extended his arms into the air. "Da?" the toddler asked. The father looked to see what had caught his son's attention. A young girl from the neighborhood was walking her dog. "Oh, it's the dog," the father replied. "Da! Da!" the son exclaimed while bouncing with excitement.

With the use of a "word," tone of voice, and gestures, this child begins to use language to ask a question, make a statement, and indicate interest. The father accepts the attempt at language as meaningful, even though it only approximates a word in its adult form. He uses the situational context and the child's gestures and emotional tone to support his interpretation of his son's meaning. It becomes obvious that the child is using "da" to mean "dog" and not "dad," "man," "teddy," "juice," or any of the other things that the child has previously referred to with those sounds. The father's response to his son turns an attempt at a word into a

**Communication develops before children use their first words.**

conversation, to the enjoyment of both. As we will see, not all attempts at communication are equally successful, leading to frustrating or amusing outcomes.

> Sixty-four students sat in a lecture room, one without any windows, listening to their professor. The professor, who had taught the course nine times before, was lecturing: "One might question, uh, the relational meanings that best describe, uh, the language of young children. Remember, that Bloom said (as well as Sinclair or, uh, and Bowerman) that it is possible to put in a logical order the kind of language experiences that occur in a typical order of uh, let us say, emergence."

Some of the poorest communication may occur in the classroom. This lecturer's convoluted word order and interruptions due to word-retrieval pauses interfere with effective communication. The meaning of the subject matter may be difficult for the students to comprehend even without the teacher's poor sentence formulation. The students may not be listening for many reasons, such as the instructor's poor narrative, fatigue from a previous activity, worry about upcoming exams, or even the lack of ventilation in the closed room.

Effective use of language for communication is not restricted to spoken words. Humans have developed additional modalities for the expression of language. One alternative—signed language—developed because some individuals are unable to perceive spoken language.

A 23-year-old student was hired as a classroom interpreter for a 19-year-old deaf engineering student. The interpreter had limited knowledge of the highly technical content of the engineering classes. To this was added the strain of translating the heavily accented and often broken English spoken by the foreign-born instructor into the completely different grammatical organization of American Sign Language. The engineering student, who had a pronounced playful streak, took advantage of these conditions for a little good-natured ribbing of the interpreter. At one point during the lecture, a fly was buzzing around the interpreter's nose and she swatted at it in mid-sentence. The student leaned forward, looked at her face, and repeated the gesture of swatting the fly, indicating he needed the gesture defined as if it were a word he did not know. When the interpreter ignored this obviously facetious request, the student only repeated it with increasing elaborations of the gesture and facial expressions. This act finally caught the attention of the instructor, who stopped the class to see if there was a problem. Thoroughly embarrassed, the student and interpreter finished out the lecture without further interruption.

American Sign Language (ASL) uses a system of manual gestures instead of spoken words to convey information. In ASL, hand and arm positions, facial expressions, and movements in space are used to express vocabulary and a grammatical structure that is different from that of spoken and written languages. Like other languages, however, ASL has a normal developmental sequence when learned as a first language. No matter the mode, all languages can be used for a variety of purposes, such as communicating, thinking, and learning, as well as teasing and humor.

Like signed language, written language also uses the visual modality for communication. The written word may be used to inform, entertain, and regulate behavior.

While traveling in the Southwest, we had occasion to visit the Ghost Ranch Living Museum in northern New Mexico. This center includes a small zoo of animals indigenous to the area. Signs in front of each animal habitat warned, "Do not feed your fingers to the animals. Their diet is carefully monitored."

This clever sign conveyed at least two important pieces of information. The animals should not be fed by visitors, and the animals will bite. In this case, the sign's creator used a humorous approach and indirect language to convey the message. The tone of the written message was particularly appropriate to the setting, because it contributed to, rather than detracted from, the visitor's enjoyment of the sights. The use of indirect language is interesting here, in that much more is communicated than the words actually denote.

Normal communication encompasses verbal and nonverbal elements that, in combination, are used for a variety of purposes. Communication is successful when information is accurately transmitted from a sender to a receiver. Some aspects of communication, such as nonverbal elements, are not always intentional. Sometimes our bodies "give us away." For example, our posture, facial expression, and voice quality may combine to indicate fatigue, even when we may be very interested in the topic of conversation. Other elements, such as proximity and gestures, communicate the speaker's status, attitudes, and emotions.

Many of the nonverbal elements of communication are culturally regulated. For example, Anglo listeners tend to provide speakers with periodic feedback by nods and vocalized signals of affirmation. A Navajo audience provides fewer overt signs of attention; polite listeners attend unobtrusively. Some cultures maintain constant eye contact when listening; for others, "staring" at a speaker is rude. Even an aspect such as the length of pauses between utterances is culturally determined. Although this may seem to be a minor component of communication, violations may have profound effects on the listener. A speaker who pauses too long may appear to be withholding and unsociable. One whose pauses are too short may appear to be impertinent and domineering. Most individuals are able to monitor and use an ongoing stream of nonverbal information for effective communication. However, these nonverbal skills are dependent on normal development and can be disrupted in some individuals, just as spoken and written communication can be impaired.

## SIX INDIVIDUALS WITH COMMUNICATION IMPAIRMENT

The need or desire to communicate permeates much of our daily lives, including family interactions, written and spoken communication at work, and recreational activities. However, those who have difficulty making themselves understood or understanding others may be acutely aware of their limitations. There may be no better way for us to appreciate the impact of these limitations than to review a few stories of individuals with various forms of communication impairment.

As we will see from these cases, communication disorders affect both children and adults, and they do not discriminate by ethnic background or economic status.

*Beth Feldman*[1] is a 23-year-old student teacher who developed bilateral vocal nodules, or bumps on both vocal folds. By noon every day, she lost her voice completely, making it impossible to control the twenty-six children in her fourth-grade class. She was warned by her supervising teacher that she could not continue as a student teacher if she did not improve her voice. Seeking help in a voice clinic at a

---

[1]We have changed the names of all individuals whose communication disorders are described in this book. In some instances the case history reflects a blend of several individuals.

university hospital, she was told that she speaks at the bottom of her pitch range, clears her throat excessively, speaks with excessive effort and tension in her throat, and exhibits other behaviors detrimental to her vocal health. She consulted two ear-nose-throat physicians (otolaryngologists), and each of them told her that she had two small nodules, one on each vocal fold, that were not big enough to explain the severe voice symptoms she was experiencing. Both doctors recommended voice therapy. Ms. Feldman's initial attempts to schedule voice therapy were thwarted by her busy schedule, and her voice problem persisted. After several months, she finally made a return visit to the voice clinic to initiate treatment.

*Jim Fields* is a 43-year-old promoter who arranges concerts for rock and pop musicians. His wife convinced him to have his hearing checked when she noticed that he was no longer hearing his wristwatch alarm and that he had difficulty understanding her over the telephone. His evaluation by an audiologist revealed a moderate to severe hearing loss of the type associated with noise exposure. The audiologist learned that his history of noise exposure dated back to his teens, when he sang in a band that in his words "substituted volume for talent." Since that time, there had been many occasions when he remembered leaving a performance with "ringing ears" or "fuzzy hearing." The audiologist explained the relationship between exposure to loud sound and the hearing loss Mr. Fields was experiencing. Mr. Fields now uses hearing protection when exposed to loud music (and other loud sounds) to slow further hearing loss. He has enrolled in a speechreading (lipreading) course to help compensate for the loss he already has. In addition, he returns for regular hearing checkups to monitor his hearing acuity. He has elected to forgo a hearing aid at this time but understands that one may become a necessity in the future.

*Rodolfo Torres*, age 13 months, was evaluated by team members of a university oro-facial disorders clinic. He was born in Mexico with a bilateral cleft lip and palate. Although his cleft lip was surgically repaired within a few weeks of his birth, the roof of his mouth remained unrepaired. All of his attempts at speech (or when crying) appeared to come out of his nose because there was open coupling of his oral and nasal cavities. He was examined by the plastic surgeon, who recommended immediate surgery to finish the repair of his cleft. Both the audiologist and otolaryngologist found that the boy had a middle-ear infection, which was producing a moderate hearing loss. The speech-language pathologist felt that Rodolfo exhibited normal language comprehension for Spanish and urged early surgical intervention in an attempt to minimize his severe hypernasality. The boy and his mother were going to live temporarily with his uncle in Tucson so the first stage of surgery could be started. The social worker on the team met with the speech-language pathologist, the plastic surgeon, and the boy's mother to arrange the temporary move from Mexico to Tucson.

*Bruce Murrich*, age 69, is a retired executive who suffered a stroke in his sleep, awakening with right-side paralysis (hemiplegia) and aphasia (loss of language). His sudden symptoms transformed him from a golf-playing, fun-loving, Arizona retiree to a man unable to speak except for occasional profanity. He was also powerless to move his right arm and leg. He and his wife reacted initially to the severe disability with disbelief and denial, hoping that, with proper medical attention, his symptoms would go away after a few days. After several weeks of continued impairment, Mr. and Mrs. Murrich sought rehabilitation, which included speech-language pathology services. Mr. Murrich began receiving weekly group therapy and individual speech-language therapy (plus physical and occupational therapies). His wife attended a weekly spouse group and received individual counseling from a social worker in the rehabilitation center. As Mr. Murrich's language improved to the point where he could communicate many thoughts and needs in two- to three-word utterances, with less profanity, his overall spirits improved dramatically. Now, about eighteen months after the stroke, both Mr. Murrich and his wife seem to accept the relative permanence of his disability.

*Devon Douglas* was 17 when we first met him. His younger brother, Andrew, had been diagnosed with a rare genetic condition that often affects development. The family lived in a remote town and traveled two hours each way to reach our clinic, where they participated in a research study to determine the communication aspects of Andrew's genetic disorder. When we first talked with the boy's mother, she had more concerns about Devon than about Andrew, despite the fact that Devon did not have the genetic disorder. She reported that he had struggled throughout his entire school history to maintain average grades. Over the years, starting when Devon was in second grade, she had repeatedly asked the school system to evaluate him for a learning disability. Each time, the school staff indicated that they did not see Devon as having any educational handicaps, so he was never evaluated. Devon himself reported that teachers had told him that he was lazy and could do better if he tried. His mother was now worried that school was such a struggle that he might drop out. As part of our research program, we were able to evaluate Devon's cognitive and linguistic skills. Testing revealed that his general cognitive abilities were in the high-average range. However, he had great difficulty putting together grammatically correct sentences, following spoken directions, and understanding what he read. In fact, his overall language skills were quite weak. At age 17, we diagnosed a language-based learning disability for the first time in this young man's life.

*Mary Kim* is an animated 5-year-old girl, the youngest of three children. When she was born, in a Los Angeles hospital, she appeared healthy in all respects, but she did not pass the newborn hearing screening test. Her parents were referred to an audiologist, who performed a diagnostic evaluation and confirmed that Mary had a profound hearing loss in both ears. Her parents were taken by surprise, because their two other children had normal hearing; however, Mary's mother had both a sister and an aunt who were deaf from birth. The deafness appeared to be a hereditary form of hearing loss affecting the development and function of an inner-ear structure, the cochlea. The audiologist fitted Mary with hearing aids on both ears and referred the family to an otolaryngologist to consider a cochlear implant, which would provide electrical stimulation to the auditory nerve. The Kims learned that Mary was a good candidate for implantation, and when she reached 12 months of age, surgery was performed. Six weeks later, when the implant was activated, Mary heard sound for the first time. She reacted initially by crying but then became alert to sound, widening her eyes and turning her head in response. The family received speech-language therapy for the next several years to enhance Mary's communication development. Now, at age 5, she is starting kindergarten, and her speech and language development are within the range of typically developing children. The

Kims informed the classroom teacher that Mary has difficulty hearing in noisy environments so that accommodations could be made to maximize Mary's opportunity for success.

These cases represent the diverse challenges encountered by professionals in the field of communication disorders. Each case demonstrates how difficulty in just one aspect of communication can affect daily life. Ms. Feldman's vocal nodules had a direct impact on her effectiveness as a teacher. Mr. Murrich's stroke forever altered both his and his wife's plans for retired life. Devon's difficulty with language had a significant effect on his school success.

## CLASSIFICATION OF COMMUNICATION DISORDERS

Communication requires the transmission of information from one person to another. Breakdown in communication may be understood by looking at the components of this process. Information can be conveyed through tone of voice, facial expression, posture, and gestures. Language, however, is the medium of choice when we wish to communicate specific ideas. **Language** involves the coding of meaning into a system of symbols that are recognized by members of the community. All the words that we use or comprehend comprise our mental dictionary, or lexicon. Like a printed dictionary, the lexicon is more than a mere list of words. It stores information about word forms, including the pronunciation of each entry, and each word has a unique meaning.

The ways in which sounds are combined into words and words into sentences is arbitrarily determined across languages. For example, in English, words may begin with an "st" combination, as in *stairs,* but not with a "ts" combination. However, Navajo includes words that start with the "ts" combination (e.g., *tseí,* meaning "rock"). These conventions within each language are completely arbitrary; English speakers are capable of producing the "ts" combination (e.g., "its") but do not use it at the beginning of words. Other rules govern how words are combined into sentences. These rules of grammar are also arbitrary and vary among languages. For example, English requires the use of nouns or pronouns to specify the subject of a sentence (e.g., "I am hungry"). In Spanish, however, the pronoun can by dropped from the sentence without any resulting confusion (e.g., "Tengo hambre"). We will explore the nature of language in more detail in Chapter 7.

For most individuals, language is communicated from speaker to listener through an oral-to-auditory pathway. The voice, tongue, lips, and other oral structures are used to produce the individual sounds of language that we recognized as **speech**. Mere changes in tongue placement result in different speech sounds, such as "k" versus "t." The addition of vocal fold vibrations changes the "t" to a "d." In other languages, additional manipulations of sound contribute to speech. For example, Chinese is considered a tonal language because changes in the pitch of the voice distinguish specific speech sounds. Our vocal mechanism also allows us to vary the pitch and loudness of speech to convey emotion and emphasis. For the average person, these aspects come together seamlessly to produce a smooth flow of words. We introduce the physical structures that support speech in Chapter 2 and follow with a discussion of the sounds of speech in Chapter 3.

Because of their knowledge of the anatomy and physiology of the oral structures, speech-language pathologists have become involved with treatment of certain disorders that do not strictly involve communication, such as swallowing and feeding. Swallowing disorders often result from the same types of disease processes and acquired damage that can affect communication. Evaluation and treatment of swallowing have become prominent components of many speech-language pathologists' work in health-related settings. Swallowing disorders are discussed in Chapter 6.

Spoken language is received by the listener through the aural modality. This requires an intact auditory system. **Hearing** includes the awareness of sound, the ability to distinguish among sounds, and the ability to process sounds that occur at a rapid rate. These abilities are essential for decoding speech. By hearing spoken language, we learn the rules of our native language, the sounds of speech, and even the accent and intonation patterns that characterize our regional dialect. When we speak, we monitor our own production and modify or correct our speech as we talk. The mechanisms of hearing, on which all these skills rely, are addressed in Chapter 10.

## Impairments of Speech

When impairments of communication occur, they typically involve a breakdown in one or more of the elements involved in speech, language, or hearing (see Table 1.1). Impairments of speech may occur in children and adults. These disorders may include aspects of **articulation**, or the way the sounds of words are produced. Some disorders of sound production are caused by structural abnormality, as in

**TABLE 1.1  Definitions of the Central Components of Human Communication (Speech, Language, and Hearing) and Examples of Communication Disorders**

|  | DEFINITION | EXAMPLES OF COMMUNICATION DISORDERS |
|---|---|---|
| Speech | Sound production for communication | Disorders of speech sound production <br> Voice disorders <br> Stuttering |
| Language | A symbol system for communication | Delayed language development <br> Autism <br> Aphasia |
| Hearing | The perception of sound | Sensorineural hearing loss <br> Conductive hearing loss |

the case of a child born with a cleft palate. For Rodolfo, his cleft palate altered the oral structures needed for speech articulation. If left unrepaired, he would have little chance to develop normal speech. In other children, developmental articulation disorders may appear without a known cause. Children may also exhibit phonological disorders, in which they are able to produce all speech sounds but combine them incorrectly in words. In many instances, children simply are slow to develop speech. All of these developmental speech sound disorders may appear without a known cause. In other cases, the disorder may be associated with a more generalized delay in development, such as occurs with mental retardation. Speech sound disorders also may be acquired following accident or disease. Disorders of speech sounds are reviewed in Chapter 4.

Speech disorders may involve the vocal mechanism. **Voice** disorders may alter the pitch, quality, or loudness of the voice, as discussed in Chapter 6. We saw in the case of Ms. Feldman that poor speaking practices may lead to physical changes in the vocal mechanism that interfere with speech over time. In her case, the voice disorder affected her professional life. In other cases, an overly breathy or harsh vocal quality or a loss of voicing may signal a health concern that requires immediate medical intervention.

Finally, a disorder of speech may involve the fluency of speech production. Fluency disorders occur when the normal, smooth flow of speech becomes interrupted, as in the case of stuttering. The individual may struggle to produce words or sentences that come effortlessly for others. For most individuals, stuttering begins during childhood, and many of those who stutter eventually overcome this difficulty. Those with persistent stuttering have to monitor their fluency indefinitely. Stuttering and other fluency disorders are reviewed in Chapter 5.

## Impairments of Language

Language impairments may include conditions that emerge as a child develops. These *developmental* language disorders may first appear during childhood but can persist into adulthood. This was the case with Devon, who had difficulties throughout his school years. In contrast to developmental language disorders, acquired language disorders occur when an individual suffers an injury or disease that causes a loss of language skills. Mr. Murrich's case presents one type of *acquired* language disorder called aphasia. Although acquired language disorders can occur at any time during life, the majority of individuals with acquired language disorders are adults. Disorders involving language skills in children and adults are discussed in Chapters 8 and 9, respectively.

## Impairments of Hearing

Disorders of hearing may arise from factors that block the conduction of sound into and through the hearing mechanism. These are referred to as **conductive hearing loss**. A common cause of conductive hearing loss in young children is fluid in the middle ear due to infection, which is called otitis media. In contrast to conductive hearing loss, **sensorineural hearing loss** refers to a hearing loss caused by disease of the inner ear or the neural transmission of sound. In Mr. Fields's case, exposure to loud sound over time produced a sensorineural hearing loss. In other cases, an individual may be born with a sensorineural hearing loss, as in the case of Mary. Although we classify hearing disorders as conductive or sensorineural, in some instances, hearing loss may involve a mix of both types. We will discuss disorders of hearing in Chapters 11 and 12.

### Personal Stories about Communication Disorders

The cases described above provide a brief look at the way in which speech, language, and hearing might be impaired at various times throughout the lifespan. It is evident that some communication impairments can have a dramatic impact on the lives of affected individuals and their families. In fact, quite a few people have written personal accounts of living with a disease or disability that affected their ability to communicate. Such stories are part of a relatively new literary genre called *pathography*. Pathography refers to literature that recounts personal stories about living with illness or disability. Such accounts include autobiographies and biographies written by the affected individual, family members, friends, physicians, or other involved parties. Although most pathographies are written as first- or third-person accounts of true events, a few are fictionalized stories. As various communication disorders are introduced in this book, we will list relevant pathographies at the end of the chapter under the heading **Readings from the Popular Literature**. These books often capture the true impact of communication disorders, whether they are present from birth or acquired later in life. Although the impairment may not be the primary focus of the story, considerable insight is offered in the context of these personal stories. For example, Mitch Albom's best seller *Tuesdays with Morrie* recounts the lessons that he learned from his former college professor, whose health was declining due to the progressive neurological disease known as amyotrophic lateral sclerosis (ALS or Lou Gehrig's disease). In the midst of this poignant story about appreciating life, the reader gains insight into the consequences of reduced motor control for the production of speech and for swallowing. We agree with the observation made by our colleague Raymond Kent, who wrote, "What often emerges in the best of these accounts is not preoccupation with a bad turn of life, but rather lessons in endurance, resourcefulness, and overcoming" (Kent, 1998, p. 22). Professionals in the field of communication disorders have the privilege of sharing in these life lessons with their clients or patients, and they often find it one of the most rewarding aspects of their work.

## CAREERS IN COMMUNICATION DISORDERS

As described in the cases at the beginning of this chapter, most individuals with speech, language, or hearing disorders can improve their communication. The professionals who provide services for the remediation of communication disorders are **speech-language pathologists** and **audiologists**. These clinical professionals rely on the information provided by research conducted by speech scientists, language scientists, and hearing scientists, as well as researchers in related fields. The professional organization for speech-language pathologists, audiologists, and scientists in the field of communication disorders is the American Speech-Language-Hearing Association (ASHA). In 1989, ASHA passed a resolution that specified the fields of **audiology** and **speech-language pathology** as separate professions. Because of the common concern for human communication impairments and the historical association of these two professions, most individuals in either field have some knowledge and training in areas served primarily by the other. At the present time, for example, the undergraduate curriculum in most training institutiones does not divide the two fields. Instead, students specialize in one or the other profession as part of their graduate school training. Although there are some job opportunities for individuals with less training (see Chapter 13 for a discussion of support personnel), a graduate degree is required for certification as an audiologist or speech-language pathologist.

An aspiring speech-language pathologist must complete all graduate courses (typically thirty-six credit hours) for a master's degree (or its equivalent) awarded from an accredited program. In addition, ASHA requires a minimum of 400 hours of supervised clinical practicum. Upon completion of the degree, a clinical fellowship year is completed under the supervision of a certified speech-language pathologist (ASHA, 2005). In the field of audiology, clinical certification require-

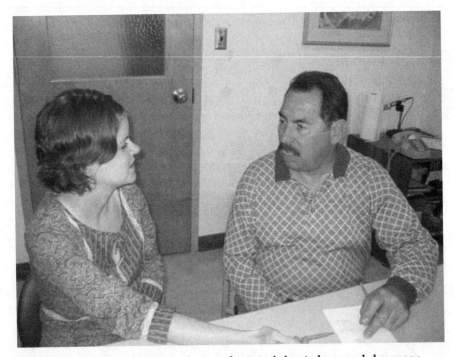

In addition to academic preparation, students training to be speech-language pathologists or audiologists conduct a supervised clinical practicum with individuals with communication disorders.

ments have recently transitioned from a master's degree to a clinical doctorate, the AuD. This degree requires a minimum of seventy-five credit hours of postbaccalaureate study, with the clinical fellowship training enfolded into this training. In 2012, a clinical doctorate will be the entry-level degree for audiologists. In addition to academic and clinical training, both audiologists and speech-language pathologists must pass a national certification examination before becoming certified to work independently in any of a wide variety of clinical settings.

Those who are interested in pursuing a research career or an academic position in a college or university typically obtain doctoral-level training for a Doctor of Philosophy (PhD) or a Doctor of Science (ScD) degree. A primary goal of doctoral-level training is to prepare individuals to conduct independent research. Such research may focus on normal aspects of speech, language, and hearing or on the nature and/or treatment of communication disorders. Many of the scientists in this field obtained research training after completing their clinical training, but some researchers pursued a research track from the outset, and did not obtain clinical training.

There are over 123,000 professionals with careers in communication disorders and sciences. This includes over 106,000 speech-language pathologists, close to 13,000 audiologists, and 1,300 individuals with dual certification in speech-language pathology and audiology (ASHA, 2005). In addition, there are about 3,600 individuals whose primary employment involves research and/or teaching at the college or university level regarding the nature and treatment of communication disorders. Like the U.S. population, these professionals represent all major racial and ethnic groups: White, African American, Hispanic, Asian/Pacific Islander, and Native American. A survey of the ASHA membership indicated that most audiologists and speech-language pathologists (73 percent) are employed full-time. For audiologists, the most common place of employment is in a health care facility (72 percent), which includes hospitals, clinics, private practices, and as part of a physician's practice. Other employment settings for audiologists include school systems (9 percent), industrial facilities, and colleges or universities. In contrast, 55 percent of the speech-language pathologists report working in a school system. Other common employment settings for speech-language pathologists are healthcare facilities, colleges or universities, and private practice offices.

The results of the ASHA membership survey provide an overview of those who work in the field of communication disorders. To get a more personal view, we asked audiologists and speech-language pathologists from around the country to share their perceptions about their careers. Our informants included individuals who represent nearly all segments of the demographic groups that comprise the professions. We interviewed thirty-five individuals, who had over 350 combined years of experience within the field.

## Clinical Careers

We began by asking our colleagues why they chose a career path in communication disorders. As one might imagine, some were first introduced to the field because they knew someone with a communication disorder. That was the case for

Nancy, who lives in Arizona and is a relative newcomer to the field, with two years of experience. Nancy wrote, "I worked for a gentleman who had Parkinson disease, and he piqued my interest in the rehabilitation fields. He persuaded me to 'lose interest in the law' (a previous pursuit) and to become involved in a 'helping profession.' After doing some research, I found speech-language pathology to be the most interesting." A few colleagues had received clinical services themselves or knew someone who was working in the field. Kim, a speech-language pathologist from Colorado, reported that she had received articulation therapy as a young child. She wrote, "I decided one day on my way to my daughter's day care to be a 'speech therapist.' At the time, I only knew the 'r,' 'l,' and 's' part of the field." In her six years in the profession, Kim now has extensive experience working in both school and hospital settings. Donna is an audiologist with thirty-five years' experience who is employed as the director of a university clinic. She reported that a relative was a teacher of the deaf and that this sparked her interest in deafness. As an undergraduate, she was in the enviable position of having three fellowships—in theater, linguistics, and audiology—to choose among. She chose audiology and said, "I have *never* regretted this decision."

Those with direct exposure to the professions were in the minority. Many of our colleagues noted a desire to enter a field where they could "make people's lives better." This sentiment was echoed by Jennifer, who wrote, "I always knew I wanted to work with children, but I wasn't sure how until I saw some speech pathologists work with language-impaired preschoolers at a local hospital. Watching them, I realized how much impact a person could have in a child's life." Jennifer has had many opportunities to rediscover this impact in her own hospital-based position as a pediatric speech-language pathologist. Others were attracted because of a specific interest area that was encompassed by the field. Paula reported that she had an initial interest in languages and language development. "Then I took an audiology course and became fascinated with the process of hearing and what can happen when people—especially children—are unable to hear." She has combined these interests for fifteen years as an audiologist. Many who come to the field of speech-language pathology have a background in psychology or linguistics. Celia chose to become a speech-language pathologist after obtaining a PhD in linguistics. Although the two fields are similar in many ways, Celia realized that she wanted more of a clinical focus, which she now enjoys in her work with adults with acquired language disorders.

Increasingly, individuals come into the profession after having worked in another field. Zarina was a bilingual second-grade teacher before deciding to go back to school. In her years of teaching, Zarina said, "I noticed that there were a lot of Spanish-speaking kids with language difficulties. I decided to go into speech-language pathology to help bilingual children. I also wanted the option of working in other settings in addition to schools." Erin was a public relations accounts executive before returning to school for a master's in speech-language pathology. "What it all came down to was more meaningful work. I wanted a job helping people instead of just helping a company make money." She picked speech-language pathology because it allowed her to combine her interests in languages (she speaks

English and French) and health. Bret wrote, "I've had a long-standing interest in how we communicate (my BA is in speech communication). I was advised by a family friend to investigate speech-language pathology . . . and learned just how varied the field is and that it could provide a lifelong, stable career." He now works as a speech-language pathologist in a rehabilitation center. Sue discovered speech-language pathology after a diverse career path that included water-quality testing, small business ownership, creative writing, and publishing. She told us, "I wanted to work more closely with people, and my background in language is directly relevant to my work with clients who have reading and writing impairments."

There is also what we like to think of as the "luck factor" that led people to discover the field. Consider Anne, who has been practicing for two years in Missouri. "I didn't really know what I wanted to do," wrote Anne. "I had several friends who talked me into taking a speech-language pathology course, and I decided then and there that I was in the right field." Carol, an audiologist of ten years in California, had a similar reaction to her initial academic exposure. "I found the course-work interesting and challenging. There didn't seem to be a single course in the program I wasn't interested in taking." For Ellen, who has now been practicing for eleven years in Tennessee, a problem with her own voice led to a career in speech-language pathology. "I wanted to work with voice disorders, as I was a voice major in music and experiencing problems. I took a class in phonetics and loved the content."

We were impressed by the variety of reasons that led our colleagues to enter the field. This may be because the professions accommodate a wide range of personality traits and backgrounds. We saw this when we asked our colleagues to tell us about the traits they considered important in their job. Here are a few of the recurring themes they expressed: Lane's experience in hospitals and skilled nursing facilities in Arizona taught him that "a speech-language pathologist needs to be flexible, adaptable, a team player, a good communicator, and very clear about personal and professional integrity. These characteristics are crucial for survival in a rapidly changing healthcare system." Another trait identified by our colleagues was an orientation toward solving problems. Ellen commented, "Task analysis is at the center of what we do: identify problems, then determine the best method of improving function." Not surprisingly, she feels that traits such as analytical skill, inquisitiveness, enthusiasm, and an action-oriented nature apply to her. Rebecca, a speech-language pathologist of twenty-one years and the director of a hospital-based center for communication disorders in New York, adds qualities such as persistence, self-confidence, maturity, and generosity to the list.

Among the most frequently mentioned traits was independence. Angie, a speech-language pathologist from Tennessee, commented, "I believe you must be assertive in this field. People's quality of life is at stake, and you must do whatever you can to help." Independence characterized clinicians in private practice, university clinics, schools, hospitals, rehabilitation centers, and skilled nursing facilities This is not surprising, in that clinicians in most settings have a great deal of autonomy in how they manage their caseload, develop programs, and provide quality service. The complementary position was expressed by Mike, a Colorado resident with twenty-three years' experience, who wrote, "I think patience may be the key to my success as an audiologist, especially when working with families with young hearing-impaired infants. They need the gift of *time* to accept their child's impairments and to implement the many recommendations we make." In fact, patience was mentioned as an important trait by almost all our respondents. Regardless of clinical setting or clientele, the field demands individuals with the motivation to identify areas of need and seek out information in this ever-advancing field.

We were also curious about what keeps these professionals in the field year after year. Some cited specific aspects of their jobs, such as the experience of developing a new program for service delivery or working with cutting-edge technology. Donna works with new advances such as programmable hearing aids and cochlear implants (see Figure 1.1). She wrote, "Patients who are realizing dramatic functional gains keep me going!" "I love the diagnostic process," writes Shara, a speech-language pathologist of eleven years. "To be able to identify strengths and weaknesses and provide explanations for behavior is very challenging. Also to be able to change those behaviors, to see them 'get it,' is exciting." Shannon, a Michigan-based speech-language pathologist, echoed several common themes: "It's the versatility of being able to work with children or adults. I also like having a solid base of knowledge in a variety of disorders. And there's also the advantage of always being able to find a job!" Angie expressed the sentiments of many of our colleagues. She wrote, "It's a fast-paced field. I am always encountering new situations that allow me to learn." Lou, a speech-language pathologist of three years, wrote, "The most exciting thing for me to experience is children's first words—the look in their eyes when they realize they are able to impact their environment using words." When asked what keeps her going, Jennifer put it succinctly, "Two words: the kids. Two more words: their smiles."

All clinicians have stories about particular clients who stand out, punctuating their careers like exclamation points along the way. This was the case for Angie, who wrote about a difficult case involving a man who had had a stroke. "He once told me, 'You remember those old movies where there are slaves rowing the boat, and there is a man standing on deck cracking his whip. That is what you were for me. I never could have done it without you.' I never gave up on him, nor he on me." Ellen writes that one of her staff was able to identify an important medical issue for a patient that had been previously missed by several other professionals. "This speech-language pathologist referred the patient back to the ear, nose, and throat physician and highlighted her findings. The ENT diagnosed the actual cause of the swallowing disorder and was able to surgically repair it. The patient resumed a regular diet." Sometimes the smallest gains are the most important to the clinician. Susan, a speech-language pathologist in Minnesota, wrote of a severely autistic child who for the first time communicated a specific desire by selecting a picture of an activity. "We were so excited for him and what this skill will do for him in the future." She is now working to expand that child's first step toward building the skills to communicate with others through the use of pictures. The im-

FIGURE 1.1   Audiologists are responsible for the selection and fitting of hearing aids. Hearing aids are programmed using specialized equipment to suit the hearing loss of each individual.

pact of these cases is captured by Lane, who commented that "the emotional rewards and the opportunity to powerfully impact and connect with people during a difficult time in their lives" are primary advantages to a career in the field of communication disorders.

## Research Careers

Audiologists and speech-language pathologists impact lives through direct clinical services. But this is not the only avenue to effect change within the professions. The desire to advance the field beyond its current boundaries inspires professionals to incorporate research into their career. Whereas direct clinical intervention improves the lives of one client at a time, research has the potential to improve the lives of many, as new discoveries further the profession's understanding, diagnosis, and treatment of communication disorders. Although opportunities for research exist in almost all job settings, less than 1 percent of the professionals see themselves primarily as researchers. Another 3 percent are college or university professors, for whom research is a typical component of their careers (ASHA, 2005). Researchers include not only those with a clinical interest but also those

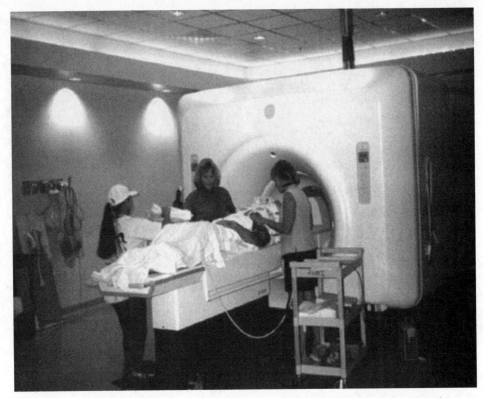

**FIGURE 1.2    Research careers in communication disorders involve the study of normal and disordered communication processes. Functional magnetic resonance imaging provides a means to examine how the brain supports speech and language.**

who focus on the scientific aspects of the human communication system (see Figure 1.2). For most of these individuals, their education included doctoral studies, which provide core training in research methods. The majority of these researchers work in university settings. We asked some of these individuals to tell us why they elected this career path and what it is like to be a researcher in the field of communication disorders.

Amy Skinder had just begun her doctoral studies at the University of Washington when we first talked with her. Prior to her enrollment, she had worked as a speech-language pathologist for four years, part of that time as a traveling clinician in a variety of settings around the country. "My goal when I finished my master's was to be able to work with a broad range of disorders. After a while, I decided that instead of knowing a little about a lot, it would be nice to focus on one area. At the same time, I was working with a client in the public school system who had severe developmental apraxia of speech as well as attention deficit disorder and other learning disabilities. I went to a seminar. . . and asked lots of questions. I found out there weren't a lot of answers. After talking with the speaker [a noted researcher], I felt encouraged to go on for my doctorate. Doctoral studies are an opportunity to indulge in trying to answer all your burning questions."

When we next caught up with Amy Skinder, she had obtained her doctorate, married, and taken a faculty position at the University of Minnesota–Duluth. Dr. Skinder-Meredith filled us in on what it is like to start an academic and research career. "I enjoy my faculty position very much. It's good to be teaching. I work with wonderful people who value my work as a colleague, a teacher, and a researcher." She emphasized the importance of her clinical experience to her teaching and research endeavors. Besides conducting research in childhood apraxia, a communication disorder she encountered as a clinician, Dr. Skinder-Meredith can draw on her clinical background to supplement her teaching. In addition to continuing her own research, she has been forging contacts with others who work in her area of interest in order to foster collaborative research.

This motivation has been echoed by many researchers we have talked with over the years. Anne Cordes Bothe, PhD is on the faculty at the University of Georgia, where she conducts research in the area of stuttering. She realized during her master's program that she wanted to go on for a doctorate. "The things that were catching my interest during my coursework and with my practicum clients were the things that we as a field didn't know or didn't yet understand. It wasn't the answers that I thought were interesting, it was the QUESTIONS! And the PhD is a research degree, which is about questions, so it became pretty obvious that this is where I belonged."

Nancy Helm-Estabrooks, ScD, wrote, "In many ways I think I was always an informal researcher—trying new approaches, developing new materials, regarding every case as a case study—even before my doctoral studies, which I pursued in my thirties. I decided to get a doctorate to further my knowledge and to write grant proposals as a Principal Investigator so I could explore and test some ideas I had for new treatment approaches."

Steven Camarata, PhD, has been on the faculty at Vanderbilt University for fifteen years. He wrote, "I wanted to teach at a university and was interested in clinical research. Being able to follow my curiosity for research [is an exciting component of the job]. This freedom is a very precious gift. I knew that research would involve a lot of mundane work, but the discovery is worth it. Plus, I want to help children with speech and language problems and realized early on that I could best do this not only by seeing patients (which I still do) but also by developing better treatments."

For our colleagues, the commitment it takes to get a doctorate was definitely worth the time and effort. Barbara Lewis, PhD, of Rainbow Babies and Children's Hospital and Case Western Reserve University, has been conducting research for fifteen years. Her work on the genetic basis of phonological disorders has drawn her into collaborations with psychologists, pediatricians, epidemiologists, and geneticists. She wrote to us, "I like the challenge of asking difficult research questions and finding results that do not always correspond to my prediction."

This was also apparent to Dr. Skinder-Meredith when she was just beginning her research career. "It is not easy to answer those big, burning questions. It's surprising how small you have to start out with your research. It's a lot more complicated than you anticipate." The profession benefits from the work of such scientists, who systematically follow a line of research, resulting in incremental advances in knowledge.

Dr. Cordes Bothe wrote, "I love to pick up a new journal and read the report of a study that flowed from a creative idea or from a creative way of approaching an old problem. If the method is good and sound, so that the results are believable, then it is such fun to enjoy the new findings and enjoy that sense of 'Well, of COURSE! Why hadn't anybody ever thought of that?' For the same reason, I love seeing a reference to my own published work in something that's almost unrelated, because somebody else saw a connection that I never even thought of." But the final impact of research is on clinical practice. We are one of the few therapeutic professions for which research advances are provided by its own membership, a situation that adds to the strength and autonomy of the professions as a whole.

Audiologist and hearing scientist Theodore Glattke, PhD, expressed the importance of researchers within the profession when he said, "If we fail to develop new knowledge, we will face extinction as service providers." Leslie Gonzalez Rothi, PhD, added, "We are the professionals best suited to perform this applied research—a bridge between basic research and clinical application."

Many of the most active researchers in our field hold an academic position. This brings with it the opportunity to interact with students. Dr. Cordes Bothe related some of her favorite aspects of teaching. "I like being able to sit with one student and figure out where she is and what her needs are and be able to point her in the right direction. I get a kick out of phrasing something just right in class so that I can see twenty light bulbs come on over the students' heads. And every so often, I get a kick out of the sudden realization that I DO know how to solve some problem after all." Dr. Glattke, on the faculty of the University of Arizona, has held an academic position for thirty years and has extensive experience mentoring students in research experiences. "It is a pleasure to witness the genuine excitement that the students express when they share their work. Sometimes they discover something about themselves as a result of the effort they put into writing about their research or synthesizing the literature base." He also had this to say about working in an academic environment: "Contributing to the development of new knowledge, integrating the new knowledge into the curriculum, and adapting mentoring styles to respond to the needs of the students are invigorating activities. It is a privilege to be allowed to teach in a university setting."

Others conduct research within health care settings. Among the leading non-university research sites are some of the Veteran's Administration (VA) Medical Centers. Dr. Gonzalez Rothi is program director of the Brain Rehabilitation Research Center at the Veteran's Administration Medical Center in Gainsville, Florida, where she combines clinical practice with cutting-edge research. She wrote that "my research background offers me a willingness to open doors that are not yet available to most. Second, no day is ever the same. Each time I come into the hospital, I find that new challenges are facing me, testing the limits of my abilities, and always inspiring me to know more." Dr. Helm-Estabrooks has also worked in the VA system and has extensive experience conducting research in clinical settings. "Research appeals to my detective instincts, developing new assessment and treatment methods appeals to my creative instincts, and clinical research allows me to work directly with patients. Also, there are many aspects to my work—patient evaluations and therapy sessions, writing, teaching, mentoring, etc.—so that I'm always challenged and never bored."

Research careers present their own unique challenges. "One of the main challenges has been to remain focused on my primary interest: genetics of speech and language disorders," Dr. Lewis expressed. "There are many temptations to digress into related but very interesting areas. You have to realize that you can't do it all." Dr. Cordes Bothe agrees. "Balance and organization [are challenges]. My job gives me at least twice as many options as any one human being could reasonably keep track of. . . . An academic position is described as 'teaching, research, and service,' but what that really means is that the challenge is to find time for good teaching, good research, and a reasonable amount of service. It often seems that each day has about two days' worth of little stuff that has to get done. The challenge is to keep track of what's really important for the long term."

What advice do these individuals have for a new generation of potential researchers? Dr. Lewis advises that "a student interested in research should learn as much as possible about research methodology and statistics while keeping a strong tie to the clinic. Most important is to identify an area of interest and explore related disciplines." Other research colleagues emphasize the value of interdisciplinary collaboration. Dr. Gonzalez Rothi urges students to "look for a program where you have an opportunity to look at a wide variety of perspectives. Set up an advisory committee that reflects this diversity. Take courses outside of your [major area of focus] that might be able to contribute to your knowledge base." Finally, Dr. Camarata provides this perspective: "Look into your heart and mind to determine whether satisfying your curiosity will sustain you. The key requirement for research is not 'intelligence' per se, but an interest in problem solving (with a large dose of persistence thrown in). If you like asking questions, a research career might be the most satisfying option."

## CLINICAL PROBLEM SOLVING

We have introduced some of types of communication disorders that concern the professions of audiology and speech-language pathology and have heard from some practicing professionals regarding their insights about the field. The ensuing chapters will lay the groundwork necessary to understand normal and disordered communication processes in children and adults. We will consistently introduce the reader to clinical cases that bring to life the realities of the communication disorders. These individuals will help the reader appreciate the diagnostic and treatment processes that are at the heart of the professions.

Audiology and speech-language pathology are, by nature, fields in which memorization of facts is not enough for success. They require the application of knowledge to real-life problems. For this reason, we will end each chapter with a section in clinical problem solving. This is an opportunity to take the information covered in a chapter and apply it to a case. We saw in this chapter how individual components of communication can break down in cases of disorder. Many communication disorders involve a combination of difficulties within the areas of speech, language, and hearing. Consider the following case:

*Bonnie*, age 8, was born with a severe hearing loss in both ears that was detected in the hospital when her hearing was screened as an infant. She could hear some low-frequency sounds in the environment and detect when someone was talking, but she could not perceive the differences in speech sounds. Bonnie was fitted with hearing aids to help her capitalize on the little hearing that was preserved, and she was placed in a preschool program that combined the use of hearing aid amplification with sign language and speech. Despite this early help, her spoken language skills were two years behind other children her age, and most people could not understand her speech when she entered first grade. She has made gains in speech and language but still struggles with spoken and written grammar. Her use of sign language has far outpaced her spoken and written language abilities. Bonnie's speech is still difficult to understand, because she makes many articulation errors involving sounds that are outside of her hearing range. Her voice has an effortful quality and sounds like she is speaking from the back of her throat. Bonnie continues to receive academic tutoring and speech therapy.

1. What aspects of speech, language, and hearing are affected in Bonnie's case?
2. Would Bonnie's communication disorder be classified as developmental or acquired?
3. Which professionals are likely to be involved with Bonnie to maximize her communication potential?

## REFERENCES

American Speech-Language-Hearing Association (ASHA; 2005). Background information and standards and implementation for the certificate of clinical competence in speech-language pathology. Available at http://www.asha.org/members/deskrefjournals/deskref/default

American Speech-Language-Hearing Association (ASHA). (2005). Highlights and trends: ASHA member counts. Retrieved November 12, 2006, from http://www.asha.org/about/membership-certification/member-counts.htm

Kent, R. (1998, Summer). Renewal and rediscovery: Insights from memoirs of illness and disability. *Asha Magazine*, p. 22.

# CHAPTER TWO

# THE BIOLOGICAL FOUNDATIONS OF SPEECH AND LANGUAGE

**PREVIEW**

Knowledge of the biological underpinnings of normal speech, language, and hearing is central to understanding the many ways in which communication can be disrupted. In this chapter, we will first examine respiration and the vocal mechanism, which provide the power source and voicing for speech. The articulators shape the sound into individual consonants and vowels to form words. Those words are perceived by the listener through the auditory system. Finally, they are comprehended by the language system in the brain, where the information is processed and stored, and a response may be formulated. These physical mechanisms work together to support communication. When communication is disrupted by developmental disorder or acquired pathology, the breakdown can often be traced to one or more of these basic biological systems.

Speech-language pathologists and audiologists are confronted daily with clinical cases that require an understanding of the physical and neurological underpinnings of communication and how impairments to these systems lead to communication disorders. Consider the following child:

> *Alicia*, age 3, was born with Down syndrome. This developmental disorder can be traced to a genetic abnormality that results in an extra copy of chromosome 21. The resulting alteration in brain development causes some degree of mental retardation and is likely to affect the capacity for normal language development. For this engaging 3-year-old girl, the occurrence of this genetic abnormality could impact her communication skills in several additional ways. Low muscle tone associated with the disorder might restrict her ability to move and explore her world, and abnormalities of her oral-facial structure could interfere with speech articulation. Her hearing might be affected because structural characteristics of the ear in children with Down syndrome make them prone to hearing loss. A multidisciplinary assessment team, consisting of a speech-language pathologist, an audiologist, a special educator, a psychologist, a physical therapist, and an occupational therapist, will work together to determine how the effects of Down syndrome manifest in this child. The team will then devise a plan intended to maximize her overall development, including communication skills. In the following sections, we will explore the biological systems that support normal communication and consider how they might be affected in clinical cases such as Alicia's.

## THE VOCAL MECHANISM

It is said that communication is an "overlaid function" that makes use of structures that have other primary functions. The same muscles and organs that allow us to breathe also provide the driving force behind sound production for speech. The larynx, which keeps us from choking food or liquid that might otherwise be misdirected into the airway, also contributes to sound production. The structures of the mouth and throat that allow us to eat and drink also permit us to change the vocal tract to produce the various sounds that make up words and sentences.

## The Respiratory System

The main function of the respiratory system is to sustain life through the continuous exchange of gases, primarily the exchange of carbon dioxide for oxygen. The human body requires a continuous renewal of its oxygen supply, usually accomplished by twelve to eighteen breaths (inspiration-expiration cycles) per minute. For the majority of people without respiratory disease, breathing occurs with little conscious effort.

Breathing is achieved by movements of the rib cage and the **diaphragm**. The rib cage can be raised slightly by contraction of skeletal muscles. The diaphragm, a large muscle that separates the chest from the abdomen, is shaped like an inverted bowl. When it contracts, it flattens and descends toward the abdomen, as shown in Figure 2.1. Because the lungs adhere to the inside of the rib cage and diaphragm, the lungs are stretched when the muscles of inspiration contract and cause the rib cage to elevate and the diaphragm to descend. This increase in lung size results in a decrease in pulmonary pressure relative to air pressure outside the body. With the airway open, air flows into the lungs through the mouth or nose (or both) in order to balance the air pressure, and we inhale. Exhalation simply results from relaxation of the muscles of inhalation. The rib cage falls back to its resting state and the diaphragm ascends as it returns to its inverted-bowl shape. The lungs then decrease in size, causing an increase in pulmonary pressure relative to the atmosphere, and air rushes out. This cycle, shown in Figure 2.1, repeats itself continuously as we breathe in and out.

The natural recoil forces of the lungs and muscular contraction function in a natural, synergistic way as we breathe at rest and during sleep. Our "in" breath is about as long as our "out" breath. When we sing or talk, however, we engage volitional forces that change the normal in-and-out pattern, enabling us to take a quick inspiration and follow it with a prolonged expiration, which we use for phonation. Research conducted by speech scientists provides a detailed understanding of the aerodynamics of speech and voice (Hixon & Abbs, 1980; Kent, 1997; Zemlin, 1998).

The muscles of the torso that support respiration serve another function important to the support of speech breathing—that of postural control. These muscles support the body so that the lungs have room to expand. A person who lacks control of these muscles may have difficulty maintaining a stable posture for efficient speech breathing.

Many disorders can disrupt the musculoskeletal system that underlies control of speech breathing. Let us refer back to Alicia's case from the perspective of the respiratory system. When the evaluation team works with Alicia, several professionals will look at her musculoskeletal system. The physical therapist will examine postural support and gross motor movements. The occupational therapist

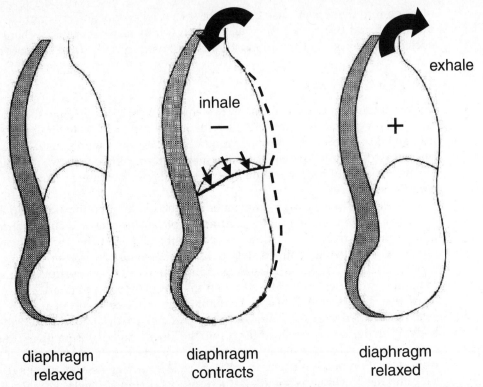

diaphragm
relaxed

diaphragm
contracts

diaphragm
relaxed

**FIGURE 2.1   Schematic drawing of the torso during quiet breathing. Note that, for inhalation, the diaphragm moves downward and the rib cage lifts up and forward so that the lung volume increases and a negative pressure is created. For exhalation, the diaphragm relaxes and returns to its dome shape and the chest wall falls back to its resting state so that the air in the lungs is compressed, causing a positive pressure.** Adapted from Hixon (1973).

will examine fine motor control, particularly in relation to age-appropriate play activities. The speech-language pathologist's primary concern will be whether Alicia has sufficient control over the muscles that support posture and respiration to permit connected speech. Alicia's muscle tone, although lower than normal, is adequate to support spoken communication. However, there are concerns about her motor skills and ability to support her body.

## The Phonatory System

Voice (or phonation) is produced by the vibration of the two vocal folds within the larynx. Although phonation is a vital part of speech production, the primary function of the larynx is to guard the airway against **aspiration**, the inhalation of fluids or other matter into the airway. The larynx sits at the top of the trachea, where it plays this primary "watchdog" role. When we swallow, the larynx elevates and muscles contract to protect the airway. The average person, for example, is unaware of the protective function of the larynx, and when asked what the larynx (or "voice box") does, may answer, "We make sound with it." In some individuals with structural damage to the vocal folds (a result of cancer, for example) or with muscular impairment of laryngeal function (perhaps part of a degenerative neuromuscular disease), the valving function of the larynx can be compromised and the patient may experience life-threatening choking spells.

The human voice represents perhaps the most elegant and complex function of the larynx in mammals. To appreciate the perspective that the human voice may well not be an evolutionary accident, one has only to listen to the sheer beauty and control of a trained singer performing an operatic aria or popular ballad, or the vocal interpretations of an accomplished actor. The communicative and artistic functions of the larynx take it well beyond its basic valving responsibilities.

The back (posterior) and front (anterior) views of the larynx can be seen in Figure 2.2. The ring-shaped **cricoid cartilage** forms the base of this structure and the **thyroid cartilage** sits above the cricoid. The thyroid cartilage is shield shaped and forms the anterior wall of the larynx. In many individuals (especially young men), we can see the prominent thyroid cartilage, which is often referred to as the Adam's apple. You can feel your thyroid cartilage by placing your fingertips on your throat, and feeling for the V-shaped notch in the front, which is called the thyroid notch (see Figure 2.2). If you are not sure whether you are touching the thyroid

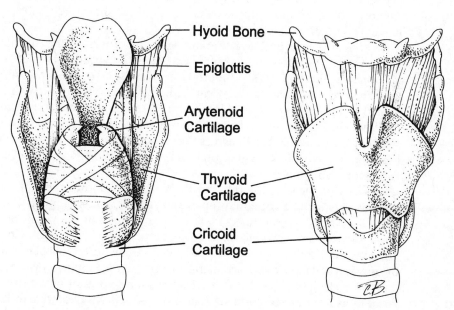

Hyoid Bone

Epiglottis

Arytenoid
Cartilage

Thyroid
Cartilage

Cricoid
Cartilage

**FIGURE 2.2  Structures of the larynx shown from the back (posterior) view on the left and front (anterior) view on the right. Note that the larynx is suspended from the hyoid bone (at the top). The V-shaped "thyroid notch" is evident in the anterior view of the thyroid cartilage.**

cartilage, it will become evident if you prolong an "ah" while you warble the pitch high and low. You will feel the cartilage move up and down with changes in pitch.

The vocal folds lie in a horizontal orientation and are attached in the front to the thyroid cartilage just below the thyroid notch. The vocal folds extend posteriorly from the thyroid cartilage to the base of two pyramid-shaped cartilages called the **arytenoid cartilages**. In order to see the vocal folds, it is necessary to view the larynx from above, as shown in Figure 2.3. In this figure, we can see the left and right vocal folds and the arytenoid cartilages in a typical position for taking in a breath. The area between the vocal folds is known as the **glottis**, which has a V shape because the vocal folds are attached at a common point in the front of the larynx and they diverge in the posterior aspect by the action of the arytenoids. During voicing, the arytenoids move to the midline, closing the glottal opening. In Figure 2.3 the view of the thyroid cartilage is blocked by another structure within the larynx called the **epiglottis**.

As shown in Figure 2.2, the arytenoid cartilages sit on top of the posterior cricoid cartilage. The arytenoid cartilages move and rotate atop the cricoid cartilage by the action of several muscles within the larynx. For example, when certain muscles contract, they move the arytenoid cartilages in such a way that they pull the vocal folds apart. The muscles that accomplish this movement are known as laryngeal *ab*ductors (they separate the folds). Laryngeal *ad*ductor muscles rotate the arytenoids in such a way that the folds come together. This muscle action is extremely quick, permitting a speaker to produce the rapid changes in voicing needed for continuous speech.

When the vocal folds are brought together (adduction), they are in the phonating position. The outgoing air builds up below the vocal folds, causing increased air pressure, referred to as **subglottal air pressure**. When this pressure is greater than the pressure holding the vocal folds together at the midline, it blows them apart. A puff of air is released between the open folds, which then return to the midline. The closure results from the elastic recoil of the vocal fold tissue and is assisted by the movement of air across the surface of the folds. This opening and closing produces what is known as one cycle of phonation. Repeated cycles produce sound, or phonation.

What we hear as the pitch of the voice relates directly to the rate, or frequency, at which the vocal folds open and close. The normal pitch of the speaking voice is primarily determined by the size and mass of the vocal folds. The tiny vocal folds in babies produce high voices because their vocal folds vibrate quickly. Nine-year-old children typically produce speaking voices just above middle C on the musical scale. We can describe this in terms of the number of vibrations per second, or cycles per second (**hertz**). The speaking voice of an adult male, whose vocal folds have increased in size since puberty, is about an octave lower than it was when he was 9 years old. The adult female, whose larynx is usually half again as large as it was when she was 9, typically speaks at a pitch that falls between that of a male adult and a child.

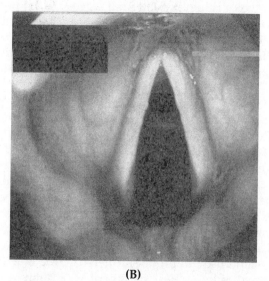

FIGURE 2.3  A drawing (A) and photograph (B) of the vocal folds viewed from above. The front of the larynx is at the top of each figure, and the back of the larynx is at the bottom. The vocal folds are apart in a V-shape as is typical during inspiration.

Because outgoing airflow causes the vocal folds to vibrate, changes in intensity, or loudness, of the voice are produced by changes in subglottal air pressure. This pressure can be raised by increasing the muscular force that holds the vocal folds together or by increasing the air pressure from the lungs (i.e., the respiratory drive). When the airflow finally breaks through the vocal folds, they are blown apart with greater force than when a less intense sound is produced. This, in turn, produces greater lateral excursion of the vocal folds, resulting in greater air displacement. In this way, a speaker can increase the intensity, and the perceived loudness, of the voice.

Just as we can regulate the loudness of our voice, we can also change the pitch by making adjustments to the vocal folds. Contraction of certain laryngeal muscles serves to lengthen the folds by stretching and tensing them or shorten the folds by relaxing and thickening them. When stretched, the vocal folds become thinner, and they vibrate more quickly, producing higher frequencies (perceived as higher pitches). Likewise, when muscle action causes the vocal folds to become shorter and thicker, they vibrate more slowly and produce lower frequencies. Speech scientists study these dynamics of vocal fold function as well as the physical characteristics of the vocal mechanism (see for example, Kent, 1997; Weismer, 1988; and Zemlin, 1998).

## The Resonance System

Although the source of the voice is the larynx, sound waves are modified by the other structures within the throat, mouth, and nasal cavities. This is analogous to the way the hollow body of a guitar modifies the sound produced by plucking the string. The sound waves that we recognize as the human voice result from both the sound produced by the larynx and the filtering of that sound by the resonance system.

The first area of the vocal tract through which the sound waves travel lies immediately above the larynx. This tubelike cavity is called the **pharynx** (see Figure 2.4). The pharynx can be studied with **videoendoscopy**, which uses an illuminated lens to look down the back of the throat toward the larynx. The structures and their movements can then viewed on a video monitor. Videoendoscopy reveals that the pharynx is constantly changing shape during speech as the tongue moves forward and backward and the pharyngeal walls move inward. The length of the pharynx also changes as the larynx rises (shortening the pharynx) or lowers (lengthening the pharynx). A fascinating videoendoscopic tape distributed by the Voice Foundation (1985) of two famous impersonators, Rich Little and Mel Blanc, revealed that much of the muscle action used to produce different voice impersonations takes place in the pharyngeal cavities. The pharynx plays an important role in shaping vocal resonance, although it obviously plays another vital role as a conduit for the passage of air and food.

In addition to the pharynx, the oral cavity also shapes the resonance characteristics of the voice. The opening within the mouth constantly changes size and shape during speech. The overall size of the oral opening is primarily determined by the position of the **mandible**, or lower jaw, which is continually lowering and elevating during speech. As the jaw drops for saying a low vowel, such as "ah," the tongue drops with it. In contrast, the tongue rides high in the mouth when producing the long "e" vowel. The tongue itself has the greatest flexibility of any muscle group in the body, constantly changing its shape and position during articulation, thus altering the overall shape and size of the oral cavity. Together, the continuous oral and pharyngeal cavities determine the shape of the vocal tract. Speech scientists study the vocal tract shape using magnetic resonance imaging

Nasal cavity

Maxilla

Hard palate

Velum

Tongue

Mandible

Epiglottis

Vocal folds

Thyroid cartilage

Cricoid cartilage

Trachea

**FIGURE 2.4   Sound produced at the larynx is modified by the resonance characteristics of the vocal tract, which consists of the pharynx and the oral and nasal cavities. At rest, the velum allows air to flow into the nasal cavity.**

(MRI) while a person holds a vowel position, as shown in Figure 2.5 (Story, Titze, & Hoffman, 1996, 1998).

The roof of the oral cavity is formed anteriorly by the bony hard palate and posteriorly by the soft palate (also known as **velum**). The velum is a muscular structure, noticeable for its dangling appendage, the uvula. The velum hangs down during normal breathing so that air can flow between the nasal cavity and the oral cavity. When eating or drinking, the opening between these two cavities is closed as the velum raises and the pharyngeal wall constricts around it. During the production of most speech sounds, the velum is raised to close off the nasal cavity from the oral cavity. This allows for oral resonance of all the vowels and consonants in the English language except for the sounds "m," "n," and "ng"). When these three nasal sounds are produced, the velopharyngeal port is open, allowing sound waves to enter the nasal cavity from the oral cavity, known as nasal-oral coupling. During normal speech production, the velum raises and lowers quickly as you produce oral and nasal sounds. For example, if you say the word *banana*, the

**FIGURE 2.5** **A side view of the articulators showing the differences in tongue and jaw position during the production of the vowels "ee"(/i/) on the left and "ah"(/a/) on the right. Note that the tongue and jaw are elevated for "ee" (/i/), whereas they are lowered for "ah" (/a/).**

initial "ba" requires a raised velum. The "n" requires a rapid drop of the velum, and the next vowel, "a," requires closure again, only to be followed by another rapid drop for the next "n," ending with an elevated velum again for the vowel "a."

Failure to move the velum rapidly enough to match the demands of the particular utterance can result in excessively nasal speech, called **hypernasality**. Many problems that involve hypernasality are caused by faulty velophryngeal closure, which could be related to a number of factors, such as cleft palate, short velum, injured palate, or paralysis or weakness of the velopharyngeal muscles (disorders that are discussed in subsequent chapters). A less common resonance disorder is *hyponasality,* which is insufficient nasal resonance often due to excessive velopharyngeal closure. Hyponasality also occurs when the nasal cavity is blocked by swollen tissues due to allergies or colds that dampen sound waves and block the airflow through the nasal cavities. Excessive tonsil and adenoid tissue will sometimes create enough obstruction to give the voice a **denasal** vocal quality that has a marked lack of nasal resonance.

The resonance system gives each voice its distinctive quality. Changes in the quality of the voice can signal vocal pathology, as we will see in Chapter 6. Let us now look at the resonance system in the case of Alicia, the child with Down syndrome.

Down syndrome can involve congenital malformations of the pharynx (specifically the naso- and oropharynx), which can result in altered voice quality. In the case of Alicia, the speech-language pathologist noted some instances of hypernasality. This might result from poor control of the velopharyngeal mechanism or from a defect in the articulatory mechanism, explained below. To differentiate between these two possible causes, the speech-language pathologist evaluated both the oral structures and velopharyngeal functioning.

## THE ARTICULATORY MECHANISM

### The Tongue

It may be surprising to realize that the tongue occupies most of the space of the oral cavity, as is evident in Figure 2.4. The tongue body is composed of a number of intrinsic muscles that run both the length and width of the structure. These muscles enable us to change its shape easily (curled, pointed, and so on). Other muscles of the tongue originate from various sites outside the tongue, such as the hyoid bone (shown in Figure 2.2). These extrinsic muscles allow the tongue to be elevated, lowered, protruded, and retracted. The way in which the tongue is postured influences the overall sound and resonance of the voice and is critical for the production of individual speech sounds. Vowels are produced primarily through changes in the shape and movement of the tongue (and elevation of the jaw). Precise movement and positioning of the tongue is necessary for many of the consonant sounds, which involve vocal tract constriction that restricts airflow. Without the precision of tongue movements, there could be no articulate speech.

### The Lips

The lips are the most visible structure of the mouth and are easily shaped and altered to produce various facial expressions. They are made up primarily of facial muscles that can be variously contracted, to pucker, retract, protrude, or form a circle. They also play a vital role in oral behaviors such as sucking, chewing, smiling, and kissing. The lips form the end of the oral vocal tract, so their position can also contribute to the resonance of the voice. You can demonstrate the effects of the lips on vocal resonance by prolonging an "eee" for five seconds while you alternately pucker and then relax the lips. The distinct changes in the resonance that occur with each pucker reflect the lengthening and shortening of the vocal tract. The lips also play a primary function in the production of several consonants. Sounds such as "m," "p," "b," and "w" are produced by movements of the lips, whereas "f" and "v" are produced with the upper teeth on or against the lower lip.

### The Mandible

The movement of the mandible, or lower jaw, allows for quick opening and closing of the mouth. Some mandibular movement contributes to change in the shape and size of the oral cavity needed for the production of different vowels. The normal speaker moves the mandible in quick synergistic movements with the lips and tongue during normal speech production. If, however, a speaker were to talk with a pen clenched between the teeth, the mandible would stay fixed to trap the pen, and immediate compensatory adjustments of the tongue and lips would be made to maintain speech articulation. Optimal speech production and vocal resonance require continuous mandible movement. Occasionally, we see patients with voice problems who speak with a clenched jaw much of the time, requiring the tongue to make all the muscle movements needed for vowel differentiation. Speaking this way is inefficient and often results in a muffled voice and imprecise articulation.

## The Palate

The bony hard palate and the muscular soft palate make up the structures of the roof of the mouth, or **palate**. The underlying bone of the hard palate is the maxilla. It is an arched structure with a vaulted ceiling that contributes greatly to oral resonance. The portion of the palate just behind the front teeth is the alveolar ridge, which is a point of contact for the articulation of several speech sounds, such as "t" and "d." Attached to the posterior hard palate just beyond the last molars is the muscular soft palate, called the velum. As discussed earlier, when the velum makes contact with the pharynx it separates the oral cavity from the nasal cavity, allowing for oral resonance of sounds.

## The Teeth

The teeth play a primary role in the chewing of food, while their contribution to speech articulation is somewhat secondary. However, a few English sounds, such as "f" and "v," are made with the lower lip tucked under the upper central incisors. This placement is referred to as labiodental (lip-to-teeth) contact. The teeth are also the contact point for "th" sounds, which are produced by placing the tongue to the upper teeth (linguadental sounds). The alveolar ridge behind the base of the maxillary teeth is an important contact point for the tongue for the production of such sounds as "n," "s," "z," "t," and "d."

When speech is slow to develop or is difficult to understand, it is important to rule out possible problems with the oral and facial structures. In Alicia's case, the speech-language pathologist performed what is known as an **oral-peripheral examination**. This is an evaluation of the structure and function of the articulatory mechanisms.

Alicia's oral-peripheral exam revealed several factors that could negatively affect communication. Some of her front teeth are quite crooked, which may interfere with sounds made against the teeth, such as "th" or "s." Her hard palate is highly arched, but does not contain any clefts or holes that would allow air to flow into the nasal cavity to produce hypernasality. Although her tongue appears large for her mouth and tends to protrude a bit, it is not actually too large. Rather, it lacks the muscle tone to rest within the mouth. Alicia's face has a soft, rounded appearance, which also suggests low tone of the facial muscles. Low tone in the oral and facial muscles can interfere with the movements needed to produce the sounds of speech. All these factors may account for the perception that Alicia's words sound "thick" and imprecise.

## THE NERVOUS SYSTEM

The remarkable ability of human beings to communicate efficiently is related primarily to a complex nervous system that permits meaningful interaction between a person and the environment, other people, and other creatures. The nervous systems of other animals may have features that permit them to perform a particular behavior "better" than human beings. For example, predator birds have more acute eyesight than humans, and the porpoise has a more advanced auditory system. However, it is their complex brain that allows humans to master the complexities and subtleties of human language. The brain is part of the **central nervous system** (CNS). It works in concert with the **peripheral nervous system** (PNS), which allows information to travel to and from the body. We will consider each separately.

### Central Nervous System

The brain and the spinal cord, seen in Figure 2.6, are considered the two primary CNS structures. The brain enables humans to engage in high-level functions, such as synthesizing information gathered from the environment, making inferences, drawing conclusions, making plans for the future, and communicating about all of these things. Because of its critical role in such functions, factors that alter brain development or damage the brain underlie many types of communication disorders. Between the brain and spinal cord is the brainstem. The brainstem and spinal cord comprise the primary pathway for sensory information that comes from the body to the brain. Conversely, the brain sends motor commands through the brainstem to the spinal cord that result in our ability to support and move our bodies. Therefore, damage to the brainstem or spinal cord, with the resulting loss of muscular control, can disrupt the biological support necessary for speech.

The brain consists of the **cerebrum** and the **cerebellum** (see Figure 2.6). The cerebrum occupies the majority of the brain cavity within the head. The cerebellum sits below the cerebrum and behind the brainstem. Both the cerebrum and the cerebellum can be further divided into right and left **hemispheres**. The hemispheres of the cerebrum are joined at the midline by a large band of fibers called the **corpus callosum**, which carries information between the cerebral hemispheres (see Figure 2.7). The surface of the brain appears as a series of ridges, called *gyri*, and grooves, called *sulci*. Large sulci are referred to as *fissures*. The gyri and sulci can be individually identified by name, so that the location of both normal and pathological features of the cortex can be described in specific terms.

The cerebral hemispheres can be further divided into four lobes (see Figure 2.6), each of which contains regions that are associated with particular functions.

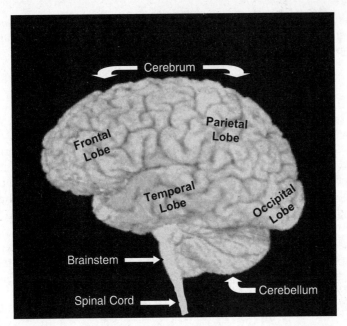

**FIGURE 2.6   Components of the central nervous system: the cerebrum, cerebellum, brainstem and spinal cord. The left cerebral hemisphere is divided into four lobes: frontal, parietal, temporal, and occipital.**

The **frontal lobes** contain the primary motor cortex, which sends neural commands, including those needed for speech, to specific parts of the body. They also contain regions that are involved with attention, impulse control, and judgment. The **parietal lobes** contain the primary sensory cortex, which receives sensory information from the body as well as other regions that support a number of cognitive functions. The **occipital lobes**, at the back of the brain, receive and process visual information. The **temporal lobes** contain the primary auditory cortex as well as regions important for language comprehension and memory.

The specialized functions of specific regions of the brain are attributed to differences in cells found within these regions. If we examine a cross-section of the cerebrum (see Figure 2.7), we can see the surface layer, or cortex. The cortex contains layers of **neurons**, which are cells that support different types of brain activity. Because the bodies of these neurons appear gray, the cortex is also called *gray matter*. The layers of the cortex within the primary motor area of the frontal lobe, for example, contain many neurons that send signals to the body for the control of movement, whereas the primary sensory cortex contains many cells that receive incoming signals from the body. If we look at the cross-section of the cerebrum (Figure 2.7), the lighter gray tissues beneath the cortex consist of nerve fibers that originate in the gray matter. These fibers connect regions of the brain, receive sensory information from the body, and send impulses to move the muscles of the body. Such fibers are collectively referred to as *white matter*.

**FIGURE 2.7**  **A midline view of the brain (on the left), a horizontal cross section of the brain (on the upper right), and a vertical cross section (i.e., coronal) of the brain (on the lower right). The cross sections allow you to see the gray and white matter distinctions and the deep subcortical structures called the basal ganglia and the thalamus. On each view, the corpus callosum can be seen bridging the right and left hemispheres.**

The brain also includes a collection of subcortical (i.e., beneath the cortex) bodies known as the **basal ganglia** (see Figure 2.7). These neural bodies are connected to the cerebellum and to cortical regions involved in movement. Disorders of the basal ganglia, such as Parkinson disease, often result in impaired movements. In the posterior half of the brain, behind the basal ganglia and close to the midline of the brain, is another collection of subcortical neurons known as the **thalamus**. This highly complex region receives and processes all types of information that is relayed between areas of the brain.

Several regions of the brain are particularly important for communication and are frequently involved when communication disorders occur. Neural impulses from the ear that occur in response to sound travel to a region of the brain called the *primary auditory cortex*. This cortex is located on the superior surface of the temporal lobe (inside the Sylvian fissure) and is sometimes called *Heschl's gyrus* (see Figure 2.8). Within the left hemisphere, the primary auditory cortex is surrounded by cortical tissue that supports higher level auditory function, including the comprehension of spoken language. Areas particularly important to this skill occupy the posterior regions of the superior temporal lobe and parts of the parietal lobe. Portions of the left inferior frontal lobe, on the other hand, are particularly important to aspects of language expression. Finally, the motor movements of speech

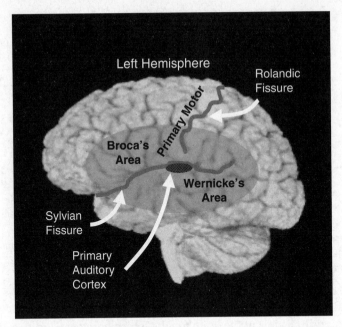

**FIGURE 2.8    Important anatomical areas of the left hemisphere. The left perisylvian region that is important for language is shaded in light gray.**

are supported by the *primary motor cortex,* which is located in the frontal lobe of each hemisphere. This area works in conjunction with subcortical structures and the cerebellum to produce the movements needed for speech.

In a normal, healthy brain, these various regions work in concert to support communication in all its complexity. However, when a brain is compromised during development or due to disease or injury, communication breakdowns can occur.

For Alicia, the effects that brought her to the developmental center began long before the day of her birth. The genetic anomaly that leads to Down syndrome affects the development of the brain. Research with this population has revealed certain brain characteristics that co-occur with this disorder. In Down syndrome, changes in fetal brain development can be detected by ultrasound between 16 and 21 weeks gestation (Bahado-Singh et al., 1992). These changes reflect neurobiologic features such as reduced brain size (particularly in the frontal lobes), fewer cells within specific layers of the cortex, and smaller cerebellar size (see Schmidt-Sidor, Wisniewski, Shepard, & Seren, 1990, for a review of the brain correlates of Down syndrome). After birth, these neuroanatomic differences can have functional correlates of concern for communication. For example, neuroimaging research has demonstrated reduced metabolic activity in the language areas of the brain associated with Down syndrome (Azari et al., 1994).

Normal brain development is characterized by overproduction of neurons and of connections between cells. After birth, the brain begins a lifetime of refining itself by pruning back excess cells and connections and strengthening those connections that are most functional. What determines which cells and connections are most functional? A large determinant of functionality is the experience the young child receives. In other words, all babies' brains are shaped by the things they see, hear, and explore. Even for a baby like Alicia, brain development is not complete at birth. Experience continues to shape the brain throughout life, and a child's early experiences are critical for realizing that child's full potential. This is one reason professionals advocate early intervention for children with or at risk for communication disorders.

In other instances of communication disorders, the brain may have developed normally, only to be damaged later by illness or injury. In fact, much of what we know about the brain's organization was learned by observing the behavior of individuals who suffered damage to localized regions of the brain. This work began in the 1800s with two landmark medical cases. Paul Broca described a case of a man who lost his ability to express himself through spoken language, but retained much of his general cognitive functioning and his ability to understand language. When this man died, Broca examined his brain and found damage to the inferior left frontal lobe, a region that has come to be known as Broca's area. This area has been closely associated with processes important for expressive language. Conversely, Carl Wernicke described a case of a man who lost the ability to comprehend spoken language and whose brain lesion was in the posterior part of the left temporal lobe. This general area, associated with language comprehension, has come to be called Wernicke's area.

The work begun by Broca and Wernicke gave rise to the **cerebral localization** perspective on brain functioning. The premise of a localizationist approach is that certain regions within the brain appear necessary for a particular skill or function. For most people, the left hemisphere is specialized for language. In particular, the regions of the left hemisphere that surround the **Sylvian fissure** are critical language areas. This so-called **perisylvian region** includes the primary auditory cortex and the primary sensory and motor regions for the face that are located on either bank of the **Rolandic fissure**, which is roughly at right angles to the Sylvian fissure (see Figure 2.8). It also includes both Broca's and Wernicke's areas and additional cortex in the region. Damage within this broadly defined perisylvian region can lead to various types of language disorders, as we will see in Chapters 8 and 9.

The localization perspective focuses on brain regions that contribute to particular functions. However, we have become increasingly aware that brain areas do not act in isolation. Rather, systems composed of various brain structures and the connections between them act together to support behavior. This insight has given rise to a *connectionist* perspective, which emphasizes the interconnectedness of functionally related brain regions. Current connectionist models of language are implemented with computer programs intended to simulate how the brain works

(Plaut, McClelland, Seidenberg, & Patterson, 1996; Rumelhart & McClelland, 1986). Information from these computational models provide understanding that complements that learned from the study of the effects of damage to critical brain regions.

For most individuals, language is a left hemisphere function; however, effective communication relies on many regions within both hemispheres of the brain. For example, listening to a lecture can involve all lobes simultaneously. As each person in attendance concentrates on the speaker, he or she tries to ignore other distractions (using frontal and parietal lobes), take in the auditory and visual speech signal (temporal and occipital lobes), interpret its content (left temporal lobe), and visually monitor the facial expressions and affect of the speaker (occipital and right parietal lobes). It is the integrated function of all these brain regions that allows the listener to receive the verbal and nonverbal information and comprehend its meaning.

## Peripheral Nervous System

To be functional, the brain must be connected to the body and the outside world. This connection is made through the peripheral nervous system. The upper portion of the peripheral nervous system includes twelve pairs of nerves that enter or exit the CNS within the cranial space occupied by the brain and brainstem. These are known as the **cranial nerves** (see Table 2.1).

As one can see from Table 2.1, most of the cranial nerves play some role in communication. Therefore, injury or disease that affects individual nerves may also impair specific aspects of communication. It is not surprising, then, that speech-language pathologists and audiologists include assessment of cranial nerve function when evaluating individuals with communication disorders.

Below the level of the cranial nerves are thirty-one pairs of nerves that enter or exit the spinal cord, referred to as the **spinal nerves**. The **spinal cord** is made up of ascending and descending nerve tracts. There are anterior and posterior nuclei (clusters of cell bodies) at thirty-one levels of the spinal cord. The motor nerves that innervate the muscles of the chest, the abdomen, and the limbs exit the anterior (front) portion of the spinal cord, and sensory information from the body is received in the posterior portion of the spinal cord. Sensory nerves come into the posterior spinal nuclei from various peripheral sites, such as glands, tissues, joints, and muscles. Some of the peripheral sensory information is processed directly at the spinal level, where various sensorimotor reflexes may occur. In other cases, the sensory information travels to the central nervous system through the **brainstem** and cerebellum, where sensorimotor adjustments may be made. The sensory information may also travel to the thalamus, where it is processed and relayed further. Some sensory impulses from the spinal nerves probably project directly (with some filtering or adjustment along the way) to the sensory cortex.

**TABLE 2.1   The Cranial Nerves**

| CRANIAL NERVE | NAME | PRIMARY FUNCTION | ROLE IN COMMUNICATION |
|---|---|---|---|
| I | Olfactory | Sense of smell | — |
| II | Optic | Vision | Face-to-face communication<br>Reading<br>Writing<br>Sign language |
| III | Oculomotor | Eye movement | Reading<br>Writing<br>Sign language |
| IV | Trochlear | Eye movement | Reading<br>Writing<br>Sign language |
| V | Trigeminal | Movement of jaw<br>Sensation from face | Speaking |
| VI | Abducens | Eye movement | Reading<br>Writing |
| VII | Facial | Movement of facial muscles<br>Sensation from tongue, velum | Speaking |
| VIII | Auditory | Hearing and balance | Listening |
| IX | Glossopharyngeal | Movement of pharynx<br>Sensation from posterior tongue, pharynx | Speaking |
| X | Vagus | Movement of larynx, pharynx, velum, diaphragm, heart, abdominal viscera<br><br>Sensation from larynx, pharynx, inner ear, other body organs | Speaking |
| XI | Accessory motor | Movement of large muscles of the head, neck, shoulders | Speaking |
| XII | Hypoglossal | Movement of tongue, supralaryngeal muscles | Speaking |

## CLINICAL PROBLEM SOLVING

Consider the following clinical case:

*Mr. Blades, age 71.* In an acute-care hospital, a speech-language pathologist is asked to evaluate the speech and language of a 71-year-old man named Mr. Blades. He had been admitted to the hospital the day before, following a car accident in which he was a passenger. He had several broken bones and had hit his head and lost consciousness for an hour. Although alert on the following day, he seemed to have difficulty understanding what was said to him. The clinician was concerned that the blow to the head damaged regions of his brain that support language, but also needed to consider other reasons for his language comprehension difficulty.

1. Why would the clinician suspect that the car accident may have produced the language comprehension problem?
2. What other biological system(s) could also be the source of poor comprehension?
3. If Mr. Blades also had difficulty speaking, what other biological system(s) could be involved? Why?

## LEARNING ACTIVITY

The respiratory system provides the power source for speech, but we barely notice how it functions.

1. How many breaths do you take in a minute as you rest quietly? Find out by counting them.
2. How many breaths do you think you take in a minute when you are talking? Find out by reading aloud and having a partner count how many breaths you take. Is it more or less than you took when breathing at rest? Why is it different?
3. How long can you sustain phonation on one breath? Find out by taking a deep breath and holding an "ah." Use a stopwatch to measure the duration.

## REFERENCES

Azari, N. P., Horowitz, B., Pettigrew, K. D., Grady, C. L., Haxby, J. V., Giacometti, K. R., & Schapiro, M. B. (1994). Abnormal pattern of cerebral glucose metabolic rates involving language areas in young adults with Down syndrome. *Brain and Language, 46,* 1–20.

Bahado-Singh, R. O., Wyse, L., Dorr, M. A., Copel, J. A., O'Connor, T., & Hobbins, J. C. (1992). Fetuses with Down syndrome have disproportionately shortened frontal lobe dimensions on ultrasonographic examination. *American Journal of Obstetrics and Gynecology, 167,* 1009–1014.

Hixon, T. J. (1973). Respiratory function in speech. In F. D. Minifie, T. J. Hixon, & F. Williams (Eds.), *Normal aspects of speech, hearing, and language* (pp. 73–126). Englewood Cliffs, NJ: Prentice Hall.

Hixon, T. J., & Abbs, J. H. (1980). Normal speech production. In T. J. Hixon, L. D. Shriberg, & J. H. Saxman (Eds.), *Introduction to communication disorders.* Englewood Cliffs, NJ: Prentice Hall.

Kent, R. D. (1997). *The speech sciences.* San Diego: Singular Publishing.

Plaut, D. C., McClelland, J. L., Seidenberg, M. S., & Patterson, K. (1996). Understanding normal and impaired word reading: Computational principles in quasi-regular domains. *Psychological Review, 103,* 56–115.

Rumelhart, D. F., McClelland, J. L., & The PDP Research Group (Eds.). (1986). *Parallel distributed processing: Explorations in the microstructure of cognition: Volume 1. Foundations.* Cambridge, MA: MIT Press.

Schmidt-Sidor, B., Wisniewski, K. E., Shepard, T. H., & Seren, E. A. (1990). Brain growth in Down syndrome subjects 15–22 weeks gestational age and birth to 60 months. *Clinical Neuropathology, 9,* 181–190.

Story, B. H., Titze, I. R., & Hoffman, E.A. (1996). Vocal tract area functions from magnetic resonance imaging. *Journal of the Acoustical Society of America, 100*(1), 537–554.

Story, B. H., Titze, I. R., & Hoffman, E. A. (1998). Vocal tract area functions for an adult female speaker based on volumetric imaging. *Journal of the Acoustical Society of America, 104*(1), 471–487.

Voice Foundation. (1985). *The voice of the impersonator.* (Videocassette developed by R. Feder.) New York: Author.

Weismer, C. (1988). Speech production. In N. J. Lass, L. V. McReynolds, J. L. Northern, & D. E. Yoder (Eds.), *Handbook of speech-language pathology and audiology.* Philadelphia: B. C. Decker.

Zemlin, W. R. (1998). *Speech and hearing science: Anatomy and physiology* (4th ed.). Boston: Allyn and Bacon.

# CHAPTER THREE

# SOUNDS IN COMMUNICATION

■ ■ ■ ■ ■

## PREVIEW

Sounds are the currency of auditory-oral communication. Speech-language patholo-gists and audiologists, as well as speech and hearing scientists, are concerned with the acoustic elements of sound. This includes an understanding of the basic physical na-ture of sound, how speech sounds are produced, and how such sounds can be mea-sured and described. Given the complexity of the sounds of language, it is amazing that young children master the language of their environment with such ease. We will examine this process in a young child who is acquiring English as his native language.

Auditory functioning supports communication at many levels. A short bark at the back door lets us know that the dog wants to come inside. The telephone's ring tells us someone is trying to reach us. With speech, humans are able to use sound to express an infinite variety of ideas, moods, and attitudes. We will examine sound first at its most basic level, as an acoustic signal, and then as the signal is modified to form human speech.

## ACOUSTIC ASPECTS OF SOUND

The essence of sound is motion. When someone talks to you from across the room, the vibrations created by his or her voice and articulation are carried through the air to your ears. Sound energy "travels" because air molecules that are adjacent to a source of vibration bump up against neighboring molecules and push them a bit. Those molecules likewise displace their neighbors, and so on, so that the vibration is propagated. The individual molecules do not move far before they rebound back in place, but they set off a chain reaction of motion that radiates from the source. As depicted in Figure 3.1, the disturbed molecules alternately bunch close together (causing areas of *compression*) and spread apart as they return to their original lo-cations (causing regions of *rarefaction*). This vibratory motion produces a sound wave that travels through the air but can also be carried through other media, in-cluding liquids, such as water, and solid structures, such as dormitory walls. One way to represent the transmission of sound is to graph the moment-to-moment po-sition of the sound source (or a molecule that is moving in response to the force ap-plied by the source). Such a graph is a **waveform**, as shown in Figure 3.1. The horizontal axis indicates time, and the vertical axis reflects displacement from a resting point.

### Frequency

The rate of vibration of the sound source is the **frequency** of the sound. It is the number of complete cycles of to-and-fro motion that occur in one second. The units

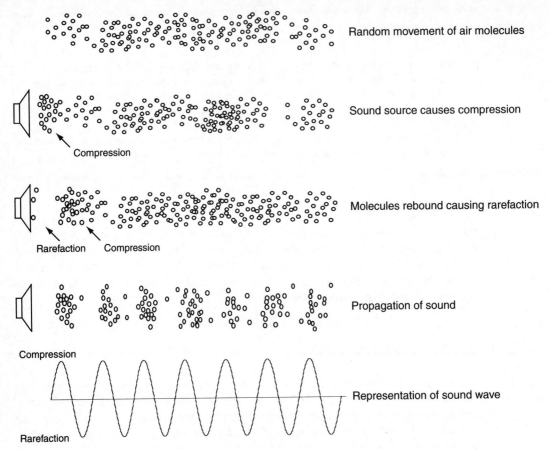

Random movement of air molecules

Sound source causes compression

Compression

Molecules rebound causing rarefaction

Rarefaction    Compression

Propagation of sound

Compression

Representation of sound wave

Rarefaction

**FIGURE 3.1    Illustrations of compressions and rarefactions of air molecules, which serve to propagate sound. The waveform at the bottom of the figure depicts the sound.**

of measurement for frequency are named Hertz to honor a scientist who made important contributions to the development of the radio. The waveform in Figure 3.2 (A) shows a pattern of vibration with three complete cycles during three-hundredths of a second (or three milliseconds). Over the course of a full second, the vibratory cycle would repeat one hundred times, so that it is a 100 Hertz (Hz) tone. Because the vibration is at only one frequency, it is called a **pure tone**, a pure tone is also called a *sine wave*. Pure tones do not occur naturally but can be produced in the laboratory and are used to test hearing at specific frequencies. Sounds in the environment are not pure tones but rather are produced by energy located at more than one frequency.

Children and young adults with normal hearing are able to hear sounds that range in frequency from about 20 to 20,000 Hz. Sounds at different frequencies are each perceived as having a different **pitch**. In other words, frequency refers to that actual number of vibrations per second (an acoustic property of the sound), whereas pitch reflects how those frequencies sound to us.

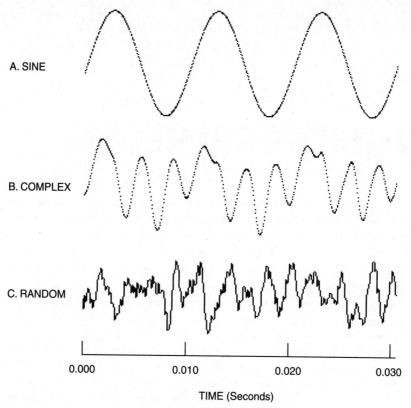

**FIGURE 3.2    Examples of simple and complex waveforms.**

The notes on a piano keyboard span a frequency range of about 20 to 4000 Hz. As shown in Figure 3.3. this frequency range includes much of the energy produced by people's voices and speech sounds. Middle C on the piano corresponds to a frequency of 256 Hz, which means that, when the piano string is struck, it vibrates 256 times in one second. This frequency is typical of the fundamental frequency of the voice of an adult woman. The average male voice has a fundamental frequency of 128 Hz, or half the frequency of a typical woman's voice. When the frequency of sound is doubled, it increases by one octave, so a woman's voice is about one octave higher than a man's voice. Additional information in a speaker's voice is carried at higher frequencies. The most important frequencies for speech sounds range from about 500 to 4,000 Hz.

## Intensity

What we perceive as the loudness of a sound is determined primarily by its **intensity**, or the pressure produced by the vibrating motion. Sound pressure level (SPL) is typically measured using a **decibel** (dB) scale. The decibel was named to honor

**FIGURE 3.3  Frequency of sound in Hertz represented on a piano keyboard. Note that the frequencies that allow us to distinguish between specific vowels or consonants are higher than those that distinguish between male and female voices.**

Alexander G. Bell, the inventor of the telephone. The scale is based on logarithms of the ratio between an arbitrary reference point and the pressure, or intensity, of a sound. The reference point for hearing, denoted as 0 dB SPL, is approximately the smallest pressure that can be detected by a person with no hearing loss. In other words, 0 dB SPL can be considered the threshold for "perfect hearing." The actual range of sound pressure from the threshold of hearing to a sound that is so loud that it causes discomfort is about a million to one (Kelly, 1985), but on the logarithmic scale the difference between these two levels is only about 120 dB. The sound pressure levels for some common sounds are shown in Table 3.1. If you compare the loudness of the human voice to various environmental sounds, you see that conversational speech falls in the middle range of intensities. It is obvious that it is easier to hear speech when we are not also confronted with louder environmental sounds.

## Complex Sounds

Most sounds in the world are not pure tones with energy restricted to one frequency; they are complex sounds with energy at more than one frequency. For example, the waveform in Figure 3.2(B) was generated by an adult male producing the vowel "ah." It is an example of a *complex waveform,* which means that more than one frequency is produced by the source. The motion pattern is complicated, with several peaks and troughs. Nonetheless, it is possible to see that the pattern is repeated three times within the time frame illustrated in Figure 3.2. In other words, the repetition rate of the complex pattern is the same as that of the 100 Hz pure tone shown in the figure. The lowest of the frequencies that make up this complex tone is 100 Hz. This is called the *fundamental frequency.*

The waveform illustrated in Figure 3.2(C) is also complex, but it does not reveal any regular or repeated pattern of motion. This type of motion pattern represents *noise,* such as that produced by a waterfall or jet engine or simply the sound

**TABLE 3.1   Possible Sound Pressure Levels of Common Environmental Sounds**

| | |
|---|---|
| 10–20 dB | Whispering heard from over five feet away |
| 40 dB | The ambient noise in a quiet room |
| 50 dB | A dog burping |
| 57 dB | The dial tone of a phone |
| 60–70 dB | Conversational speech |
| 74 dB | A door closing |
| 79 dB | A dog barking |
| 89 dB | A door slamming |
| 100 dB | A household fire alarm |

made by producing "sssss" or "shhhh." When noise is produced by motion that is completely random, it is called *white noise* because it contains all frequencies. This is analogous to white light, which contains all colors. We hear white noise on the television when we try to tune in a channel that is not broadcasting or that is not available through the cable company. Noise can be produced also by abrupt or brief sounds, such as consonants produced without voice (e.g., /p/, /t/, /k/).

Speech sounds can also be displayed in terms of the intensity of their energy at various frequencies over the period of time that they are spoken. This display is known as a **spectrogram**. The spectrogram in Figure 3.4 shows the differences among the words *bit, bat,* and *bait* that are readily apparent to the listener. These words differ in the two parameters of sound that we have already discussed: frequency and intensity. For each of these words, we can see the distribution of sound energy (intensity) at different frequencies. The energy appears as horizontal bands on the spectrogram with greater intensities shown as darker bands at particular frequencies. The lowest dark band of energy is the fundamental frequency of the speaker's voice.

For each of the words in Figure 3.4, we see differences in the relative intensity and duration of each sound that makes up the word. The portion of speech corresponding to vowel sounds contains regions of strong acoustic energy. When we listen to words, we pick up information about the speaker's voice primarily from vowels because of the relatively long duration of voiced sound production. In contrast to the vowels, the unvoiced consonant "t" produces a short and relatively weak burst of energy, which is represented by a much lighter shade of gray on the spectrogram. These differences in the frequency and intensity of speech sounds may seem subtle when examined visually. However, they are adequate to distinguish between words, for those with normal hearing.

The spectrogram also reveals a third parameter that differentiates the sounds of speech: time. It is the combination of the distribution of sound energy over certain frequencies and the particular timing patterns that lead to the perception of three different vowels and, thus, three different words, in the case of *bit, bat,* and *bait*. Changes in the spectral energy and timing also help differentiate consonants, as in the words *pot, got,* and *not*.

FIGURE 3.4   Complex speech sounds can be analyzed to show the component frequencies that we hear as different speech sounds. The words shown in this spectrogram are *bit, bat,* and *bait.*

## THE SPOKEN SOUNDS OF COMMUNICATION

### Vocalization

As we learned in Chapter 2, the production of speech sounds relies on the coordinated action of many physical elements, including muscles of the larynx, throat, face, and oral structures. **Vocalization** requires a sound generator—the larynx—and a force to drive this generator—air. During normal breathing, the vocal folds of the larynx are open, allowing air to flow in and out unobstructed. For speech, the vocal folds are open during the production of voiceless sounds and are closed to produce voiced sounds. When exhaled air hits the closed (or closing) vocal folds with sufficient force, the folds blow apart and the exhaled air pushes against the stationary air above the folds, setting in motion a sound wave.

The frequency of the sound created by the vibrating vocal folds depends on the mass and length of the folds. Larger vocal folds tend to vibrate fewer times per second and therefore produce sounds at a lower frequency. Thus, men's voices tend to be lower than women's, and women's voices are lower than children's.

Table 3.2 shows some frequencies of different voices for comparison. The fundamental frequency of the voice is carried by the vowel sounds in speech. The frequency of consonant sounds is much higher than the fundamental frequency of the voice.

## Speech Sounds

As clinicians, we need a precise system for differentiating among the sounds that people produce. The written word, as produced with the English alphabet, is inadequate for this task because one letter can correspond to more than one sound. Consider the "o" in *off* versus in *over,* or the "c" in *cat* versus in *certain.* For other consonants, two or three letters represent the sound (e.g., "th," "sh," "ng," "tch"), and the same sound can be represented in more than one way (e.g., "f" and "ph"). Further complicating matters is the occurrence of "silent letters" (e.g., "p" in *ptomaine,* "gh" in *weight*) in English orthography. For these reasons, those who study speech use the *International Phonetic Alphabet* (IPA). The IPA symbols for consonants appear in Table 3.3, along with their corresponding sounds in words, and the IPA symbols for English vowels are depicted in Figure 3.5. Some additional symbols are used for specific vowel sounds; in all, more than forty different symbols are needed to specify the sounds of English, compared with the twenty-six letters of our alphabet. These symbols allow us to specify the meaningful sounds, or **phonemes**, of the English language. A unique IPA symbol is associated with each phoneme in a manner that avoids the confusion caused by a single letter having more than one pronunciation (e.g., the letter "c" can be produced like a "k" or an "s"). The actual production of a sound by a speaker is referred to as a **phone**. The term **allophone** refers to the variations in phones that are still categorized as the same phoneme. For example, we say the "t" in *tap* slightly differently than in *setting,* although both are considered versions of "t." By convention, phonetic symbols are written between two forward slash marks to indicate a phoneme with all its various acceptable allophones (e.g., /t/).

**TABLE 3.2   The Fundamental Frequency of the Human Voice**

| SOURCE | FREQUENCY LEVEL OF THE VOICE |
|---|---|
| An infant cooing | 380 Hz |
| Boys or girls, age 9, talking | 260 Hz |
| An adult woman saying "hat" | 256 Hz |
| An adult man saying "hat" | 128 Hz |
| **CONSONANT SOUNDS** | |
| s or z | 4000–8000 Hz |
| t or v | 6000–7000 Hz |
| th (as in "thick") | 7000–8000 Hz |

## Consonants

Consonant sounds are the result of precise placement and movement of the articulators. They can be characterized by three general parameters: the *place* of articulation, the *manner* in which the sound is produced, and whether the consonant is voiced. This place-manner-voicing system can be used for describing the production of specific sounds. Table 3.3 includes the consonants used in English and shows how each phoneme is distinguished by its place, manner, and voicing characteristics. The anatomical *place of production* is named for the articulator(s) involved or the contact point for the tongue. These are shown across the top of Table 3.3, ordered from front to back in the vocal tract: *bilabial* (lips), *labiodental* (lips and teeth), *interdental* (between the teeth), *alveolar* (ridge behind upper teeth), *palatal* (hard palate), *velar* (velum, or soft palate), and *glottal* (glottis). The glottis is not strictly an articulator but functions to produce the unvoiced /h/ sound, as in "hip." We see the *manner of production* on the left-hand margin. There are six consonants (/p/, /b/, /t/, /d/, /k/, /g/) classified as *stops* or **plosives**, produced by briefly obstructing the airflow and then releasing it. The consonants that are paired in Table 3.3 (e.g., /p/ and /b/; /t/ and /d/) are called **cognates**. Each pair has the same manner and place of production, differing only on the dimension of voicing in that some sounds are accompanied by voice and others are not. For example, /b/ is a voiced stop, whereas /p/ is the voiceless cognate for /b/. In Table 3.3, voiced sounds are marked with an asterisk. The **fricative** consonants (/f/, /v/,

**TABLE 3.3  The Consonants in English**

| MANNER OF ARTICULATION | PLACE OF PRODUCTION | | | | | | |
|---|---|---|---|---|---|---|---|
| | Bilabial | Labiodental | Interdental | Alveolar | Palatal | Velar | Glottal |
| Stop or Plosive | p (*pat*) | | | t (*toe*) | | k (*kick*) | |
| | b* (*bat*) | | | d* (*doe*) | | g* (*gap*) | |
| Fricative | | f (*fat*) | θ (*thin*) | s (*sip*) | ʃ (*shoe*) | | h (*hip*) |
| | | v* (*vat*) | ð* (*that*) | z* (*zip*) | ʒ* (*measure*) | | |
| Affricate | | | | tʃ (*chop*) | | | |
| | | | | dʒ* (*job*) | | | |
| Nasal | m* (*mom*) | | | n* (*nun*) | | ŋ* (*sing*) | |
| Lateral | | | | l* (*lap*) | | | |
| | | | | r* (*rare*) | | | |
| Glide | w* (*wall*) | | | | j* (*yes*) | | |

*Consonant is voiced.

/θ/ as in thin, /ð/ as in that, /s/, /ʃ/ as in shoe, /ʒ/ as in measure, and /h/) are created by articulators forming a constriction of the airway that produces some audible noise as air flows through. All of the nine fricatives are also **continuants**, because they can be continued as long as the airflow is present. The **affricate** consonants (/tʃ/, /dʒ/ are combinations of a stop and a fricative. Only three consonants in the English language are **nasals** (/m/, /n/, and /ŋ/), produced with the velopharyngeal port open. There are two commonly recognized liquid, or *lateral*, consonants. The lateral /l/, is produced with the tongue tip raised to contact the alveolar ridge while openings along the sides of the tongue allow the air stream to pass. The liquid consonant /r/ requires retraction and elevation of the tongue, with the sides of the tongue often touching the hard palate. The last consonant grouping in Table 3.3 are the glide sounds (/w/, /j/), which are often classified as semivowels.

The consonant systems vary across languages. For example, English contains only one glottal sound, the fricative /h/, whereas other languages, such as Navajo, include glottal stops. On the other hand, English contains certain consonants (e.g., /l/ and /r/) not found in some other languages, such as Chinese. Sometimes, what we perceive as the "accent" of a non-native speaker of English relates to a subtle alteration in the place, manner, or voicing aspects of the consonants.

Correct production of speech sounds requires specific positioning and movement of the articulators to achieve the ideal place of contact, shape of the oral cavity, force, airflow, and pattern of movement (Daniloff, 1973). These movements must be accomplished quickly in running speech, which requires a stream of air and continuous sequencing of articulatory movements. The sounds that precede or follow a particular sound influence the production of that sound, a process often called sound assimilation. For example, if we say, "Tea, too," the production of the /t/ phone in each word will be slightly different; the high vowel /i/ in *tea* will bring the tongue tip slightly more forward than for the production of /t/ in *too*. Assimilation provides some evidence that speech production is organized by the nervous system in larger units than the single phone. Production of a phone in running speech is often indistinguishable from the production of an adjacent phone preceding or following the target phone, a process known as **coarticulation**.

## Vowels

Like consonants, vowels are also coded using IPA symbols, as shown in Figure 3.5. Vowels are produced with the mouth relatively open, and voicing is generated by vocal fold vibration. The sound generated by the vocal fold vibration is then modified by positioning of the pharynx, soft palate, tongue, jaw, and lips to create a distinct configuration of the vocal tract. The unique sound for each vowel is dependent on the position and height of the tongue in the oral cavity as well as the configuration of the lips. For example, as shown in Figure 3.5, in the production of the /i/ ("ee" as in *beet*) vowel, the tongue is positioned high and forward in the mouth. In addition, the jaw is elevated, and the lips are slightly withdrawn. Conversely, we see that the /a/ ("a" as in *father*) vowel is produced with the jaw

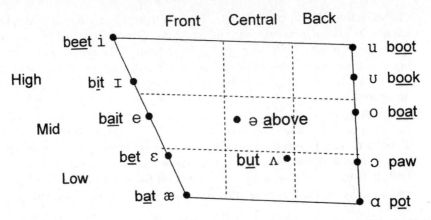

**FIGURE 3.5** The vowel quadrilateral showing twelve vowels used in English, their place of articulation in the oral cavity (front, central, back), and the relative height of the highest part of the tongue (high, mid, low).

dropped and the back of the tongue held low in the oral cavity. In addition to single vowel sounds, we also produce sounds called **diphthongs** that contain a combination of two vowels. Diphthongs, such as /aɪ/ in *buy* or /ɔɪ/ in *boy*, are assimilated blends of separate vowels that produce a two-vowel glide. Production of a diphthong requires a quick sequence of vocal tract adjustments, usually involving rapid movements of the tongue from low to high (or vice versa) and back to front (or vice versa).

Each vowel found in a particular language has its own distinctive production characteristics. For example, listening to an Australian speaker and an American speaker, one will perceive the same English language with the same consonants embedded within markedly different vowels and diphthongs. These differences may cause difficulties for the listeners as they try to understand each other. As mentioned earlier in this chapter, vowels allow us to hear the voice of the speaker. Although consonants play a primary role in how well speech is understood, or its *intelligibility*, the vowels we utter also contribute to how well someone can understand us.

## Prosody

So far, we have discussed the constituents of speech that make up the individual sounds within words (i.e., the consonants and vowels). However, additional aspects of sound are critical in conveying meaning in conversation. These aspects include the tempo, rhythm, and intonation with which the sounds and words are spoken. These elements make up the **prosody** of speech.

Prosody conveys information about the grammatical structure of a spoken sentence. For example, the speaker uses short pauses to set off a phrase embedded within the sentence (separated by commas in written text), as in "The report, which appeared to be composed by monkeys typing at random, received a failing grade."

Variations in intonation also allow us to discriminate between statements and questions. For example, the words "You liked rhubarb pie" can be expressed as a statement (meaning, "You had it before, and you liked it") or as a question (meaning "Did you really like it?"). The difference between a statement and a question is conveyed in English by the steady or falling intonation in the statement form and the rising intonation on the question form. These types of prosodic cues are referred to as *linguistic prosody,* because they provide information about the sentence structure and type.

Prosody can also convey information about the feelings or emotions of the speaker. This *emotional prosody* is how others detect, from the tones of our voices, whether we are upset, or secretly pleased, or simply neutral. In other cases, we purposefully mismatch the content of our words with the emotional tone of our speech to express sarcasm or irony. Most individuals are exquisitely sensitive to the myriad of overtones that can be added to speech via emotional prosody. In fact, when there is a mismatch between what we say (i.e., the words used) and how we say it (i.e., the emotional prosody), our listener is likely to assume that the prosodic information conveys our true meaning. That is why we hear comments such as, "She said it was OK, but she didn't seem too happy about it." The additional information conveyed through emotional prosody may be intentional or unintentional, which is why we sometimes say, "Your voice is telling on you."

## SPEECH SOUND DEVELOPMENT

A child who is born with a normally functioning hearing mechanism and raised in a speaking environment will systematically acquire the perceptual capabilities needed to understand the language he or she hears. As the baby develops, we see a corresponding development of the baby's knowledge and use of the sound system (see Table 3.4). In order to understand the development of the child's auditory and early sound production capabilities, let us look at the experiences of a single child.

### Birth

Abraham was born in the early morning of May 15. He was the first child in his family. Within days of Abraham's birth, his hearing was screened. Neonatal hearing screenings have become widely used as part of a well-baby checkup. The relative cost of widespread screenings is minor compared to the advantages gained by early intervention for children born with a hearing loss. In Abraham's case, the results confirmed normal hearing.

The development of Abraham's sound system actually began while he was still in the womb. A developing fetus responds to sound by the third trimester of gestation (Birnholz & Benacerraf, 1983). The fetus will change positions and increase heart rate in response to sound. If the sound persists, these behavioral signs of hearing will wane, only to return if the characteristics of the sounds change

**TABLE 3.4  Approximate Ages for Milestones in the Comprehension and Production of Sound**

| AGE | MILESTONE |
| --- | --- |
| 0 weeks | Startles at loud sound<br>Prefers mother's voice to strangers'<br>Produces reflexive, vegetative sounds |
| 4 months | Responds to household sounds<br>Can discriminate among many speech sounds<br>Produces differentiated cries<br>Produces vowel-like sounds |
| 7 months | Produces canonical babbling<br>Uses sound with communicative intent |
| 10 months | Produces "protowords"<br>Repeats sounds made by others<br>Produces jargon<br>Understands some words |
| 12 months | Produces words with simplified forms |

(Leader, Baillie, Martin, & Vermeulen, 1982). However, the sounds that reached Abraham in utero were probably more limited in scope than what he can now hear. First of all, his mother's body tissues attenuated, or reduced, the sounds (Walker, Grimwade, & Wood, 1971). Because the voice of Abraham's father had to travel from the air through his wife's body to reach his developing child, Abraham probably heard only a muffled version of his father's voice in the womb. The lower frequencies carried by vowel sounds and the pitch, rhythm, and intonation of the father's voice were probably heard more clearly than the higher frequency sounds that distinguished the consonants of his speech. In contrast, the mother's voice had a direct route to her fetus via internal sound vibrations that traveled through her body to the womb. This advantage makes maternal speech recorded within the womb more intelligible than the speech of others (Armitage, Baldwin, & Vince, 1980; Bench, 1968).

The influence of prenatal auditory experience can be measured in babies soon after birth. Researchers use techniques such as "high amplitude sucking," in which infants suck on a pacifier that is wired to data-recording instruments. Infant abilities are explored by conditioning babies to change their rate of sucking in response to what they hear. DeCasper and colleagues examined infant responses to sounds available in the prenatal environment and found that the infants showed preferences for recordings of an intrauterine heartbeat (DeCasper & Sigafoos, 1983) and the voice's of their own mother's (DeCasper & Fifer, 1980). Therefore, it is no surprise that Abraham is comforted by being held against his mother's body as she speaks gently to him. The warmth of her body and the sound of her heartbeat and voice are already familiar to him.

At home, Abraham is already a beginning communicator. However, much of this is unintentional on his part. As his uncle holds him, Abraham makes a series of lip smacks. In response, his uncle responds playfully as if the baby just related a shocking secret. Later, as his mother gives him a sponge bath, Abraham is fussy and emits a series of cries. His mother "explains" to him that she is bathing him and that she is trying to do this as fast as she can. She then picks him up in a towel to rock him, telling him he is okay. While dressing him, she "trades" sounds with him by repeating his short cries and other vocalizations. Soon, his parents begin to recognize the different types of cries he makes. For example, Abraham's father recognizes a cry of protest as he removes a bottle of formula from Abraham's mouth in order to reposition him. These early interactions provide the infant with important information about communication. The infant learns that vocalizations have the positive effect of parental attention and response. The close proximity of the parent's face allows the infant to see his or her parent's facial expressions. The give-and-take interchanges lay the groundwork for conversational turn-taking.

## 6 Weeks

Abraham awakens from his nap. His legs and arms stretch and move about as he makes a series of sounds. His mouth is open, and he emits a series of short, vowel-like sounds as well as lip and tongue smacks. Sometimes these sound like exclamations, comments, or complaints. Early on, infants' cries and other vocalizations often occur with the velopharyngeal port open, giving sounds a nasal quality (Oller, 1980). Infants may produce sounds on both expirations and inspirations. Each infant is quite variable in how he or she produces sounds from one time to the next. It may be that the infant is "trying out" the many combinations of positions and movements that can be used to produce grunts, cries, and other vocalizations (Boliek, Hixon, Watson, & Morgan, 1996).

Abraham's father enters the nursery and gets down to eye level with his son. When he calls his son's name, the infant turns his head and looks at his father's face. His father asks, "Are you waking up? Are you waking up now?" Abraham gives his father a big smile. These types of interactions demonstrate the infant's early response to and preference for familiar faces and voices. In return, Abraham's interest in his father's voice is rewarded by more verbal attention from his father. In fact, Abraham's parents speak to him quite a lot. They name his body parts as they wash him. They tell him about his fashion options while dressing him for the day. They recite nursery rhymes while changing his diaper. Although all this language stimulation may seem beyond his level of comprehension, it provides him with an ongoing stream of information from which he is already beginning to gain knowledge about his native language.

Like parents around the world, Abraham's parents talk to him with exaggerated stress and pitch variations, slower rate, and liberal use of repetitions. This type of speech is often called *child-directed-speech* or, sometimes, *motherese*. Adults and older children often use child-directed speech when speaking to infants and toddlers, and babies seem to prefer this type of speech. Researchers feel that the exaggerations of child-directed speech may also play an important role in helping the young child segment the ongoing stream of speech into units of phrases, words, and individual sounds (Jusczyk, 1997; Kuhl & Iverson, 1995).

## 4 to 6 Months

At 4 months, Abraham's major activity for the day is putting things into his mouth, with a secondary emphasis on drooling. He tries putting his hands, his feet, his toys, and even dry leaves into his mouth, then makes a grab for his grandmother's earrings. This is a typical mode for exploring the world at this age. Regardless of whether his mouth is full, he makes a variety of vowel sounds. Sometimes, they are abrupt exclamations (e.g., "eh!"). These sounds are not necessarily directed toward anyone, although they stop when his mother approaches. His mother gets down on the ground with him and exclaims, "How's my big boy?! How's my big boy?!" He looks at her intently and then squeals in response. Although Abraham does not yet understand just what is said to him, he is learning about the give-and-take of "conversation" and sounds that comprise his native language.

We know that infants have perceptual capabilities from very early on that allow them to begin to recognize the individual sounds of speech. As we discussed earlier, the production of individual sounds varies from one word to the next due to coarticulatory effects. Nonetheless, we perceive all the variations on the sound "b" as the phoneme /b/, and all the variations of "p" as the phoneme /p/. This trait, common to mammals including humans, is known as *categorical perception* because acoustic signals that lie on a physical continuum between sound pairs such as /b/ or /p/ are perceived as one sound or the other. A complementary situation exists for vowels, wherein a large variety of acoustic representations are perceived as one of a much smaller set of vowel sounds. This is known as the *perceptual magnet effect* (Kuhl, 1994; Kuhl & Iverson, 1995) because, when we hear an acoustic signal that is vowel-like, our perception of that signal is drawn, like a magnet, toward the prototypical vowel that is closest to the sound heard.

These early perceptual capabilities are shaped by the listener's experience with the language or languages heard. An early study by Eimas, Siqueland, Jusczyk, and Vigorito (1971) showed that infants could distinguish between such acoustic contrasts at four weeks after birth. Subsequent work (e.g., Burnham, Earnshaw, & Clark, 1991; Kuhl, Williams, Lacerda, Stevens, & Lindblom, 1992; Streeter, 1976; Werker & LaLonde, 1988) has shown that infants initially perceive contrasts that include sounds not found in their native language but later lose the ability to discriminate between non-native speech sounds. This suggests that the perceptual change reflects a developmental milestone that requires exposure to spoken language to be achieved.

## 7 to 9 Months

At 7 months of age, Abraham celebrated this first Christmas. Wearing his pajamas and a red Santa's hat, he sat on the couch and reached for the small gift that fell out of his Christmas stocking. His parents began to unwrap the gifts for him, but, once they were started, he was able to tear the remaining paper off them. He mouthed each piece of torn wrapping paper before tossing it aside. He patted an unwrapped box with his open hand and watched his parents as they held up each gift, naming and commenting about each one. This "joint reference" between parent and child provided Abraham with the opportunity to observe objects and actions at the same time that he heard the words that related to them. His breathing was rapid and loud, and he waved his arms with excitement.

During this period, Abraham reached a new milestone in the development of the speech sound system. His production of sounds no longer consisted solely of vowels. The first consonants were added to his repertoire. Abraham exclaimed "Da!" as he reached for an as-of-yet untasted piece of wrapping paper. These first consonant-vowel (CV) and consonant-vowel-consonant-vowel (CVCV) utterances are referred to as **canonical babbling**. This type of babbling is nonspecific, in that babies Abraham's age do not use these CV or CVCV combinations to refer to specific objects or intentions. However, Abraham, like other babies, produced these sound combinations with the prosody of speech, so that it seemed as though he was speaking even though no true words were produced.

Abraham's initial production of canonical babbling at 7 months was about average for developing infants. Eilers and Oller (1994) reported that normally hearing infants may enter the stage of canonical babbling as early as 3 months or as late as 10 months. Auditory experience seems critical for the development of this milestone. Hearing-impaired infants are delayed in canonical babbling, with the onset occurring after 11 months of age. In contrast, infants with other developmental problems but no hearing loss may show little or no delay in reaching this milestone (Eilers & Oller, 1994).

At 6 and 7 months of age, babies continue to make vowel-like sounds, and they also produce consonant-vowel (CV) combinations. They make these sounds regardless of whether another person is interacting with them. However, there are qualitative changes in sound production at this stage as well. For example, Abraham often seemed fascinated with his own babbling. He seemed to play with variations of his own babbling, producing a string of sounds and then repeating them with a slight change in the overall pattern. For example, while playing, he produced "di da . . . di da . . . daaaaaah . . . da." As at earlier ages, these sounds appeared to be a form of vocal play, without reference to any object in particular.

Another change is the emergence of communicative intent behind Abraham's use of sound. This preverbal use of sound is typical among babies at this age. Parents recognize their baby's use of sounds to direct their attention to an object, to request actions ("give me"), or just as a social interaction. At this age, Abraham used sounds to signal refusal, for example. His mother offered him a spoonful of strained peas, which appeared to be out of favor at the time. He exclaimed his disgust and turned his face away from the offending food. These first intentional vocalizations are quite probably precursors of linguistic behaviors yet to come. In fact, babies at this stage begin to comprehend a few spoken words, signaling the onset of the first true linguistic stage of development.

## 10 to 14 Months

Abraham learned to walk before his first birthday. Initially, he used a coffee table or the couch to lift himself up and then "cruised" around the room, holding on to the edges of the furniture. Then he walked without support. But often, he was able to take only a few steps before landing on his seat. His most efficient mode of locomotion was still crawling.

Abraham also expanded his sound repertoire. In addition to the single syllables that were heard at 7 to 9 months, he learned to produce consonants in combination. As he stood ready to walk to his mother's outstretched arms, we heard "yee yeah adee di hee." Then Abraham's father, holding a video camera, caught his attention. His mother asked, "Do you want to walk to Daddy?" Abraham piped in with an enthusiastic "da! dee!" Although this approximated the word "daddy," it was not yet a true word for Abraham. In fact, a few minutes later, we heard Abraham utter a chorus of "da dees" when attempting to walk toward his mother and also when attending to neither parent. In this particular case, "da dee" reflected a different milestone in the development of speech sounds: the ability to repeat sound strings produced by others. We saw this new ability to repeat more explicitly when Abraham's mother was encouraging him to show off for the camera. She told him, "Wave to the camera. Wave! Wave!" He echoed back "ey . . . ey" as a shortened form of "wave." Then he waved his hands, first one hand and then both. Next, his mother told him, "Say 'Hey!' You know how to say 'Hey!' Say 'Hey!'" And he repeated "Hey!"

At this stage, we often hear a chain of syllables with sentencelike inflectional patterns, such as "ba to aa aa na?" We refer to these speechlike sound strings as *jargon*. Such an utterance is directed toward a listener, with the baby often searching to make eye contact, causing the listener to feel almost obligated to answer the jargon question with "yes" or "no." Abraham appeared to demand an object from the listener, give it back, and then demand it again. He changed his role within the communicative exchange, alternating between asker and giver. The sound of his voice carried as much of the message as the reaching gestures or looking at the object.

Jargon includes many combinations of consonants and vowels, and there does not appear to be a one-to-one representation for a particular object or desire. That is, the baby is not using the same combination of sounds to represent particular words. Although many of the consonant-vowel combinations are repeated, others are unique. The intention of the utterance is carried more in the inflection and prosody than in the consonant-vowel combination. At earlier ages, vocalizations flowed easily, and there was no demand that babies produce any specific sounds. When they use vocalized jargons as intentional communication, however, babies begin to use the inflectional patterns that have been heard in their native language that represent particular needs and wants. At this stage, we hear front, middle, and back vowels sandwiched between many different consonantlike sounds.

Around the age of 11 months, Abraham entered a stage characterized by "nonreduplicated or variegated babbling" (Schwartz, 1984), meaning the jargon sounds were individualized and not often repeated. At this stage, the infant begins to show real control over the stress and intonation of vocalization, with the jargon pattern closely resembling the language the baby has been hearing. Ingram (1976) presented a number of diary studies that described particular babies at 11 to 12 months who were beginning to repeat the same vocalization pattern in a given situational context. There was still enough phonetic variability to preclude the utterance from being classified as true words. Many of the utterances at this age sound more like phrases than single words.

A baby this age produces phonetically consistent forms that are the immediate precursors to true words. Schwartz (1984) describes these precursors as **protowords** (primitive, early forms of an actual word). Whereas jargon vocalization appears to be more related to the affective, emotional state of the infant and is therefore rather free-flowing, protowords have much greater specificity and appear to be more object- or action-specific. Sometimes, babies this age embed a protoword in the prosodic jargon. At other times, we observe a combination of prosodic jargon, then a slight pause, followed by the production of a protoword. It would seem that the first true words that often appear at 12 to 13 months do not come suddenly but have developed gradually, from babble to jargon to protowords and then finally to a true word with relative phonetic stability.

Despite the arrival of the first few words, typical 1-year-olds seem to attempt most of their communication by continuing differentiated jargon. The first words are not said very often. The jargon pattern becomes longer, sounding more like real language and occasionally containing a real word. Although a wide variety of sounds may be heard in the jargon of children, relatively few are heard in their first words. Much of the intended message, when understood by the listener, is communicated not by the occasional word but by the general intonational pattern of the utterance and by the situational context.

When imitating the sounds of others, there is some selectivity regarding the kinds of sounds chosen for play. We also see this pattern as babies begin to produce their first words (Ferguson, 1978). Babies imitate the sounds they can physiologically produce; if a sound is too complex to make, babies will usually simplify the utterance, perhaps changing the consonant to one they can produce and preserving the vowel that was in the model. Abraham was heard doing just this when he looked at a tiger in a picture book and said, "tita." As the first words are produced, there is similar selectivity, such that the first words require less complex motor control. Many of the first words may involve similar sounds, often voiced consonants produced at the front of the mouth, such as /m/ and /b/. Babies often use the same consonant-vowel combination for several different words. For example, /ba/ may by used for words as different as *ball* and *car*. Over time, as children add to their repertoire of speech sounds, the pronunciation of these two words becomes distinct.

## 15 Months and Older

At this age, Abraham has entered the true verbal stage of communication development. We will look in some detail at his development from single words to sentences in Chapter 7. However, Abraham will continue to add to his sound system as well during this time (see Figure 3.6). As he grows, he will add sounds in a fairly predictable way. Irwin and Wong (1983) described the sequence in which typically developing children like Abraham add sounds to their repertoire between 1½ and 3 years of age. Their work shows that most children at 18 months have one or two distinct vowels and a few consonants that they use to produce approximations of their first words. By 24 months, many of the vowels are produced distinctly, and a few new consonants are added. As depicted in Figure 3.6, by the age of 3, children have expanded their consonant repertoire, which greatly aids the overall intelligibility of their speech. Over time, children learn to use their acquired sounds in different positions within words (Dyson, 1988). The job of learning the sounds of speech and using them correctly in connected speech takes years to complete. Some normal 5-year-olds, for example, may still be mastering some of the latest acquired sounds, such as /r/ and /l/ (Kenney & Prather, 1986), although these sounds begin to emerge much earlier. Likewise, normally developing children may make sound errors in some words and not in others. This is because the

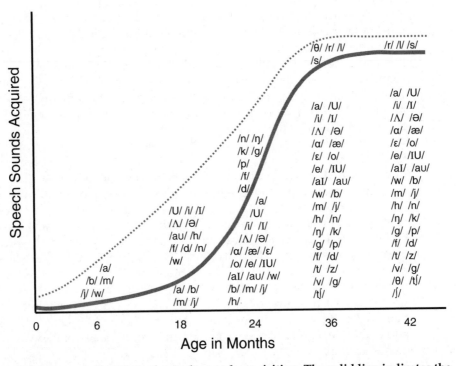

**FIGURE 3.6   A depiction of speech sound acquisition. The solid line indicates the increase of the number of speech sounds that children acquire with age. The dotted line represents additional sounds that are in the process of being acquired; that is, they are mastered by some but not all children at a given age.**

Data from Sander (1972) and Irwin & Wong (1983).

production of a particular sound is influenced by all other sounds contained in the word. As children mature, their speech is less affected by these coarticulatory effects (Nittrouer, Studdert-Kennedy, & McGowan, 1989). By age 4, most children can be readily understood, even by those who do not know them well.

## CLINICAL PROBLEM SOLVING

Kim was born with a severe hearing loss affecting both of his ears. He responded reliably to sounds of 500 to 1000 Hz at 40 dB HL; sounds at 2000 to 4000 Hz were heard at 50 to 60 dB HL; and sounds above 4000 Hz required even greater intensities (up to 80 dB HL).

1. What does this mean for Kim in terms of everyday hearing experiences? What types of environmental sounds will he hear, and what will he miss?
2. Give examples of how his experience with the sounds of speech might affect development of this aspect of communication.
3. Which components of speech (i.e., vowels, consonants, prosody) will be most difficult for him to hear?
4. Some children (and adults) who experience a hearing loss become proficient speechreaders. Which aspects of speech sound production can be best discriminated by this method and why? What aspects of conversational speech make speechreading difficult?

## REFERENCES

Armitage, S. E., Baldwin, B. A., & Vince, M. A. (1980). The fetal sound environment of sheep. *Science, 206,* 1173–1174.

Bench, J. (1968). Sound transmission to the human fetus through the maternal abdominal wall. *Journal of Genetic Psychology, 113,* 85–87.

Birnholz, J. C., & Benacerraf, B. R. (1983). The development of human fetal hearing. *Science, 222,* 516–518.

Boliek, C. A., Hixon, T. J., Watson, P. J., & Morgan, W. J. (1996). Vocalization and breathing during the first year of life. *Journal of Voice, 10,* 1–22.

Burnham, D. K., Earnshaw, L. J., & Clark, J. E. (1991). Development of categorical identification of native and non-native bilabial stops: Infants, children, and adults. *Journal of Child Language, 18,* 321–260.

Daniloff, R. G. (1973). Normal articulation processes. In F. D. Minifie, T. J. Hixon, & F. Williams (Eds.), *Normal aspects of speech, hearing, and language.* Englewood Cliffs, NJ: Prentice Hall.

DeCasper, A. J., & Fifer, W. P. (1980). Of human bonding: Newborns prefer their mother's voices. *Science, 208*(1), 1741–1776.

DeCasper A. J., & Sigafoos, D. (1983). The intrauterine heartbeat: A potential reinforcer for newborns. *Infant Behavior and Development, 6,* 19–25.

Dyson, A. T. (1988). Phonetic inventories of 2- and 3-year old children. *Journal of Speech and Hearing Disorders, 53,* 89–93.

Eilers, R. E., & Oller, D. K. (1994). Infant vocalizations and the early diagnosis of severe hearing impairment. *Journal of Pediatrics, 124,* 199–203.

Eimas, P. D., Siqueland, E. R., Jusczyk, P. W., & Vigorito, J. (1971). Speech perception in infants. *Science, 171,* 303–306.

Ferguson, C. (1978). Learning to pronounce: The earliest stages of phonological development in the child. In F. Minifie & L. Lloyd (Eds.), *Communicative and cognitive abilities: Early behavioral assessment.* Baltimore: University Park Press.

Ingram, D. (1976). *Phonological disability in children.* New York: Elsevier North Holland.

Irwin, J. V., & Wong, S. P. (1983). *Phonological development in children 18 to 72 months.* Carbondale: Southern Illinois University Press.

Jusczyk, P. W. (1997). *The discovery of spoken language.* Cambridge, MA: MIT Press/Bradford Books.

Kelly, J. P. (1985). Auditory system. In E. R. Kandel & J. H. Schwartz (Eds.), *Principles of neural science.* New York: Elsevier.

Kenney, K. W., & Prather, E. M. (1986). Articulation development in preschool children: Consistency of production. *Journal of Speech and Hearing Research, 29,* 29–36.

Kuhl, P. K. (1994). Learning and representation in speech and language. *Current Opinion in Neurobiology, 4,* 812–822.

Kuhl, P. K., & Iverson, P. (1995). Linguistic experience and the perceptual magnet effect. In W. Strange (Ed.), *Speech perception and linguistic experience.* Baltimore: York Press.

Kuhl, P. K., Williams, K. A., Lacerda, F., Stevens, K. N., & Lindblom, B. (1992). Linguistic experience alters phonetic perception in infants by 6 months of age. *Science, 255,* 606–608.

Leader, L. R., Baillie, P., Martin, B., & Vermeulen, E. (1982). The assessment and significance of habituation to a repeated stimulus by the human fetus. *Early Human Development, 7,* 211–219.

Leonard, L., Schwartz, R., Folger, M., & Wilcox, M. (1978). Some aspects of children's imitative and spontaneous speech. *Journal of Child Language, 5,* 403–416.

Nittrouer, S., Studdert-Kennedy, Y. M., & McGowan, R. S. (1989). The emergence of phonetic segments: Evidence from the spectral structure fricative-vowel syllables spoken by children and adults. *Journal of Speech and Hearing Research, 32,* 120–132.

Oller, D. (1980). The emergence of speech sounds in infancy. In G. Yeni-Kamshian, J. Kavanaugh, & C. Ferguson (Eds.), *Child phonology. Vol. 1: Production.* New York: Academic Press.

Sander, E. K. (1972). When are speech sounds learned? *Journal of Speech and Hearing Disorders, 37*(1), 55–63.

Schwartz, R. (1984). The phonologic system: Normal acquisition. In J. Costello (Ed.), *Speech disorders in children.* San Diego: College-Hill Press.

Streeter, L. A. (1976). Language perception of two-month-old infants shows effects of both innate mechanisms and experience. *Nature, 259,* 39–40.

Van Riper, C., & Emerick, L. (1984). *Speech correction: An introduction to speech pathology and audiology* (7th ed.). Englewood Cliffs, NJ: Prentice Hall.

Walker, D., Grimwade, J., & Wood, C. (1971). Intrauterine noise: A component of the fetal environment. *American Journal of Obstetrics and Gynecology, 109,* 91–95.

Werker, J. F., & LaLonde, C. E. (1988). Cross-language speech perception: Initial capabilities and developmental change. *Developmental Psychology, 24,* 672–683.

# CHAPTER FOUR

# DISORDERS OF SPEECH SOUND PRODUCTION

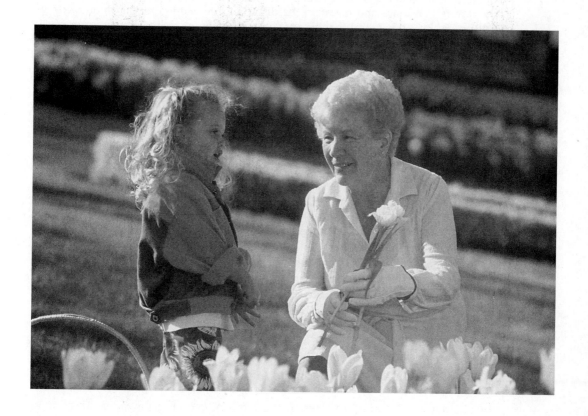

■ ■ ■ ■ ■

## PREVIEW

Disorders of articulation affect both children and adults. Speech sound errors may range from a mild lisp to nearly unintelligible speech that results from many sound substitutions, omissions, and distortions. Childhood speech sound problems may be caused by structural anomalies, such as cleft palate, but are more frequently related to faulty or incomplete learning of the sound system. Some adults show the residual signs of a childhood speech disorder. In others, speech sound errors result from damage to the central nervous system. Brain damage may produce the slurred or labored speech of dysarthria or the unpredictable errors of apraxia. In evaluating the wide range of articulation disorders, the speech-language pathologist must recognize the factors that cause and maintain the disorder. Intervention may include medical procedures, behavioral therapy, or the application of technology to improve communication.

The emergence of spoken words is one of the most important milestones in a toddler's life. We commonly hear from excited parents who report hearing "dada" or "mama" in their child's babblings, well before these sounds are used as true words. As long as the baby's word attempt contains sufficient phonemes to be recognized, the listener accepts it as the target word. In the first three years of life, parents pay more attention to the emergence of new words and overall communication, rather than the precision of articulation. If the young child's speech can be understood, there is usually little concern. During the preschool years, children's articulation improves and approximates adult sound production. However, some children persist in using immature patterns of speech, often interfering with their ability to make themselves understood. In the case of acquired articulation disorders, an adult may begin to make speech errors following an illness or injury. Persistent speech sound errors in either adults or children may warrant a referral to a speech-language pathologist.

## TYPES OF SPEECH SOUND ERRORS

In Chapter 2 we studied the speech mechanisms required for the production of normal speech, and in Chapter 3 we considered the consonants, vowels, and diphthongs of English. We also learned that sounds are strung together to form words in connected speech. We say these sounds very rapidly. It is often in the rapid production of sounds required for normal speech that speech sound errors become most noticeable. Whether heard in a single syllable, a single word, a phrase, or sentences, such errors are known as **misarticulations**. There are four forms of misarticulation: **substitution errors** (*fith* for *fish*), **omission errors** (*fi'* for *fish*), **distortion errors** (a lisped "sh" in *fish*), and **addition errors** (*fisha* for *fish*). These error types can be easily remembered by the acronym SODA (substitution, omission, distortion, addition).

## Substitutions

Substitutions are a common speech sound error in young children. Preschool children often substitute one phoneme for the target phoneme, with a certain logic or predictability. In many cases, the incorrect sound is similar to the target sound in terms of the place and manner of articulation and voicing characteristics of the sound (see also Chapter 3). For example, the child who says, *I tee the wabbit* has used two common substitutions heard in the speech of young children with articulatory errors of substitution. Like the /s/ in *see*, the substituted /t/ is a voiceless sound that is made near the same spot in the front of the mouth; the /w/ has many production similarities to the target sound /r/ that it replaces. In other cases, the incorrect sound shares similarities with other sounds within the word. For example, when a child says *bate* for *bake*, the /t/ replaces /k/ because /t/ is produced forward in the mouth, closer to where /b/ is produced.

Until children acquire a particular sound of the adult phoneme system, they often replace it with a sound they have some success in making. Many of the substituted sounds are ones that are acquired by children at earlier ages than the target sound. For example, if 4-year-olds cannot say an /s/, they might well substitute a sound that they can say, such as /t/. Substitution is perhaps the most common articulatory error in the child who is learning to talk. However, these errors may persist or be far more frequent in a child with a speech disorder.

## Omissions

When speakers omit sounds from words, their speech is difficult to understand. Consider the following exchange between a 28-month-old boy and his father:

DAD:   Look at all that stuff!

CHILD:   I bri a boo. A bir boo. [I bring a book. A bird book.]

DAD:   (Looks at book.) Is it a bird book?

CHILD:   I ge thi un, you ge tha un. [I get this one, you get that one.]

DAD:   Oh. Ok, I get this book about shells.

CHILD:   I a pi un. [It's a pink one.]

DAD:   It's a pretty pink shell.

As we can see, it is difficult to tell what this child is saying from his words alone. If not for the father, who provides a running translation, we might not know what this child was actually saying.

Shriberg (1980) noted that the omission of consonants, known as a syllable-simplification process, is a natural part of phonological development. A particular sound or a whole class of sounds may be omitted. Occasionally, a young child will leave all endings off words. For some children, simplification processes can lead to the omission of an entire syllable, which is what occurs when the young child says *nana* for *banana* or *amblance* for *ambulance*. In each case an unstressed syllable has been omitted from the word. These omissions of either sounds or syllables occur frequently in the speech of toddlers and become less common as the child grows older. However, when a 4-year-old child persists in making sound omissions, or an adult begins to produce them after years of normal speech, these omissions signal an articulation disorder.

## Distortions

As we saw in Chapter 3, the production of a sound must be relatively close to the target to be perceived by listeners as correct. Slight variations of a sound that still sound like the target sound are acceptable *allophones*, but marked variation in sound production is classified as a distortion. With a distortion error, the target sound is produced with some change of the sound, although not enough to be classified as a sound substitution or an addition. One of the most common distortions is the lateral lisp, in which the target /s/ or /z/ phonemes sound slushy (the /s/ or /z/ sounds as if it has an unvoiced /l/ as part of its production). Adults may produce sound distortions if they have a neurological condition that affects their speech.

## Additions

A fourth type of articulatory error involves an addition of a sound. We might hear an individual with an addition error saying *boata*. In other cases, an extra vowel may be inserted between the two consonants of a consonant blend (e.g., *galass* for *glass*). As in these examples, the addition error is often an unstressed vowel. Unlike other types of articulation errors, addition errors are not typically seen as a part of normal development. They can occur when an individual adds additional voicing dimension to a word or is unable to stop the flow of air (voiced or voiceless) at the end of it. Occasionally, an individual with a disorder such as cerebral palsy or other physical disability affecting motor control will make voicing additions.

## SPEECH SOUND DISORDERS IN CHILDREN

Disorders affecting the speech sound system affect approximately 3.8 percent of 6-year-old children (Shriberg, Tomblin, & McSweeny, 1999). Boys are identified as having difficulty with speech sound production slightly more frequently than are girls. Some children experience difficulty because of structural abnormalities that affect the speech system. Others seem to make speech sound errors despite the lack of any obvious cause. We will consider both types of speech sound disorders in this chapter.

## Structural Impairments in Children

In Chapter 2, we saw that sound production relies on a number of physical systems. If one or more of these systems are compromised, due to genetic disorders, birth defects, or injury, the ability to produce speech sounds may also become impaired. For children, there may be a collection of structural anomalies that fit a broader pattern of anomalies known collectively as a **syndrome.** A syndrome is identified when a certain number of features co-occur across individuals. For example, a child may be classified as having the Treacher Collins syndrome, characterized by a lack of mandibular growth, downward-slanting eyes, notched lower eyelid, and microtia (a lack of external ear development). This syndrome is genetic in origin and may often be observed in several members of the same family. A syndrome is often named after the physician(s) or other professional who first described the group of signs that co-occurred in their patients. Other syndromes, such as fetal alcohol syndrome, are named for the factors that cause the condition. Besides oral-facial abnormalities, a symptom complex may include hearing loss, language delay, mental retardation, or problems in speech sound production.

Sometimes we see children who were born with facial or tongue muscles that lack neural innervation. One girl, age 8, was unable to smile because the necessary facial muscles had no innervation; by extensive neuro- and plastic surgery, some of the nerve fibers used to move the jaw were transplanted to innervate the muscle fibers used in smiling. The operation was successful, giving her a smile and enough functional control of her lips to improve her speech.

Occasionally, tongue problems may contribute to articulation difficulty. The tongue may appear to be too large (macroglossia) or too small (microglossia). Macroglossia, seen with certain developmental syndromes, has been thought to contribute to poor articulation. At one time, tongue reduction surgery was recommended for these children, but follow-up studies have failed to document improved articulation (Lynch, 1990). Sometimes the tongue appears to be too large because it is riding forward in the mouth and protruding, possibly because of abnormalities in the back of the oral cavity, such as enlarged tonsils. In other cases, a forward tongue carriage may be the result of muscle weakness and inadequate neural innervation of the tongue muscles. These types of problems will be discussed with dysarthria later in this chapter.

A tight lingual frenulum is another feature of the tongue that has been blamed for articulation problems. The lingual frenulum is the small band of tissue on the base of the tongue's underside. When it is too tight, forward and upward movement of the tongue tip is restricted. In rare cases, this could interfere with the production of sounds, like /l/, for which the tongue tip must be elevated. When protruded, the tongue will often appear to be heart shaped, indented at the tip. This condition is sometimes called "tongue tied." Most "tongue-tied" children, however, experience no difficulty with articulation. In the rare case when this condition interferes with speech some parents may elect to have the lingual frenulum clipped by a surgeon. However, this practice is declining because the necessity of surgical intervention in these cases is open to question.

Dental abnormalities have also been blamed for articulation problems. Shelton and colleagues (Shelton, Furr, Johnson, & Arndt, 1975) looked closely at the influence of various dental abnormalities on improvement in articulation therapy, concluding that even children with severe malocclusion could learn to articulate normally. Sometimes the orthodontic correction of malocclusion, the wearing of braces or bands, will interfere with tongue precision, creating a possible articulation problem. Such problems are temporary, however, and the child usually learns to adjust speech movements to accommodate the orthodontia.

**Cleft Lip and Palate.**    Among the more common structural anomalies are cleft lip and palate. Clefting occurs when different sections of the embryo first form, between the fifth and twelfth weeks of pregnancy. Clefts may occur to either side of the midline of the upper lip, to the right or left of the bone that holds the upper front teeth (the **alveolar ridge**), and along the midline of the velum or hard palate. These predictable locations for clefts relate directly to the fact that these structures grow as separate segments that must fuse together during embryonic development.

Estimates of the incidence of cleft lip or palate range between 1 in 500 to 1 in 750 babies (Peterson-Falzone, Hardin-Jones, & Karnell, 2001). Clefts vary widely in severity. A small defect may involve a partial division in the uvula and a gap within the soft tissues of the velum. Severe facial clefts may involve both sides of the lip and alveolar ridge (in which the top front teeth are rooted). A cleft may also extend from the velum forward into the hard palate so that the nasopharynx is open to the mouth. For many children, the cleft is part of a syndrome that affects additional aspects of development (Shprintzen, Siegal-Sadewitz, Amato, & Goldberg, 1985). For example, a child born with velocardiofacial syndrome may have other facial anomalies and heart defects in addition to cleft palate. These children frequently have problems with language development as well. For other children, the cleft lip or palate is the only problem.

Perhaps we can best appreciate the impact of a cleft on the life of a child by considering the case of Andres.

*Andres* is an engaging 3-year-old who was born with a left unilateral cleft lip and palate. In the country of his birth, his mother lacked the resources to feed and care for her child, and Andres was brought to an orphanage. When he was adopted at 14 months, he was small for his age, weighing only 14 pounds. In addition, his language skills lagged well behind age expectations. Whereas children of 14 months are typically producing some words, Andres was not yet producing anything that even sounded like the speech sounds of his native language. His adoptive parents were a U.S. couple who brought him to the United States. Andres's adoptive mother was a speech-language pathologist who had special expertise in cleft palate.

Because Andres's parents adopted him knowing he had a cleft palate, they did not experience the initial emotional shock that most parents who discover their baby has this condition must contend with. Moreover, Andres's parents had a much better understanding of the implications of raising a child with a cleft palate from a medical and communication standpoint. For example, they were aware that some of the corrective surgery that Andres should have would need to be scheduled quickly. In fact, many babies born with cleft lips and palates have already had a repair of the lip well before Andres's age. Therefore, Andres's parents arranged for an initial evaluation with an ear, nose, and throat (ENT) doctor and a plastic surgeon soon after arriving home. By 16 months, Andres had his first surgery, during which his lip cleft was closed and preliminary work was begun to close the palate. In addition, tubes were inserted through Andres's eardrums so that the fluid that frequently accumulated inside the middle ear could drain.

Much to his parents' delight, the day after his first surgery, Andres produced his first speech sound, an /m/. As his mother related, "His eyes just lit up." He seemed to recognize that this sound was an important development, and he produced several more in succession. His first word approximations, *more, mom,* and *milk* built on this early appearing sound. Subsequently, he added /h/, /n/, /p/ and a nasal-sounding /b/, along with several different vowels. These additional sounds allowed him to expand his repertoire of words to include social routines like *hi* and an approximation of *please.* He also produced some vocalizations that were unidentifiable as English sounds.

Andres made a return trip to the hospital for a second round of surgery at 18 months. This time, surgery targeted repairs of the soft and hard palate. Andres and his parents stayed overnight, which was required by the hospital staff to assure that he was alert and able to drink independently before he was released. After an episode the next day in which he ran down the hall with his mother gamely attempting to keep up with his IV pole and tubing, the staff decided he could go home. Another postsurgery challenge was that Andres was fitted with arm splints to prevent him from reaching his stitches. However, these did not always remain on this active boy. On several occasions, Andres handed the splints to his mother to indicate she should put them back on.

It is safe to say that Andres's cleft lip initially had an impact on every aspect of his life. However, we also see how quickly intervention with these children can improve both their communication skills and the quality of their lives. As we see with Andres, a good home environment and medical and behavioral treatment transformed a child who had delayed development along with a cleft lip and palate into an active little boy whose cleft was just one more fact of his life.

Andres's case illustrates that treatment of the child with cleft palate typically involves both medical and behavioral interventions. Indeed, Andres's treatment to date has involved his parents, a plastic surgeon, an ENT, and a speech-language pathologist. The cleft palate team may also include additional members, such as a pediatrician or orthodontist. An audiologist may be called upon to evaluate hearing loss that can occur with structural anomalies involving the auditory system. In Andres' case, tubes that allow middle-ear fluid to drain will help him maintain normal hearing. Hearing loss due to middle-ear infection (see also Chapter 11) is common in children with cleft lip and palate (Handzic-Cuk, Cuk, Gluhinic, Risavi, & Stajner-Katusic, 2001). In Chapter 13, we will see how the various professionals on a cleft palate team function together.

By 23 months, Andres was producing two-word utterances, but his spoken vocabulary was still quite limited. In addition, the words he did use were difficult to understand because they only approximated the adult form. For example, he rarely used sounds that required contact of the tongue to the alveolar ridge. He also did not use "back" consonants (i.e., /k/, /g/). His sound preferences probably reflected a combination of factors, some related to his cleft and some that may have been compensatory. Children with complete clefts often have difficulty producing the tongue-to-palate contact and movement of the soft palate for back consonants, and thus they may avoid them. His mother also wonders whether his tendency to hold his security blanket in his mouth limited his opportunity to produce alveolar sounds like /t/ and /s/. If so, this would be another example of a physical impediment that affected speech sound development. In contrast, he seemed to understand very well for his age. At 28 months, his parents made the decision to enroll him in language therapy with the goal of expanding his vocabulary and increasing his utterance length. This focus was intended to help him achieve parity with his preschool classmates, whose skills were somewhat more advanced.

The configuration of the oral and nasal structures of children with cleft lip and palate often leads to abnormal resonance (see Chapter 2 for an explanation of resonance). These altered oral structures also may affect the child's ability to produce certain sounds. For example, a cleft palate would preclude a normal-sounding /k/ or /g/ because placement of the back of the tongue against the cleft velum does not stop the air stream completely.

## Neuromotor Impairments in Children

Children may develop a motor impairment after injury or disease that affects the nervous system. For example, a child who suffers a head injury in a car accident may have difficulty controlling the oral structures necessary for producing speech sounds with precision. Other children may display motor impairments from the time of birth. Some of these children are diagnosed as having **cerebral palsy**. These children tend to have motor impairments that involve the speech musculature and other body systems. Children with apraxia or dysarthria of speech may show delays in the development of speech without the involvement of other motor systems that frequently occurs with cerebral palsy. We will examine each of these forms of neuromotor speech impairments.

**Cerebral Palsy.**    Cerebral palsy is not a disease *per se*, but rather a term used to label a number of conditions that result from damage to or imperfect development of the central nervous system. According to McDonald and Chance (1964), about 3 in every 1,000 newborns could be classified as having cerebral palsy. This neurological impairment may occur before birth, during birth, or during the first three years of life. Therefore, a delay in motor skills including crawling, sitting, standing, walking, chewing/swallowing, self-feeding, and talking may be evident. The finer the motor skill required, such as in talking, the more likely the child will have a problem. In cerebral palsy, motor deficits may be grossly divided into four types:

*Spasticity.* **Spasticity** is characterized by severe tightness of the muscles. Speech prosody is often interrupted by respiratory and voice breaks. Articulation is often severely defective.

*Athetosis.* **Athetosis** is characterized by a series of involuntary muscle contractions, with flailing of extremities and much facial grimacing. Lack of respiratory control causes a monotonic voice, often lacking sufficient loudness. There are many phonemic distortions.

*Mixed.* This type of cerebral palsy, sometimes called tension athetoid, represents a mixture of both tight spasticity and flailing athetosis.

*Ataxia.* **Ataxia** is characterized by a lack of balance and severe problems in coordination of movements. Ataxic speech sounds like the slurred, arrhythmical speech of someone inebriated.

The motor speech problems of the child with cerebral palsy can be classified as a type of dysarthric speech. (Dysarthria also occurs in adults who suffer brain damage and is discussed in greater detail later in this chapter). Cerebral palsy implies a motor disorder of speech that is developmental in nature. If the condition is severe, the affected child enjoys few normal developmental experiences and a marked delay in speech. The treatment of the dysarthria for the child with cerebral palsy, therefore, may be quite different from that of one who acquires dysarthria after normal speech patterns have been established.

Often the child with cerebral palsy is so physically active with muscle contractions or unstable head and trunk posture that speaking appears almost impossible. The speech-language pathologist may work closely with other treatment specialists, such as the orthopedic surgeon, the physiatrist (a physician specializing in physical or restorative medicine), the physical therapist, the occupational therapist, and the special educator in order to address speech goals in concert with these other issues. For other children with cerebral palsy, articulate speech is not a realistic goal; for these children, some form of nonvocal communication system must be introduced. A manually or electronically operated communication board can be an effective alternate communication system (see Figure 4.1). Thanks to modern technology, there are assistive communication devices available to meet the basic communication needs of the most severely handicapped child with cerebral palsy.

**Developmental Dysarthria and Apraxia.** Some children exhibit signs of speech disorders typically associated with brain damage in adults. These are children with signs of developmental dysarthria or apraxia of speech. Children identified as having developmental dysarthria typically have abnormal muscle tone in facial muscles, which may be worse on one side than the other. Low muscle tone may result in a soft, somewhat drooping facial expression. Muscle tone that is abnormally high may produce a taut appearance or contribute to facial distortions and grimaces. Some children with dysarthria may have trouble with drooling or eating. Children with dysarthria have difficulty producing rapid speech or nonspeech

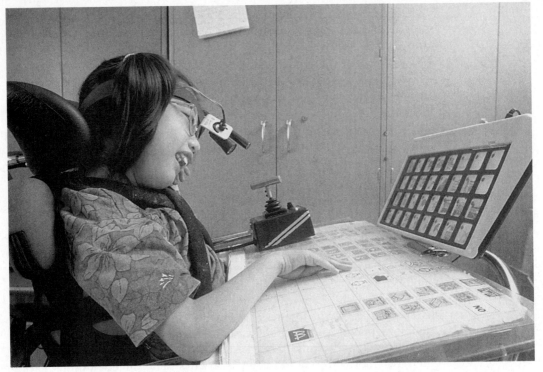

**FIGURE 4.1    A child with cerebral palsy uses a head-mounted electronic pointer to select pictures, allowing her to communicate simple messages.**

movements. Affected children typically are late in acquiring their first words. As they grow older, their speech often remains very difficult to understand. Dysarthria may be associated with conditions such as cerebral palsy but may also occur in the absence of a more pervasive disability.

Children with developmental apraxia of speech are somewhat more difficult to identify. Often, they lack the more apparent motor signs that characterize developmental dysarthria. Apraxia has been defined as an impairment in the ability "to program, combine, and sequence the elements of speech" (Jaffee, 1984, p. 166). A child with a pure apraxia of speech would demonstrate relatively normal comprehension of language but be unable to imitate a simple spoken word, despite having no muscular weakness or paralysis. A case presentation of a 6-year-old girl with apraxia of speech illustrates the problem:

> *Esme* was a friendly and enthusiastic 6-year-old enrolled in a public school kindergarten. From her first day, it was apparent that her speech skills were well below average. Esme was nearly impossible to understand. Her kindergarten teacher was also concerned about Esme's language skills. The kindergarten program was largely built around language arts, and Esme had difficulty participating in many

of the classroom activities. The kindergarten teacher asked the school's speech-language pathologist to observe Esme in the classroom. The speech-language pathologist noted that Esme was rarely understood by her teacher or classmates and often showed signs of frustration and distress while trying to communicate. Immediate intervention was needed.

The speech-language pathologist contacted Esme's mother to obtain permission to see Esme for a formal evaluation and for therapy. Esme's mother confided that her child had been evaluated once before. At the age of 2, Esme had been seen at the county's developmental disabilities center because she had not yet started to speak. At that time, based on her poor motor and speech development, she was diagnosed as mentally retarded. Her mother was so distressed at this diagnosis that she refused all preschool services and refused to release the records of that diagnosis to anyone. She was sure her child was bright and feared Esme would be stigmatized and held back by a diagnosis of retardation. Instead, the mother kept Esme at home and spent a great deal of time taking her on field trips and engaging in other creative activities with her. The mother waited until Esme was 6 to enroll her in kindergarten, hoping that the extra year would give her a developmental advantage to compensate for her poor communication. Although still wary of therapists and special education professionals, after some discussion she agreed to allow the speech-language pathologist to see Esme again.

A formal evaluation revealed that Esme rarely pronounced any words correctly, even when speaking only single words. She often made errors on initial sounds in words and omitted endings altogether. Her sentences tended to be short, with an average of three words per sentence. A battery of language tests indicated that her receptive language skills were slightly above average and her expressive language skills were poor.

During subsequent therapy sessions, Esme made slow and inconsistent progress. The speech-language pathologist began noticing signs suggesting that Esme may have had more than the typical phonological disorder. She sometimes showed facial tension while speaking. Once, when trying to imitate a /d/ sound, she used her fingers to move her tongue into position. Sometimes she would reach for a card and grab the wrong one while telling herself "no!" These behaviors suggested problems with planning and sequencing speech movements. The speech-language pathologist made a diagnosis of developmental apraxia of speech. Esme's mother was convinced, after much counseling, to take her child back to the developmental disabilities center so that she could be evaluated by a physical therapist. The physical therapist confirmed that Esme had a mild limb apraxia in addition to apraxia of speech. With this information, the mother, school staff, and therapists met to discuss how classroom materials and procedures could be modified to minimize the effects of Esme's apraxia. The speech-language pathologist provided a teacher in-service on the expected impact that Esme's apraxia would have on her academic progress, including writing, test taking, and oral skills.

Apraxia of speech is more of a motor speech problem than an overall language problem; however, apraxia creates a marked discrepancy between receptive language and the ability to express language through speech. Often the affected children are forced to struggle at the single-word level. Even when they can produce multiword sentences, their speech lacks the normal prosody. Children with apraxia require intensive individual therapy as well as language-based intervention in which efforts are made to encourage the development of a variety of communication skills.

## Phonological Disorders

Some children's poor articulation skills are not readily attributable to structural abnormalities. Parents become concerned when their child's speech seems to lag behind their playmates. For some children, speech articulation errors are limited to just a few sounds. In other cases, articulation errors are so numerous that the young child's speech is nearly impossible to understand.

When a child is referred for an articulation disorder, a speech-language pathologist will attempt to characterize the child's sound errors. Some children will mispronounce only a few sounds, such as /r/, /l/, or /s/. Since children tend to master these sounds relatively late (4 years old or older), the speech-language pathologist may recommend a "wait and watch" approach. Intervention may be limited or deferred while the child is given a chance to self-correct articulation through normal maturation. For school-age children, even a few sounds produced in error is unusual. A 10-year-old boy's lisped /s/ rarely interferes with his ability to communicate his ideas. It can, however, negatively affect the way other children view him (Hall, 1990). Such children are typically candidates for therapy and are often quite motivated to correct their speech.

The phonological approach to speech sound disorders recognizes that the child has difficulty mastering the adult phonology, or speech sound system, of the child's native language. All children, in their early attempts to use spoken language, make simplifications of speech sound patterns (Ingram, 1981). As Dunn (1982) wrote, "The term phonological process . . . is frequently used as a way to describe the systematic simplifications observed in child speech" (p. 147). Children with phonological disorders, however, continue to use these simplification processes long after their peers have ceased using them (Grunwell, 1980). Some common **phonological processes** are shown in Table 4.1.

Because phonological processes represent systematic error patterns, therapy concentrates more on correcting the processes than on treating individual sound errors. Robbie is one such child.

At age 4, Robbie was brought to a university speech-language clinic by his concerned parents. Robbie's parents, most other family members (including three older siblings), and neighbors had difficulty understanding him. He had normal hearing, normal cognitive ability, and a normal speech mechanism at the time of the speech evaluation. His articulation errors were abundant. He could correctly say /m/, /p/, /b/, /t/, /d/, /n/, when these were the initial sounds in a word. He correctly said /m/, /p/, /b/ when they occurred in the middle of words. He produced no final consonants correctly. Most of his consonant errors were omissions, although he made a few consonant substitutions: t for k, d for g, t for f, b for v, t for θ. Of all the English consonants, he said only six correctly; most of his vowel sounds were produced correctly. His overall attempts at conversation were restricted to two- or three-word utterances, many of which were not intelligible. He appeared to limit his mean length of response to two or three words as a conscious gesture to accommodate his listeners; he apparently had learned that, if he said more than that, no one would understand him.

Because Robbie could say six consonants correctly in the initial position, a phonological approach to his problem focused on making him aware that many words had consonant endings that he could say. At the start of therapy, the stop consonants that he could produce correctly (/p/, /b/, /t/, /d/) were presented at the beginning and the end of a word; and he was cued to say these sounds in both word positions. In therapy, he was soon able to produce most of the six target sounds (the ones he could say at the evaluation) at both the beginning and the end of a word, such as *pop, top, mop, Bob, tub, mom, Pam* (his sister), and so forth. Later therapy sessions included working on phonetic sounds that Robbie should have been making correctly by focusing on the processes that characterized his sound substitutions.

Studies of children with phonological disorders reveal that they frequently have features in common, including impairments in other domains (Ruscello, St. Louis, & Mason, 1991; Shriberg, Kwiatkowski, Best, Hengst, & Terselic-Weber, 1986). About two-thirds of children with disordered phonology are boys. Frequently, there are signs of general neuromotor problems, including mild muscle weakness and incoordination. A phonological disorder is often accompanied by a developmental language disorder (see Chapter 8), in which expressive language is

**TABLE 4.1   Phonological Processes**

|  | EXAMPLES | |
| --- | --- | --- |
| *Phonological Processes* | *Adult Word* | *Child Word* |
| **SYLLABLE-SIMPLIFICATION PROCESSES** | | |
| Deletion of the final consonant | ball | "ba–" |
| Deletion of the unstressed syllable | away | "–way" |
| Cluster reduction | stop | "–top" |
| **ASSIMILATION PROCESSES** | | |
| Regressive (backward) assimilation | doggie | "goggie" |
| Progressive (forward) assimilation | television | "televivon" |
| **SUBSTITUTION PROCESSES** | | |
| Stopping—fricatives are replaced by stops | shoes | "tood" |
| Fronting—palatal and velar sounds are replaced by alveolar sounds | bake | "bate" |

Used with permission of Prentice Hall. From L. D. Shriberg, Developmental phonological disorders, in *Introduction to Communication Disorders*, ed. T. Hixon, L. Shriberg, and J. Saxman (Englewood Cliffs, NJ: Prentice Hall, 1980).

more commonly impaired than receptive language. Half of all children with speech sound disorders also have difficulty learning to read. Problems with academic skills may persist long into the school years, even after speech is no longer obviously impaired (Shriberg & Kwiatkowski, 1988). Sometimes a family history of phonological as well as other speech or language disorders can be documented for these children (Lewis, 1990).

## Tongue Thrust

Several generations of Americans have been evaluated and treated for **tongue thrust** as part of an orthodontic management program. Children with tongue thrust use an unusual sequence of oral movements when swallowing. The tongue pushes forward against the anterior teeth (particularly the upper incisors). This forward tongue movement while swallowing has led some to refer to tongue thrust as reverse swallowing. The forward tongue movement is accompanied by high tension in the muscles controlling lip movement, which is needed to prevent the tongue from protruding as it pushes forward during swallowing. This abnormal and inefficient pattern of swallowing tends to make children with tongue thrust messy eaters. In addition, the frequent forward pressure of the tongue forces the teeth out of alignment. For this reason, many orthodontists are reluctant to fit a child with braces until the tongue thrust habit has been overcome. This problem frequently requires direct intervention with special procedures known as **myofunctional therapy** to develop optimal intraoral tongue postures for swallowing (Barrett & Hanson, 1978).

Some children with identified tongue thrust also have an associated articulation disorder, most commonly heard by others as a lisp because the anterior sibilants (particularly /s/ and /z/) are mispronounced. Speech-language pathologists who have been trained in myofunctional therapy techniques may choose to treat the articulation disorder and tongue thrust simultaneously. When there is tongue thrust but no articulation disorder, the speech-language pathologist may elect to administer myofunctional therapy to correct abnormal tongue and lip postures and movements (ASHA, 1991).

## Hearing Loss

In Chapters 10 and 11 we will see the importance of the hearing mechanism in the development of normal communication. Human communication is primarily an oral-aural interaction. A conductive or sensorineural hearing loss can seriously impair the aural reception of language. Hearing loss is a frequent cause of a developmental communication problem (articulation and language). Some children simply cannot hear certain phonemes. When children lack the ability to hear spoken sounds, it is difficult for them to learn to produce them. Common causes of hearing loss and its effect on speech sound development are described at length in Chapter 11.

# EVALUATION OF SPEECH SOUND DISORDERS IN CHILDREN

Many times, children (and adults) are referred for speech sound disorders because others find their speech difficult to understand. Formal evaluation of these disorders may involve several steps that are designed to determine whether errors are part of normal development or consistent with a speech disorder that warrants therapy. A complete evaluation may include testing to determine which individual sounds or patterns of sounds are affected and whether there is any physical reason (e.g., a oral-facial anomaly, hearing loss) that these speech errors are occurring.

## Speech Sound Screening

A screening measure is not designed to determine whether a disorder exists, but whether additional testing to make this kind of determination is warranted. Screening programs for children are common in the public schools, particularly in kindergarten and the first few elementary grades. Such programs are typically set up in the fall, and all new children in a school district (kindergarten and other grades) meet with the speech-language pathologist or a speech-language assistant (see Chapter 13) for a brief screening. The screening might focus on naturalistic dialogues with the children to observe their articulation and their overall language function, voice quality, and speech fluency. However, many young children are reticent about talking to a stranger, making a natural conversation impossible. Therefore, it is usually necessary to structure the screening so that a maximum amount of information can be obtained from a relatively brief speech sample.

It should be noted that certain speech sounds are stressed in the screening program—usually those that young children typically mispronounce throughout the early years. Ideally, the screening test should differentiate between those children who will outgrow their problem with maturation and those with articulation problems that need remediation.

## Assessing Children with Speech Sound Disorders

Formal evaluation of speech sound disorders may begin with simply listening to the child (or adult) in conversation. The conversation may be between the client and other children, between parent and child, or between clinician and child. This may involve discreet observation of a school-aged child at home, on the playground, or in the classroom. Other children may be seen in a clinic testing suite (which often looks like a playroom for young children) that has observation mirrors permitting the clinician to observe the child in as natural a communication setting as possible. A conversation during spontaneous play will often reveal how the child actually talks outside of the testing situation. With an older child, an actual conversation about topics of interest will reveal the communicative ability, offering information about articulation proficiency as well as about voice, language, and fluency.

The well-trained experienced and speech-language pathologist is able to observe the child's productions systematically and make a useful summary statement based on the observations relevant to the articulatory adequacy, specifying type and number of errors, place of error, and so forth. It is possible, however, that observation of play and conversation will not reveal all of the client's speech errors, nor will conversation alone provide the diagnostic information that a more structured evaluation will include. Therefore, the evaluation is likely to include conversational speech and more formal testing.

Assessing children with speech sound disorders will typically include procedures designed to assess whether physical problems are contributing to a speech sound disorder. Two common measures include a hearing screening and an examination of the oral mechanism.

**Audiometric Testing.** Audiometric testing, or at least as a screening measure, should be part of every articulation evaluation. As we will see in Chapters 11 and 12; even a mild hearing loss can affect which sounds are heard and produced. The child's ability to perceive the sounds of words is an important part of the evaluation. Therefore, audiometric testing may include evaluation of speech sound reception and discrimination levels.

**Oral Mechanism Evaluation.** A oral mechanism evaluation provides the speech-language pathologist with information about the adequacy of oral structure and function. As discussed earlier in this chapter, structural defects and incorrect movements of the articulators can all contribute to faulty speech production. An oral mechanism examination form (see Figure 4.2) lists the clinician's observations about various structural areas of the vocal tract and how well they function for speech.

The particular form pictured in Figure 4.2 could be used for either a child or an adult. It allows the clinician to note structural deviations in the oral and facial structures used for speech. It is important to note that many minor, or even some significant, deviations from normal structure may not impede correct articulation or may do so only temporarily. For example, dental malocclusions rarely cause poor speech. A child who has lost his front teeth may lisp temporarily until the permanent teeth grow in.

The oral mechanism form also requires the clinician to note whether specific speech gestures are being made with precision (e.g., lip closure to produce /pa/; lifting the tongue during production of /ta/). In addition to simple speech gestures, the ability to produce rapid alternating speech sounds (e.g., /pʌ pʌ pʌ/) is tested. Individuals who have normal control over speech articulation are able to produce these repeating or alternating syllables (i.e., /pʌ tʌ kʌ/) rapidly, smoothly, and without pauses between syllables. The ability to produce repeated syllable strings is called **diadochokinesis**. Those with neurological impairments or physical deviations of the oral structures may produce these syllables more slowly, may struggle to produce them, or may produce them with imprecise movements.

The advantage to the speech-language pathologist of using a form to summarize the data from the oral examination probably lies in the need to be complete

## ORAL MECHANISM SCREENING FOR SPEECH

| Structures | Function |
|---|---|
| **Instructions**: Visually inspect structures to complete each item. Note deviations that occur. | **Instructions**: Demonstrate item. For each item, obtain 3 trials. Note deviations that occur. |

**Facial Structures**
    facial muscle tone
    facial symmetry
    lip symmetry
    Other:_____

Lip closure achieved for /pa/
Tongue tip raised for /ta/& /la/
Rounded lips for /wʌ/
Dental-labial position for /vʌ/
Comments:_____
_____

**Oral Cavity**
    tongue
    teeth
    hard palate
    soft palate
    uvula
    faucial pillars
    tonsils
    Other:_____

Velum raised for sustained /a/ (three trials)
Comments:_____
_____

Sound quality for sustained /a/
Comments:_____
_____

**Diadochokinesis** (16 repetitions each)

| | accurate | rhythmic | time (secs) |
|---|---|---|---|
| /pʌpʌpʌ.../ | Y   N | Y   N | |
| /tʌtʌtʌ.../ | Y   N | Y   N | |
| /kʌkʌkʌ.../ | Y   N | Y   N | |
| /pʌtʌkʌ.../ | Y   N | Y   N | |

**FIGURE 4.2**　Oral mechanism screening for speech.

and systematic. The form, in effect, provides a checklist for each part of the oral mechanism in terms of its structural and performance adequacy. For the patient with dysarthria or a major structural defect (such as a cleft palate), a more detailed and supplementary examination would be required.

**Articulation Inventory.**　Many commercially available articulation tests provide the clinician with a ready inventory of speech sounds. Most tests can identify not only the actual sounds produced incorrectly but also the place in the word where the error occurs (initial, medial, or final position) and the type of error (omission, substitution, distortion, or addition). A typical articulation inventory will provide the type of information found in Figure 4.3. This form shows the results of a single-word articulation test given to 5-year-old Katie, who demonstrated a number of speech sound errors. The errors may be described individually as substitutions (e.g., p for f ) or omissions (e.g., – for f) in the initial (I), medial (M), or final (F) position in the word. In the column labeled Phonological Process, errors are ascribed

| ARTICULATION TEST | | | | |
|---|---|---|---|---|
| **Name:** Katie | | **Age:** 5.0 years | | |
| **SOUND** | **ITEM** | **I** | **M** | **F** | **PHONOLOGICAL PROCESS** |
| p | pencils, zipper, cup | ✓ | ✓ | -/p | Final consonant deletion |
| m | matches, Christmas, drum | ✓ | ✓ | -/m | F.C.D. |
| n | knife, Santa, gun | ✓ | ✓ | -/n | F.C.D. |
| w | window | ✓ | | | |
| h | house | ✓ | | | |
| b | rabbit, bathtub | ✓ | ✓ | -/b | F.C.D. |
| g | gun, wagon, flag | ✓ | ✓ | -/g | F.C.D. |
| k | cup, chicken, duck | ✓ | ✓ | -/k | F.C.D. |
| f | fishing, telephone, knife | p/f | p/f | -/f | F.C.D., Stopping |
| d | duck, window, bed | ✓ | ✓ | -/d | F.C.D. |
| ŋ | finger, ring | | g/ŋ | -/ŋ | F.C.D., Stopping |
| j | yellow | ✓ | | | |
| t | telephone, bathtub, carrot | ✓ | ✓ | -/t | F.C.D. |
| ʃ | shovel, fishing, brush | t/ʃ | t/ʃ | -/ʃ | F.C.D., Stopping |
| tʃ | church, matches | t/tʃ | t/tʃ | -/tʃ | F.C.D., Stopping |
| l | lamp, yellow, squirrel | w/l | w/l | -/l | F.C.D., Liquid Simplification |
| r | rabbit, carrot, car | w/r | w/r | -/r | F.C.D., Liquid Simplification |
| dʒ | jumping, pajamas, orange | d/dʒ | g/dʒ | -/dʒ | F.C.D., Stopping |
| θ | thumb, bathtub, bath | t/θ | -/θ | -/θ | F.C.D., Stopping |
| v | vacuum, shovel, stove | b/v | b/v | -/v | F.C.D., Stopping |
| s | scissors, pencils, house | d/s | t/s | -/s | F.C.D., Stopping |
| z | zipper, scissors | d/z | d/z | -/z | F.C.D., Stopping |
| ð | this, feather | d/ð | d/ð | | Stopping |

**FIGURE 4.3** Articulation test results for Katie, age 5 years. Note F.C.D. = final consonant deletion. Items adapted from the *Goldman-Fristoe Test of Articulation* (Goldman & Fristoe, 1986) and the *Khan-Lewis Phonological Analysis* (Khan & Lewis, 1986).

to one of three phonological processes used. *Stimulability* testing (discussed later in the chapter) would follow the formal articulation test to see whether, under the special conditions of those tests, the incorrect sounds could be produced correctly. A phonological process evaluation (described below) might follow, particularly if stimulability was unsuccessful in eliciting correct sound productions.

**Phonological Process Analysis.**   For many children, the speech sound errors are not limited to a few consistently misarticulated sounds. More often, the speech-language pathologist finds errors on many of the consonant sounds. These errors at first glance may seem inconsistent. Certain consonants may be correctly produced in a few words, whereas in others they are omitted, distorted, or replaced with another consonant. A careful examination of these speech-sound errors almost always reveals a pattern. For example, when a child says *Tuta too my tir* for *Susan took my shirt*, the errors might be classified in the two ways shown in Table 4.2. Substitution errors are shown by writing the error sound followed by a slash (/) and the target sound. Omitted sounds are denoted with a minus (–) sign.

When the sound errors are listed individually in Table 4.2, we notice that the child is inconsistent in the use of the /t/ sound. The child uses it correctly when attempting the word *took* but substitutes it for the /s/ and /z/ in *Susan* and /ʃ/ in *shirt* and omits it altogether at the end of *shirt*. This use would be puzzling if we concentrated only on the individual sound errors. However, all these errors, plus those not involving /t/, can be accounted for by two general patterns, or **phonological processes**. The substitutions of /t/ for /s/, /z/, and /ʃ/ are all examples of a process called *stopping*, in which a stop consonant (e.g., /t/, /d/, or /g/) is substituted for a continuant (e.g., /s/, /f/, or /v/). All the errors of omission occur on the final consonant, indicating a process of final consonant deletion. Many phonological processes are seen in normally developing children, but persist in children with phonological disorders.

**Stimulability.**   An important part of the articulation evaluation is assessing how well the client can produce omitted or incorrect sounds when provided help to do so. This is known as *stimulability*. After the formal articulation test is completed, the speech-language pathologist selects several incorrect sounds to determine if

**TABLE 4.2   Examples of Sound Errors in Children's Speech**

|  | INDIVIDUAL ERRORS | PHONOLOGICAL PROCESSES |
|---|---|---|
| **ATTEMPTED STATEMENT:**<br>Susan took my shirt. |  |  |
| **CHILD'S STATEMENT:**<br>Tuta too my tir. | Initial t/s  t/ʃ<br>Medial t/z<br>Final –/n –/k –/t | Stopping<br>Stopping<br>Final consonant deletion |

the client is stimulable for those sounds. Children who can correct their sound errors when given visual, auditory, or tactile cues have a better prognosis for correction than those who cannot.

**Stimulability testing** can occur at several levels. The higher the level at which the child is able to produce the sound correctly, the easier it is to correct the production of the sound. At the highest level, the clinician may ask the child to say a mispronounced word over again by prompting, "Can you say that better?" If the child does not correct word production, the clinician might ask the child to repeat the word after a model is given. If the child's attempt is incorrect, the clinician might draw attention to visual cues to aid articulation by instructing the child to "watch how I say it." If the addition of visual cues is not effective, the clinician might ask the child to produce the target sound in a consonant-vowel combination, like *la-la-la*. If necessary, visual and tactile cues may be added to help the child. These steps are taken to determine what capacity the child has for producing the sound and how much support and cueing the child needs to do so.

**Severity and Intelligibility.**    Formal testing of the sounds a child (or an adult) can produce does not always reflect the overall severity of a client's problem. For example, consider the speech of the following two children:

> MARIA:   He go bi tee [He's got big teeth]. Bu i no a he [But it's not a he]. I a she! [It's a she!]
>
> JOSEPH:   I see a amblance [I see an ambulance]. Let me see. I see an elphant [I see an elephant].

Both of these children have one phonological process that describes their speech errors. Maria tends to delete final consonants, and Joseph shows a pattern of weak syllable deletion. Although both children's errors can be described with a single process, Maria is much more difficult to understand than Joseph. This illustrates that knowledge of specific error types does not always provide accurate insight concerning overall severity. Kent, Miolo, and Bloedel (1994) reviewed the wide variety of available methods for estimating the overall intelligibility of speech. They noted that these measures tend to emphasize different aspects of speech analysis. A clinician may select among measures that emphasize phonetic contrasts, phonological error patterns, whole-word identification in isolation or in connected speech, or measures that require listeners to rate how well speech can be understood. Some of these measures were developed with the characteristics of a particular type of articulation problem in mind (e.g., speech associated with hearing impairment, dysarthria, phonological disorders). Therefore, the clinician's decision concerning which measure to select may reflect the type of client he or she needs to evaluate and even the types of speech sound errors the client shows (Kent et al., 1994; Shriberg, Austin, Lewis, McSweeny, & Wilson, 1997).

**Other Testing.**    Speech sound disorders may co-occur with other disorders. For example, children with genetic syndromes or multiple handicaps may have conditions that require coordinated evaluation by multiple professionals. In other cases, a speech sound disorder co-occurs with a language disorder. In these cases, the speech-language pathologist must try to determine the extent to which the sound errors are affecting the ability of the child (or adult) to produce elements of the language. For example, a phonological process such as final consonant deletion will eliminate parts of speech like the past tense *-ed*. Other processes like stridency deletion will eliminate the plural and possessive /s/. Because phonological disorders frequently co-occur with language difficulties, many clinicians routinely include one or more language measures in their assessment. We will consider the evaluation of language skills further in Chapter 8.

## INTERVENTION METHODS FOR CHILDREN

There are several approaches to treating speech sound errors in children. If a child has physical problems that affect his or her ability to produce speech, a team approach involving several professionals may be involved. For example, treatment may include surgical interventions to repair a cleft palate or coordinated efforts by a speech-language pathologist and physical therapist to provide support for a child whose control of his or her overall posture and muscle tone is too poor to support speech. If hearing loss is contributing to poor articulation, treatment of speech may follow fitting the child with hearing aids.

For a child whose only difficulty involves poor speech sound production, a number of methods are available for treatment. Which method is selected may depend on how many and what types of speech sound errors the child makes, and how stimulable the child is for these sounds. The least effective clinicians may be those who apply the same intervention method to all children. Therapy methods are typically tailored to meet the needs of the individual child. However, two components are important to all forms of intervention: methods to assist the child in acquiring an adultlike speech sound system and methods to assure that newly acquired sounds are used in all words and in all speaking situations.

### Acquisition Training

There are many published programs and informal programs that are designed to improve the speech of children. Here we examine general approaches to acquisition training that use different ways of obtaining correct sound production. Semantic approaches attempt to make the child realize that his or her current method of speaking is not communicating the meaning intended. This cognitive approach can motivate a child who is capable of producing correct pronunciations but does not do so. Other children may not know how to produce correct sounds and may require more direct instruction. We will consider several approaches that concentrate on correcting sound errors by helping children achieve correct movements of the speech articulators.

A *semantic* approach to articulation therapy emphasizes the changes in meaning that sometimes accompany phonological errors. Let us look at an example of a semantic approach to therapy.

> Brian is a school-based speech-language pathologist who has a group of three first-grade children with phonological disorders. All of these children make systematic substitutions of one class of sounds for another. For example, Amon, one of his students, reduces clusters like /st/ or /bl/ to one sound (/t/ or /b/). Another student, Marta, uses stop consonants in the place of fricatives (see Table 4.1 for example of phonological processes). Brian is able to address each of these children's different patterns of sound errors through a semantic approach. He has selected pairs of picture cards that contrast the error sound with the sound pattern each child needs to master. For example, one card shows a stop sign and its pair shows a toy top. The words *stop* and *top* contrast the cluster /st/ with the word that would be produced if the child reduced the cluster from /st/ to /t/. Other pairs of cards contrast the error patterns of the other children. Brian and the children play a modified game of *go fish*. There are two sets of each picture, so that a child holding one picture can ask another child for that picture in an attempt to obtain matching pairs. Each child has to show the picture he or she requests so that Brian can tell whether each child produces the target sound. Amon is holding the stop sign card, but asks "Do you have any top signs?" Brian replies, "No, I don't have any tops, but I do have a stop." This highlights for Amon the difference between what he asked for and what he meant to ask for. Likewise, when Marta asks Amon for a "tail" when she meant to say "sail," Amon has the opportunity to model the correct word. This approach works for these children because they are able to produce the sounds they are working on, but don't necessarily do so when they need to. It doesn't take long before the children realize that to get what they want, they have to produce the sound patterns that correspond to the correct word.

Many children need only a few examples of these minimal pairs before they are able to produce the target sounds in additional words (Elbert, Powell, & Swartzlander, 1991). The semantic method serves to alert the children to the fact that there is a difference between what they are saying and what they should be saying and that this difference is important. This method does not require children to think about the sounds themselves, an advantage for young children, who have little awareness of sounds as units smaller than words.

Some clients will not benefit from a semantic approach. They may see the differences in meaning between their sound errors and the correct production but be unable to produce the sound correctly without additional assistance. A *cross-modality* approach may provide that assistance. Cross-modality approaches utilize sensory information to facilitate correct articulation. For example, a client and clinician may face a mirror while the clinician demonstrates the target sound. The client may then attempt to repeat the sound while monitoring his or her movements visually in the mirror. In another case, a clinician may rub a child's alveolar ridge with a mint so that the child can feel and taste where the tongue belongs for /t/ and /d/. Or clients are instructed to put their hand over their larynx to feel the difference between /s/ and /z/. This additional sensory input can be an effective way for adults or children to monitor their performance.

For some sounds, there are few available cues that the client can see or feel. Sometimes it is possible to take advantage of the *coarticulatory context* to promote correct sound production. Coarticulatory context refers to the fact that the sounds preceding and following a phoneme will influence the way that phoneme is produced. For a phoneme like /r/, for which there are few visual cues, coarticulatory context can help in learning correct production. For example, the /g/ and /k/ in /gr/ or /kr/ blends require a high, back tongue carriage, which carries over to facilitate a correct production of /r/. Once this correct tongue placement is established in blends, it can be used in words with other sound combinations. Let's take a look at an approach that capitalizes on co-articulatory context.

Makayla has teamed with her school's art teacher to integrate her articulation therapy into her students' classes. The art teacher's lesson plan involved constructing hand puppets in the shape of dragons. Makayla sat at the table with one of her students, Emily, who was working on the production of /r/. A number of other students were seated at the table as well. As Makayla assisted these students with the construction of their puppets, she asked them what sounds dragons might make. Several children offered that they may make a sound like /grrrrr/. Makayla readily agreed that /grrr/ was a strong candidate for dragon speech. She encouraged each of the children to make their puppets imitate sentences that contained extended /gr/ blends. Soon, the children were pronouncing sentences like "Grrrr, I will grrrrab the grrrreasy grrrrrapes!" or "Grrrr, grrrasshoppers are grrrross!" By saying /grrrr/ at the start of each sentence, Emily had an opportunity to position her tongue for a correct /r/ before it came up in a full word. The use of /gr/ in words blends facilitated tongue position during running speech. Finally, by extending the /gr/ to /grrr/, Emily could slow down production of the blend to increase her chances of correct productions. Though this activity, Emily had an opportunity to work on her speech without missing out on art class. In addition, because many children were engaged in "dragon talk," she didn't feel singled out.

These different techniques can be used in conjunction with behavioral techniques. Many behavior-modification programs are commercially available for use with children with articulation disorders. These programs offer a number of attractive therapy materials designed to make the learning task interesting and fun for the young child. As a first step, the speech-language pathologist establishes a baseline of what the child is able to produce. For example, a particular target sound is selected, and the number of productions the child is able to say correctly, either spontaneously or by prompting, is established as the child's general proficiency for that sound. The treatment program for that sound then begins, following the systematic presentation of a particular program. The child is given an occasional prompt (a helping suggestion) to aid in production tasks, and as the typical program progresses, the clinician fades out support by doing less and less.

### Generalization

If clients have learned the correct pronunciation of the /r/ sound, it does them little good if they can produce it only in /gr/ blends or only in the therapy setting. The goal of articulation therapy is for clients to be able to use the newly corrected sounds in all words and in all situations. When clients are able to transfer their newly learned articulation skills to untrained words and new settings, we say that they are demonstrating generalization of articulation skills. Generalization does not always occur automatically. The therapist should incorporate activities into the therapy program that promote generalization.

Generalization goals may be broken down into categories, such as generalizations to other sound contexts, to different speaking tasks, and with different speaking partners. Research has shown, for example, that training children on developmentally late-appearing sounds facilitates more generalization to other untrained sounds than when children are trained on earlier-appearing sounds (Gierut, Morrisette, Hughes, & Rowland, 1996). Therefore, through careful consideration of which sounds to train, a clinician can see gains on other sounds "for free." In some cases, the therapist may be able to find a few words in which the client is able to correctly produce the target sound. Generalization then involves transferring this limited skill to greater numbers of words (Prather & Whaley, 1984). For example, the client may lateralize the /s/ (air escapes over the sides of the tongue) in /sl/ blends but produce /st/ blends accurately. In this case, the therapist may present /sl/ blends in conjunction with /st/ blends to facilitate generalization. If the target sound is never produced correctly, the therapist may select a small set of words that begin with the target sounds for initial training. When these are mastered, the therapist may incorporate new words containing the target sounds into the therapy sessions. This set of words is expanded to include words with the target sounds in the medial and final position. The therapist may also include combinations of sounds within words that are more difficult for the client. Different words will be included in each session to promote generalization to new words.

Single-word responses can be expanded into short phrases and sentences. Sometimes a standard carrier phrase can be used initially to facilitate articulation in longer utterances. For example, a group of children might play a game of twenty questions in which each child asks, "Is it a. . . ?" to find out what card the therapist holds. Older children and adults can practice articulation while reading sentences and short passages. The use of carrier phrases or reading tasks allows clients to practice their articulation skills without having to concentrate on the content of the message. As articulation skills become increasingly automatic, the clinician will incorporate conversational tasks into the therapy session.

As therapy progresses, children and adults become increasingly adept at monitoring their articulation during the therapy session. This self-monitoring process appears to relate to the client's ability to generalize articulation skills (Shriberg & Kwiatkowski, 1990). Outside of the therapy session, clients are typically more concerned with the content of their speech than their articulation. To promote generalization to other settings, the therapist may enlist the cooperation of others. For a child, the therapist may provide parents with tips for facilitating correct articulation at home. Teachers may monitor articulation in the classroom. A peer may be enlisted for activities outside the therapy setting. McReynolds (1982) writes that bringing other people into generalization sessions as critical listeners will sometimes accelerate generalization; however, she notes that we must caution others "not to overdo their help, so that the person does not become overly self-conscious about the problem" (p. 136). Individuals should be treated gently when they make mistakes and given realistic positive reinforcement when they produce sounds well.

## ACQUIRED SPEECH SOUND DISORDERS IN ADULTS

Adults who have developed normal speech and language abilities give little attention to how they speak. The motor patterns for speech are well established and relatively automatic under most circumstances; however, adults may acquire structural or neurological impairments that disrupt their ability to produce speech sounds. Treatment of such impairments differs from treating developmental speech sound disorders, because adults may need to change their articulation patterns, and formerly automatic processes may need to become more intentional.

### Speech Sound Disorders Due to Structural Impairments

Structural changes of the speech articulators can result from traumatic damage or surgical removal of all or portions of the larynx, tongue, jaw, teeth, or lips. Removal of the larynx results in the dramatic loss of the laryngeal voice and is discussed in Chapter 6. In some cases, portions of the tongue must be surgically removed because of cancer. The procedure is called a **glossectomy**, and it may be either partial or total, depending on the extent of the disease. Articulation is a challenge without the tongue; recall from Chapter 2 that many of the sounds of English are differentiated by movements of the tongue. The speech therapy goal following glossectomy is to adjust the placement of the remaining articulators to produce the most intelligible speech possible. There are many subtle adjustments that can be made to approximate speech produced without the tongue. For example, the sound /t/ normally requires the tongue to touch the alveolar ridge, just behind the teeth, but in the absence of the tongue, the patient might touch the lower lip behind the front teeth in a manner that stops and then releases the airflow. Because the manner of production is still a plosive and it is produced at the alveolar ridge, listeners may be tricked into thinking they heard a /t/. In fact, it is typically easier to understand the speech of a glossectomy patient if you do not look at the mouth, where some surprising articulatory placements are being made.

In some cases, structural changes of the articulators can be compensated for by specially designed artificial replacements, such as a prosthetic tongue and jaw

(Arcuri, Perlman, Philippbar, & Barkmeier, 1991; Leonard & Gillis, 1982, 1983). The artificial tongue does not move but fills in the gap resulting from tongue removal. This improves the speaker's ability to use the remaining articulators to overcome the changes in the oral structures. Some speakers adapt to their new anatomy by making appropriate articulatory adjustments. When therapy is needed, the speech-language pathologist works with the patient to come up with the most satisfactory approximation of sounds that are in error due to structural changes. In some cases the rate of speech must be slowed to allow the necessary time to articulate in a manner that is different from lifelong speech patterns.

## Motor Speech Disorders

The most commonly acquired articulation disorders in adults are due to neurological impairments that affect the motor control for speech. They are collectively referred to as motor speech disorders and include the disorders of dysarthria and apraxia of speech. As we saw earlier in this chapter, these disorders can occur in children as well. When they occur in adults, they are typically caused by damage or dysfunction of the motor control centers in the central or peripheral nervous systems, or both. The disturbances may affect any or all aspects of speech production, including respiration, phonation, resonance, and articulation.

**Dysarthria.**   The dysarthrias are a group of motor speech disorders caused by weakness, paralysis, slowness, incoordination, or sensory loss in the muscle groups responsible for speech. The muscle weakness and poor control typically result in imprecise articulation, so that speech is difficult to understand. The sounds may be distorted or involve the substitution of an incorrect sound. The specific characteristics of dysarthria tend to reflect the location of the damage to the nervous system, so that certain clusters of symptoms have been associated with certain diseases (Duffy, 1995). Some of the causes of dysarthria are stroke, Parkinson disease, Huntington's disease, amyotrophic lateral sclerosis (ALS, or Lou Gehrig's disease), and cerebellar diseases. In addition to imprecise articulation, symptoms include hypernasality because of poor motor control of the soft palate, disturbed voice quality including harshness or breathiness due to poor control of the larynx; and abnormal prosody because of poor control of changes in pitch, loudness, and timing. If motor control is so severely impaired that no understandable speech can be produced, it is called **anarthria**.

**Apraxia.**   **Apraxia of speech** differs from dysarthria in that there is no muscle weakness, paralysis, or incoordination, but there is impaired ability to plan the movements for speech production. Thus, apraxia of speech has been referred to as an impairment of the motor planning for articulation. Speech is difficult to understand because of substitution errors, sound repetitions, and some inappropriate sound additions. The errors are often inconsistent, so that repeated attempts at the same word come out differently on each attempt. In adults, apraxia of speech often co-occurs with the language impairment of aphasia, and in those cases it is difficult to separate the speech and language disorders. However, apraxia of speech can exist independently of aphasia, so that language formulation, reading, and writing are unimpaired but speech production is disturbed (Duffy, 1995).

## Treatment of Motor Speech Disorders

The goal for the management of motor speech disorders is to improve communication. This can be accomplished through therapy designed to improve the intelligibility, naturalness, and efficiency of speech production, but it may also be achieved by the use of assistive devices. There are excellent resources that provide treatment approaches specific to particular syndromes (Duffy, 2005; Moore, Yorkston, & Beukelman, 1991; Square-Storer, 1989; Yorkston, Beukelman, & Bell, 1988). Treatment may be directed toward the restoration of normal speech production processes or the compensation for impaired motor control. In some cases, adjustments need to be made to overcome the impairment. For example, Parkinson disease often results in a dysarthria characterized by imprecise articulation, decreased loudness, and flat prosody. A treatment approach called the Lee Silverman Voice Treatment trains patients to increase the effort that they exert while speaking by adjusting their loudness. With increased loudness, the Parkinson patients also increase their articulatory precision and thus remarkably improve their speech intelligibility (Ramig, Countryman, Thompson, & Horii, 1995).

Although the symptomatology of apraxia and dysarthria differs, there are similarities in some of the behavioral treatment approaches appropriate to these speech disorders. For both types of disorders, treatment involves in an orderly progression of tasks and intensive drill to reestablish and stabilize the motor movements. For example, a treatment continuum for apraxia of speech begins with the clinician saying the target word, followed by the patient and clinician producing the target together. If the patient correctly produces the response simultaneously with the clinician, then the clinician reduces support by mouthing the word along with the patient, and ultimately the patient produces the word in response to a question without support from the clinician (Wertz, LaPointe, & Rosenbek, 1984). In cases where speech production is not adequate for everyday communication, augmentative communication devices may be appropriate.

# AUGMENTATIVE AND ALTERNATIVE
# COMMUNICATION SYSTEMS

Some adults and children have physical limitations so severe that oral speech may not be an attainable goal. For these individuals, alternate methods must be found for communication. These range from a simple signaling device, like the call bell on a bedside nightstand, to sophisticated electronic devices that are tailored to the client's individual needs. The speech-language pathologist's challenge is to find the combination of features in a communication device that best matches the client's needs and abilities. A child who can identify pictures but cannot yet read may start with an electronic touch-screen device that displays and speaks the names of objects and actions common to his or her daily life. (see Figure 4.4). An adult who can read may do well with a device that can produce both synthetic speech and written output (see Figure 4.5). Adults with moderately impaired intelligibility may need to augment spoken communication with an alphabet board or other visual support to achieve successful communication.

Before a device can be selected, an initial assessment of the client's abilities must be obtained, often through the coordinated efforts of a variety of professionals, such as audiologists, vision specialists, psychologists, speech-language pathologists, and physical and occupational therapists. These individuals contribute information concerning the client's sensory, motor, cognitive, and language abilities. This evaluation is designed to determine the client's limitations as well as strengths that might be used for communication. For example, an individual with limited visual acuity may do better with simple line drawings than with glossy photos. An individual with severe cerebral palsy and limited use of the hands may have sufficient control of eye movement, head movement, or even foot movement to use a special switch with an electronic device (see Figure 4.1). Different devices may be needed to allow the child or adult to communicate from different positions,

**FIGURE 4.4   Children with severe disabilities may learn to use electronic devices to communicate by selecting a picture in order to play a recorded word or message.**

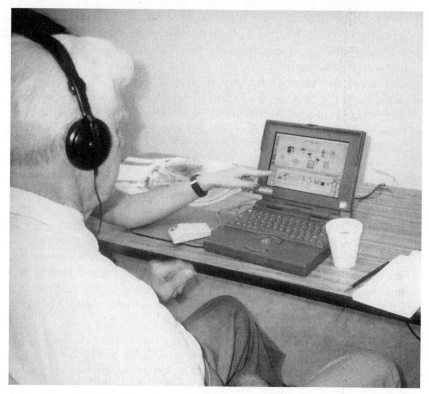

**FIGURE 4.5   An adult uses the Lingraphica® (Tolfa) system to communicate recent events in his life..**

such as sitting in a wheelchair or lying in bed. The devices selected must be able to accompany the client and be available whenever the client needs to communicate.

The decision about how the child or adult will communicate is closely related to what information will be communicated. Communication involves a code that is passed from sender to receiver. For normal speakers, this code is oral language. For a patient who is recovering from surgery to remove the larynx, the code might be written language. For a child who cannot write, the code might be a symbol system. For a child of more limited language or cognitive abilities, pictures might be used. In selecting the code, both the client's abilities and the people he or she needs to communicate with must be considered. It makes no sense to train clients to expert levels with a symbol system, for instance, if their families, teachers, and classmates prefer not to learn this system as well.

After one or more communication systems are selected, training is vital for developing successful communication. Training is geared toward the client's developmental level and daily needs. For a toddler, it may mean starting with toys and activities that develop turn-taking skills and communicative intent. For a school-aged child, it might include the use of language for academic purposes as well as for interpersonal communication. For the adult, the goal may be to reestablish communication that has been affected by illness or injury. Training often involves trial and error on the part of both the client and the clinician. Imagine the dilemma of the clinician who must try to adapt a communication system to meet the particular needs of the client before the client has the means of communicating those needs. And imagine the frustration of the client who must wait until the clinician figures it out!

A client with the desire and means to transmit a message is still only half of a successful communication exchange. Communication requires other people. Family members often receive direct training on how to use and maintain augmentative devices, but the client is also likely to encounter others who have never seen an augmentative device. Unfortunately, some people may not want to take the considerable time and effort involved in communicating through an alternative system. Communication is inevitably slower and is often less accurate. It can be tiring for both the sender and receiver. However, for many nonverbal individuals, the basic need to interact with other people provides the motivation and reward for the effort involved. This can clearly be seen in the case of Mr. Moser.

> *Mr. Moser* had been a high school science teacher until he suffered brain damage at the age of 43. An artery at the base of his brain had been thin-walled and weak. Eventually, this section of the artery ballooned out, forming an aneurysm, which ultimately burst. Immediate surgery was able to halt the bleeding, but not before sections of his brainstem and cerebellum were damaged. When he recovered from surgery, he was left with a variety of permanent deficits.
>
> Damage to the auditory tracts in the brainstem causes a rare form of acquired auditory disorder. Although he could hear sounds and tell when two sounds were different, Mr. Moser could not attach meaning to what he heard. Consequently, he could not understand spoken language, although he understood written language quite well. Damage to the motor tracts running through the brainstem and cerebellum left him confined to a wheelchair. He suffered from ataxia of movement. When he reached for objects, his hands and arms would waver back and forth. He would frequently over- or undershoot his reach for the object he wanted. His speech was similarly affected. His voice was a monotone and low in pitch. He spoke with great effort, and his face often contorted as he struggled to get out the words. He spoke only when asked specifically to do so.
>
> Because of his difficulty in producing the movements needed for speech and his inability to monitor his speech through audition, he became mute. In place of speech, he relied on an electronic communication system that allowed him to type in a message that was displayed on a small screen. Messages were typed with an ever-wavering index finger, one letter at a time. When he wished to convey a longer message, which he frequently did, the device printed the message on paper. His laboriously produced messages revealed his intelligent, inquisitive, and outgoing personality. Armed with his communication system and a large amount of persistence and charm, Mr. Moser was able to interact with others through written language.

## CLINICAL PROBLEM SOLVING

Kiesha, age 6, was brought into our research lab to participate in a language study. While she was there we taped the following conversation:

KIESHA:   Hey, Piget [Piglet]!

DAD:   There he is. You found him. There's Piglet.

KIESHA:   Shhhhh.

DAD:   Oh, is it because he's sleeping?

KIESHA:   Kaiet [quiet]!

DAD:   Ok, I'll be quiet. Are they all asleep?

KIESHA:   We da he seep [Where does he sleep]?

DAD:   What are they doing?

KIESHA:   Let's make 'em seep [sleep]. He's at home.

DAD:   Who's this guy.

KIESHA:   Gover [Grover]. And Ernie. Cookie Monser [Monster].

1. Does this speech sample indicate an articulation disorder? Would you feel the same if the child had just turned 3? (To review normal development, consult Chapter 3).
2. Using Table 4.1, can you identify any phonological processes among the sound errors? Remember that identification of a phonological process requires evidence of a pattern that affects more than one individual sound.
3. What factors would you need to rule out as causes of these speech errors before considering therapy?
4. Which therapy approaches might you consider for remediation in this case? Which would not be appropriate? Why?

## REFERENCES

American Speech-Language-Hearing Association (ASHA). (1991). The role of the speech-language pathologist in management of oral myofunctional disorders. *Asha, 33* (Suppl. 5), 7.

Arcuri, M. R., Perlman, A. L., Philippbar, S. A., & Barkmeier, J. M. (1991). The effects of a maxillary speech-aid prosthesis for the combined tongue and mandibular resection patient. *Journal of Prosthetic Dentistry, 65*(6), 816–22.

Barrett, R. H., & Hanson, M. L. (1978). *Oral myofunctional disorders* (2nd ed.). St. Louis, MO: Mosby.

Duffy, J. R. (2005). *Motor speech disorders: Substrates, differential diagnosis, and management* (2nd ed.), St. Louis, MO: Mosby-Year Book.

Dunn, C. (1982). Phonological process analysis: Contributions to assessing phonological disorders. *Communicative Disorders, 7,* 147–163.

Elbert, M., Powell, T. W., & Swartzlander, P. (1991). Toward a technology of generalization: How many exemplars are sufficient? *Journal of Speech and Hearing Research*, 34, 84–87.

Gierut, J. A., Morrisette, M. L., Hughes, M. T., & Rowland, S. (1996). Phonological treatment efficacy and developmental norms. *Language, Speech, and Hearing Services in Schools*, 27, 215–230.

Goldman, R., & Fristoe, M. (1986). *Goldman-Fristoe Test of Articulation*. Circle Pines, MN: American Guidance Service.

Grunwell, P. (1980). Developmental language disorders at the phonological level. In F. M. Jones (Ed.), *Language disability in children*. Lancaster, PA: MTP Press.

Hall, B. J. C. (1990). Attitudes of fourth and sixth graders towards peers with mild articulation disorders. *Language, Speech, and Hearing Services in Schools*, 22, 344–340.

Handzic-Cuk, J., Cuk, V., Gluhinic, M., Risavi, R., & Stajner-Katusic, S. (2001). Tympanometric findings in cleft palate patients: Influence of age and cleft type. *Journal of Laryngology & Otology*, 115, 91–96.

Ingram, D. (1981). *Procedures for the phonological analysis of children's language*. Baltimore: University Park Press.

Jaffee, M. B. (1984). Neurological impairment of speech production: Assessment and treatment. In J. Costello (Ed.), *Speech disorders in children* (pp. 157–186). San Diego: College-Hill Press.

Kent, R. D., Miolo, G., & Bloedel, S. (1994). The intelligibility of children's speech: A review of evaluation procedures. *American Journal of Speech-Language Pathology*, 3, 81–95.

Khan, L., & Lewis, N. (1986). *Khan-Lewis Phonological Analysis*. Circle Pines, MN: American Guidance Service.

Leonard, R. J., & Gillis, R. (1982). Effects of a prosthetic tongue on vowel intelligibility and food management in a patient with total glossectomy. *Journal of Speech & Hearing Disorders*, 47(1), 25–30.

Leonard, R. J., & Gillis, R. (1983). Effects of a prosthetic tongue on vowel formants and isovowel lines in a patient with total glossectomy (an addendum to Leonard & Gillis, 1982). *Journal of Speech & Hearing Disorders*, 48(4), 423–6.

Lewis, B. A. (1990). Familial phonological disorders: Four pedigrees. *Journal of Speech and Hearing Disorders*, 55, 160–170.

Lynch, J. I. (1990). Tongue reduction surgery: Efficacy and relevance to the profession. *Asha*, 32, 59–61.

McDonald, E. T., & Chance, B. (1964). *Cerebral palsy*. Englewood Cliffs, NJ: Prentice Hall.

McReynolds, L. V. (1982). Functional articulation problems. In G. H. Shames & E. H. Wiig (Eds.), *Human communication disorders: An introduction*. Columbus, OH: Charles E. Merrill.

Moore, C. A., Yorkston, K. M., & Beukelman, D. R. (Eds.). (1991). *Dysarthria and apraxia of speech*. Baltimore: Paul H. Brookes.

Peterson-Falzone, S. J., Hardin-Jones, M. A., & Karnell, M. P. (2001). *Cleft palate speech* (3rd ed.). St. Louis: Mosby.

Prather, E., & Whaley, P. (1984). Articulation training based on coarticulation. In H. Winitz (Ed.), *Treating articulation disorders: For clinicians by clinicians*. Baltimore: University Park Press.

Ramig, L. O., Countyman, S., Thompson, L., & Horii, L. (1995). A comparison of two intensive speech treatments for Parkinson disease. *Journal of Speech and Hearing Research*, 39, 1232–1251.

Ruscello, D. M., St. Louis, K. O., & Mason, N. (1991). School-age children with phonologic disorders: Coexistence with other speech/language disorders. *Journal of Speech and Hearing Disorders*, 34, 236–242.

Shelton, R. L., Furr, M. L., Johnson, A., & Arndt, W. B. (1975). Cephalometric and intraoral variables as they relate to articulation improvement with training. *American Journal of Orthodontics, 67*, 423–431.

Shprintzen, R. J., Siegal-Sadewitz, V. L., Amato, J., & Goldberg, R. B. (1985). Retrospective diagnosis of previously missed syndromic disorders among 1000 patients with cleft lip, cleft palate, or both. *Birth Defects, 21*, 85–92.

Shriberg, L. (1980). Developmental phonological disorders. In T. J. Hixon, L. Shriberg, & J. Saxon (Eds.), *Introduction to communication disorders*. Englewood Cliffs, NJ: Prentice Hall.

Shriberg, L., Austin, D., Lewis, B. A., McSweeny, J. L., & Wilson, D. L. (1997). The percentage of consonants correct (PCC) metric: Extensions and reliability data. *Journal of Speech Language and Hearing Research, 40*, 708–722.

Shriberg, L. D., & Kwiatkowski, J. (1988). A follow-up study of children with phonologic disorders of unknown origin. *Journal of Speech and Hearing Disorders, 53*, 144–155.

Shriberg, L. D., & Kwiatkowski, J. (1990). Self-monitoring and generalization in preschool speech-delayed children. *Language, Speech, and Hearing Services in Schools, 21*, 157–170.

Shriberg, L. D., Kwiatkowski, J., Best, S., Hengst, J., & Terselic-Weber, B. (1986). Characteristics of children with phonological disorders of unknown origin. *Journal of Speech and Hearing Disorders, 51*, 140–161.

Shriberg, L. D., Tomblin, J. B., McSweeny, J. L. (1999). Prevalence of speech delay in 6-year-old children and comorbidity with language impairment. *Journal of Speech, Language, and Hearing Research, 42*, 1461–1481.

Square-Storer, P. (Ed.). (1989). *Acquired apraxia of speech in aphasic adults*. Salisbury, UK: Lawrence Erlbaum Associates.

Wertz, R. T., LaPointe, L. L., & Rosenbek, J. C. (1984). *Apraxia of speech in adults: The disorder and its management*. Orlando, FL: Grune & Stratton.

Yorkston, K. M., Beukelman, D. R., & Bell, K. R. (1988). *Clinical management of dysarthric speakers*. Boston: College-Hill Press.

## READINGS FROM THE POPULAR LITERATURE

Albom, M. (1998). *Tuesdays with Morrie*. New York: Doubleday. (amyotrophic lateral sclerosis [ALS], or Lou Gehrig's disease)

Gordon, S., & Tempel, L. (1992). *Parkinson's: A personal story of acceptance*. Boston: Branden. (Parkinson disease).

Grady-Fitchett, J. (1998). *Flying lessons: On the wings of Parkinson's disease*. New York: Forge. (Parkinson disease)

Grealy, L. (1994). *Autobiography of a face*. New York: Harper Perennial. (facial cancer)

Handler, L. (1998). *Twitch and shout: A Touretter's tale*. New York: Dutton. (Tourette syndrome)

Hasse, J. (1996). *Break out: Finding freedom when you don't quite fit the mold*. Berea, OH: Quixote Publications. (cerebral palsy)

Kondracke, M. (2000). *Saving Milly: Love, politics and Parkinson's disease*. New York: Ballantine Books. (Parkinson disease)

McDermott, J. (2000). *Babyface: A story of heart and bones*. Bethesda, MD: Woodbine House. (Apert syndrome)

Montague, A. (1999). *Elephant man* (3rd ed.). New York: E. P. Dutton. (facial disfigurement)

Rabin, R. (1985). *Six parts love: One family's battle with Lou Gehrig's disease*. New York: Scribner. (ALS)

Reeve, C. (1997). *Still me*. New York: Random House. (spinal cord injury, ventilator dependency)

Robillard, A. B. (1999). *Meaning of a disability: The lived experience of paralysis*. Philadelphia: Temple University Press. (motor neuron disease).

Sacks, O. (1973). *Awakenings*. New York: E. P. Dutton. (cases of diminished movement and communication related to Parkinsonism)

Sienkiewicz-Mercer, R., & Kaplan, S. (1989). *I Raise my eyes to say yes*. West Hartford, CT: Whole Health Books. (cerebral palsy)

Stehli, A. (1995). *Dancing in the rain*. Westport, CT: The Georgiana Organization. (stories by parents of children with special needs)

Webster, B. D. (1989). *All of a piece*. Baltimore: Johns Hopkins University Press. (multiple sclerosis)

Wexler, A. (1995). *Mapping fate*. New York: Times Books: Random House. (Huntington disease)

# CHAPTER FIVE

# DISORDERS OF FLUENCY

# PREVIEW

The area of fluency and fluency disorders has been one of the most dynamic areas within the profession of speech-language pathology. Principal among disorders of fluency is the phenomenon of stuttering. The various definitions of stuttering reflect a wide range of perspectives that experts have brought to bear on trying to understand this disorder of communication. Developmental, familial, psychological, neurological, and motoric factors all appear to interact in cases of stuttering. Although stuttering is the most common fluency disorder, there are other disorders characterized by changes in fluency. We will briefly consider a fluency disruption called cluttering as well as cases of acquired stuttering in adults.

When Abraham[1] was about 3 years of age, his mother noticed that his sentences did not always flow smoothly. Sometimes he would repeat the same word several times before he was able to get the rest of the sentence out. There were pauses midsentence. In fact, at times Abraham sounded quite disfluent. This concerned both of his parents because they each had a family history of **stuttering**. The mother's brother had stuttered during most of his childhood, although he was described as completely fluent as an adult. The father's sister began stuttering as a child and continued to stutter into adulthood. Abraham's parents did not want him to struggle to communicate the way their siblings had, and they were naturally concerned when Abraham went through periods when he seemed particularly disfluent. At age 3 years, 3 months, we had the following conversation with him:

AUTHOR:   What's Wishbone?

ABRAHAM:   Um, he's one of the shows that I watch. He's a dog. The story of Wishbone is really . . . um, really a show.

AUTHOR:   He's a dog. And he has his own show?

ABRAHAM:   No, there's a . . . there's a boy in it.

AUTHOR:   What do they get to do?

ABRAHAM:   They do everything. But only in the show, they get to do . . . I don't know. (Abraham notices the barnyard toys and goes to them.)

AUTHOR:   Let me see what's in this barn. There's a lot of animals in here.

ABRAHAM:   Yeah, I . . . (Silence)

AUTHOR:   All right. Well, there's a cow. And there's a baby cow. That's a . . . that's a brown cow.

---

[1]We followed the speech and language development of Abraham in Chapters 3 and 7.

ABRAHAM:  No, that's a white cow. That's called . . . that's called . . . These two are cows.

AUTHOR:  Oh yeah? What kind of cows?

ABRAHAM:  Black ones and white ones.

AUTHOR:  Black ones and white ones. And this is a dog.

ABRAHAM:  This is . . . This is a dog.

AUTHOR:  Do you think he's a sheep dog?

ABRAHAM:  Nooo.

AUTHOR:  Do you think he's a cow dog? Does he have to watch out over the cows?

ABRAHAM:  (Nods in agreement)

AUTHOR:  Well, I've got some hay. (Picks up a cow) Do you think he's a hay eater?

ABRAHAM:  Yes he is. I'll put hay on his . . . in his . . . in his . . . in there so he can't eat anything. (Abraham puts animals in the hay loft.)

AUTHOR:  Now, we have two cows in the hay.

ABRAHAM:  Is this one the . . . the . . . the . . . the baby one?

AUTHOR:  I don't know. It's kind of small. Maybe he is a baby one.

During this brief conversation, we were able to observe a number of interruptions in the flow of communication. These included whole word repetitions ("the . . . the . . . the . . . the baby one"), phrase repetitions ("This is . . . this is a dog"), and interjections ("um"). However, Abraham seemed completely unfazed by his disfluencies. His focus was on the toys and our play, and he was probably unaware of his own speech patterns. Notice, too, that Abraham was not the only one to show speech repetition. The author repeated part of a sentence ("That's a . . . that's a brown cow") during the conversation as well. In fact, everyone experiences a minor interruption in the flow of speech at some time or another. Differentiating between "normal" disfluencies and stuttering is an ongoing challenge to those working in the area of fluency disorders.

It is not always easy to distinguish an episode of disfluency that characterizes stuttering from an episode that is a momentary lapse of fluency. This is particularly true in the case of young children. As young children are learning to put together sentences, it is very common to hear them make false starts (I . . . he did it!), revise midsentence ("He's in . . . he's on TV"), hesitate over the next word to come ("I want . . . juice") We often get the sense that these interruptions in fluency have more to do with the child's partial grasp of the language than any struggle to get the words out. Likewise, we have all heard a child so excited that word or phrase repetitions came pouring forth ("Mommy! Mommy! Mommy! Mommy! Mommy! Can I, can I, can I have one?!"). For most children, these episodes reflect normal development, rather than the onset of stuttering. In fact, for Abraham, this proved to be the case. As he continued to develop speech and language skills, the episodes of disfluency decreased. By 4½ years, no one, including his parents, had any concerns about his speech fluency.

## NORMAL DISFLUENCIES VERSUS STUTTERING

Conture (1990) noted that deciding who is and who is not stuttering is a relative rather than an absolute decision, in that there is no behavior that children who stutter display that normal children never exhibit. Although normally developing children (and adults on occasion) sometimes experience breakdowns in these speech parameters, the child who stutters exhibits those behaviors to a greater degree. For example, normal children such as Abraham may repeat words or phrases at the age of 3. However, by the age of 4½, children usually repeat utterances only when they wish to emphasize something (Curlee, 1980).

### Early Signs of Stuttering

Although no method is foolproof for identifying the young child who will persist in stuttering, a number of behavioral signs are considered to be "red flags" (see Table 5.1). In true developmental stuttering, speech is characterized by changes in duration, rate, and rhythm, with frequent interruptions of fluency from sound to sound and from word to word. One distinction that has been suggested involves the unit of speech in which the disfluency occurs (Andrews et al., 1983; Wall, 1988). Normal disfluencies typically occur on whole words, phrases, or sentences; stuttering is more likely to affect single sounds and syllables. A child showing normal disfluency may say, "I want . . . I want it," whereas a child who stutters may say, "I wwwwwwant it." The frequency of disfluent episodes is also different for children with normal disfluencies than for those who stutter. Wingate (1962) found that nonstuttering children seldom make repetitions for more than 3 percent of their total speech utterances; children who stutter were found to have a frequency of syllable disfluencies ranging from 7 to 14 percent.

The signs of stuttering are not restricted to interruptions of speech. Conture and Kelly (1991) reported that young children who stutter could be differentiated

**TABLE 5.1   Signs Often Associated with Normal and Stuttered Speech**

| NORMAL DISFLUENCIES | |
| --- | --- |
| Word repetitions | I like that . . . that book. |
| Phrase repetitions | I want a . . . want a big one! |
| Sentence repetitions | Watch me! Watch me! Watch me! |
| Hesitations | He took . . . my juice. |
| Interjections | We, um, got to go too. |

| STUTTERING | |
| --- | --- |
| Syllable repetitions | We saw a vi-vi-vi-video. |
| Sound repetition | I g-g-g-got it from school. |
| Sound prolongations | Wwwwwwait for mmmme. |
| Sound blocks | [starts word but no sound comes out] |
| Nonspeech behaviors | [e.g., blinks, facial tension, limb movement] |

from nonstuttering children by the types of facial behaviors they exhibit. For example, children who stutter were likely to look away, blink their eyes, raise their upper lip, or press their lips together during periods of disfluency, whereas their fluent peers showed these behaviors less frequently. Stuttering children may show signs of struggle or tension while attempting to speak, whereas children with normal disfluencies typically seem unaffected by the disfluent episode.

Several investigators (Schwartz, Zebrowski, & Conture, 1990; Yairi & Ambrose, 1992) have examined the earliest signs of stuttering by studying the behaviors of young children whose parents reported stuttering of a recent onset (within the previous twelve months). Yairi and Ambrose (1992) interviewed parents concerning the age of their children and the characteristics of their disfluent speech when stuttering began. Parents reported that their children were sometimes quite young, between the ages of 20 months to 5 years of age, when stuttering was first observed. Just under half of the parents reported that their children began to stutter suddenly, whereas other parents remembered the onset as evolving gradually over the course of several weeks. Schwartz and colleagues (1990) recorded the speech of such children on videotape to assess the behaviors associated with the earliest stages of stuttering. The investigators reported that the disfluencies of these children included many sound prolongations (33 to 60% of all disfluent episodes). The children also exhibited frequent nonspeech behaviors, such as eye movements or eye closings during disfluent episodes. Somewhat surprisingly, the stuttering behaviors of children who were at the younger end of the age range did not differ remarkably from those at the older end. Although prolongations were somewhat more frequent for children who had been stuttering longer, the authors emphasized that there were more similarities than differences among the behaviors of children at different ages.

The signs that suggest the onset of stuttering, as opposed to developmental disfluencies, can vary between children and even within a single child. However, we have seen that there are some early indications that a child is struggling with more than just the normal disruptions of fluency that all children experience. These signs can be seen in the case of a young boy who was brought to the clinic for a fluency evaluation.

> *Jackson* was 6 years old when he was first seen in the clinic. His mother brought him in because "he stutters." She reported that he had started stuttering two years before, but she had always assumed that he would grow out of it. Now that Jackson was in school, however, she was concerned that other children were teasing him. She had already noticed that Jackson seemed aware that his speech was different from other children. She reported that he sometimes got frustrated when trying to talk. As far as she knew, no one in her family had ever stuttered, and she couldn't recall anyone having had any kind of developmental problems at all.
>
> When we talked with Jackson, it was apparent that his speech showed more than the typical amount of disfluency. In fact, sometimes it seemed as if he could hardly get his thoughts out. His speech was frequently disrupted by sound prolongations and blocks, when no sound came out at all. During these episodes, his mouth seemed to lock into a tense position from which he was unable to break free.

His brows knit together, and sometimes he would blink or contort his face until the disfluent period passed and speech resumed its normal flow. When asked why his mother brought him to the clinic, he replied, "I-i-i-t's . . . because I t-t-t-t-t . . . alk . . . I can't talk."

In contrast to his disfluency, a formal assessment of Jackson's language showed average to above average skills. When he was not stuttering, he did not show problems with speech articulation. An examination of his oral mechanism (see Chapter 4) revealed normal structure, muscle tone, and nonspeech movements. Likewise, he could repeat nonsense words and say entire sentences in a fluent, sing-song cadence, which indicated he possessed the physical mechanisms to support normal speech.

## Persistent Stuttering

A majority of children who show early disfluencies will eventually develop fluent speech. However, some children will not. Yairi and colleagues reported that children destined to recover from early stuttering-like behaviors may initially show more disfluencies than children who continue to be disfluent. However, the children who recover typically show reductions in the number of disfluencies within the first year after their stuttering-like disfluencies began. In contrast, children who failed to recover were relatively stable in their rate of disfluency (Yairi, Ambrose, Paden, & Throneburg, 1996). Although there is a chance that some of these children will recover still later in childhood, they are at risk for struggling with fluency throughout their lives. Let us look at the case of one such man:

> *Mr. Andrews*, age 32, has stuttered since childhood. Although he had received therapy several times, he continued to show a variety of stuttering signs. His stuttering consisted primarily of silent blocks, during which his mouth and face contorted as he struggled to speak. Occasionally, he also experienced part-word repetitions, in which the first sound of a word was repeated over and over. He had recently contacted the clinic because he thought that his stuttering was preventing him from advancing in his career. He expressed, "T———eam work is very important in my c-c-c-c-ompany, and I knnnnnnnnow that the others would rather not have me on the team b———cause of my stuttering. When I present m———y ideas, they d———on't take them as ssssseriously." He reported that he was able to speak fluently "most of the time" after his last experience with therapy in high school. However, to maintain fluency, Mr. Andrews felt he had to concentrate harder on how he was speaking than on what he was actually trying to say. Over time, his disfluency had slipped back to pretherapy levels. He was willing to try again to reduce his stuttering severity.

Adults who stutter may show some of the same characteristics of childhood stuttering. They may continue to produce sound repetitions and prolongations, along with silent interruptions, called blocks, in the flow of speech. "Secondary" characteristics of stuttering, which may have been present during childhood, may be more pronounced. These characteristics include facial tension, facial contortions, and extraneous movements during the stuttering episode. In addition, these adults typically have had years of frustration about being unable to communicate ideas with the ease that comes naturally to others. This frustration can become as problematic as the actual episodes of fluency breakdown.

It is not uncommon for nonstuttering individuals to stereotype those who stutter as having a variety of negative traits, including being anxious, tense, insecure, or nervous (Kalinowski, Lerman, & Watt, 1987). Indeed, several studies have examined physiological correlates of stress and found evidence of increased levels of stress and anxiety among those who stutter (Blood, Blood, Bennet, Simpson, & Susman, 1994; Weber & Smith, 1990). An alternate explanation is that stuttering stress and anxiety are a consequence of repeated negative experiences with communication. Several studies suggest that this is the case. For example, Miller and Watson (1992) reported that their subjects who stuttered were no more anxious overall than nonstuttering subjects. However, the two groups differed in terms of their attitudes toward communication, with attitudes worsening with increased stuttering severity. Craig (1990) showed that, prior to treatment for stuttering, adults who stutter were significantly more anxious during a communication task than control subjects. After their level of disfluency was decreased through treatment of stuttering behaviors, their anxiety was reduced to a level characteristic of nonstuttering adults. Such findings have led to a shift in clinician perceptions concerning the role of personality traits such as anxiety or other negative affective states (Cooper & Cooper, 1996).

One of the more puzzling features of persistent stuttering is that speech can be completely fluent under certain speaking circumstances. Let us consider the following case:

> *Mr. Tirai,* age 27, was a graduate student who had come to this country to study engineering three years earlier. Although he spoke two other languages with native proficiency, he had only rudimentary English at that time. He spent his first academic year in the United States studying primarily for his English language proficiency exam. He needed to pass this exam to continue his program in engineering. An outgoing man, he also spent his time going to campus and community cultural events, through which he developed a number of American friends. Through his determined study, his circle of English-speaking friends, and a measure of talent for learning languages, he steadily gained proficiency in English. Other than his accent, his English seemed largely unremarkable. He had long since acquired the common grammatical forms of English. His vocabulary had grown to a point where he rarely needed to search for words in conversation. However, in his final years of study, he was beginning to show occasional episodes of stuttering-like disfluencies. Although "stuttering" was not a word he had acquired in English, he managed to convey that he had escaped from stuttering by speaking English, but that it appeared to have caught up with him just as he was feeling comfortable with his new language.

Mr. Tirai was fluent for an extended period of time while he was learning English. Others have discovered they can induce short-term fluency by adopting foreign accents or imitating voices. Fluency may be achieved under conditions of **delayed**

**auditory feedback**. This involves use of instrumentation that presents the speaker's own voice, through headphones, at a slight time delay. So, as the speaker is talking, what he or she hears lags behind what is currently being said. Choral reading or speaking, during which people speak in concert, also tends to promote fluency. Likewise, intentional changes in the rhythm of speech, such as in chanting or singing, will produce fluency. All of these speaking conditions, from learning a foreign language to chanting, involve a change from the normal pattern of speech production. It appears that such changes may "override" whatever mechanisms may lead to disfluent episodes in regular speech. Unfortunately, as Mr. Tirai found, when speakers grow proficient with these "unusual" speaking conditions, stuttering may reappear.

## STUTTERING IN THE POPULATION

The **prevalence** of a disorder is the number of people in the population who have a particular problem at any given time. There have been several prevalence studies of stuttering over the years. The National Institute of Deafness and Other Communication Disorders (NIDCD; 1992) of the National Institutes of Health (NIH) estimated that approximately 2 million Americans stutter. This corresponds to a prevalence of approximately 0.8 percent. This figure is comparable to estimates of 0.8 percent derived by Hull, Mielke, Willeford, and Timmons (1976), 0.7 percent by Young (1975), and 0.8 percent by Morley (1952).

Although less than 1 percent of the population may be identified as stutterers at any given time, the percentage of people who stutter varies across the lifespan. Morley (1972) followed approximately 1,000 children in Newcastle-Upon-Tyne for fifteen years to examine various aspects of development. In this particular study, the **incidence** of stuttering, or the number of new cases identified during a period of time, was about 4 percent, or 1 in 25 children. NIDCD estimates that 1 in 30 children will go through a period of disfluency that lasts a minimum of six months.

Stuttering is typically first identified before the age of 5 and many resolve to normal fluency before puberty (Morley, 1972; Wingate, 1976). Wingate (1976) summarized fourteen studies and concluded that approximately 80 percent of children recover from stuttering. Although there has been some dispute about the exact number, it appears that for the majority of children who stutter at an early age stuttering will disappear before they graduate from high school. Curlee (1980) came to the following conclusion: "if the incidence of stuttering among the general population does approximate 4 percent, a recovery rate of 80 percent would account for a 0.7 percent prevalence of stuttering" (p. 281).

In some respects, stuttering is an "equal opportunity" disorder. It affects people of all racial and socioeconomic backgrounds. However, it does appear that some individuals are at higher risk than others for developing the disorder. Stuttering affects more boys than girls. NIDCD (1992) estimated that four times as many boys stutter as girls. Others have placed the male-to-female ratio at 3:1 (Hull et al., 1976) or 2:1 (Morley, 1972; Yairi & Ambrose, 1992). These differences may reflect, in part, the different age groups examined in these studies. The male-to-female ratio tends to increase with older ages, which has led some to suggest that girls may show higher rates of recovery with age than boys (Yairi, Ambrose, & Cox, 1996).

In addition to the surplus of males among individuals identified as stutterers, a family history of stuttering increases an individual's risk for the disorder. Although the population prevalence for stuttering is thought to hover around 0.7 to 0.8 percent, the prevalence among the relatives of an individual who stutters is much higher (Andrews & Harris, 1964; Howie, 1981; Kidd, 1980; Yairi & Ambrose, 1992; Yairi, Ambrose, & Cox, 1996). Yairi and Ambrose (1992) reported that almost half (46.6%) of their sample of young children who stutter had parents or siblings who also stuttered at one time. If blood relatives in the extended family were considered, two-thirds (66.3%) of the children had a positive family history for stuttering. The pattern of family aggregation for stuttering may signal the presence of a single major gene that contributes to expression of the disorder (Yairi et al., 1996). However, the actual components that contribute to the development of stuttering may be more complex. Some have suggested that genetic factors may confer a risk for stuttering, but that certain environmental factors are needed to trigger the disorder (Andrews et al., 1983; Howie, 1981).

Family history for stuttering may account for some of the variability seen among individuals who stutter. Janssen, Kraaimaat, and Brutten (1990) examined a variety of traits in subjects who stuttered with reference to family history for stuttering. One group had a positive family history for stuttering; the other did not. Those with relatives who stuttered had more sound prolongations and silent blocks in their speech. They also showed differences on measures of duration and variability in the acoustic stream from those without a positive family history. In contrast, the two stuttering groups did not differ on measures of reading, autonomic nervous system response, or responsiveness to therapy. Janssen and colleagues suggest that these results indicate that familial or genetic contributions to stuttering may have a greater impact on the motoric aspects of stuttering than on other associated features of the disorder.

## DEFINITIONS

Definitions of stuttering are many and varied. Let us consider a few of the definitions that have appeared in the literature over the years.

> *1955, Johnson*: "Stuttering is an anticipatory, apprehensive, hypertonic avoidance reaction" (p. 23). According to Johnson, stuttering is what speakers do when they expect stuttering to occur: dread it, tense in anticipation of it, and attempt to avoid doing it.

> *1977, World Health Organization*: Stuttering includes "disorders in the rhythm of speech, in which the individual knows precisely what he wishes to say, but

at the time is unable to say it because of an involuntary, repetitive prolongation or cessation of sound" (p. 227).

*1978, Wingate*: "Stuttering is characterized by audible or silent elemental repetitions and prolongations. These features reflect a temporary inability to move forward to the following sound" (p. 249).

*1980, Perkins*: "Stuttering is the abnormal timing of speech sound initiation."

*1987, Speech Foundation of America*: Stuttering is defined as "a communication disorder characterized by excessive involuntary disruptions or blockings in the flow of speech, particularly when such disruptions consist of repetitions or prolongations of a sound or syllable, and when they are accompanied by avoidance struggle behavior" (p. 183).

*1991, Perkins, Kent, and Curlee*: "Stuttering is a disruption of speech experienced by the speaker as a loss of control" (p. 734). They differentiate stuttering from nonstuttered forms of disfluencies by identifying the latter as "abnormal as well as normal sounding disfluency not experienced as loss of control" (p. 734).

*1995, Cooper and Cooper*: "Stuttering . . . is a clinical syndrome characterized by abnormal and persistent disfluencies in speech accompanied by characteristic affective, behavioral, and cognitive patterns" (p. 126).

There is no one definition of stuttering that is uniformly accepted by experts in the field. The differences among these and other definitions available in the literature reflect the fact that stuttering is a complex disorder that is not simply characterized. These definitions highlight the differences in perspective among stuttering experts. Several of the definitions are limited to the description of stuttering behaviors (e.g., prolongations, repetitions) from a listener-based perspective. Three include the perspective of the individual who stutters by including his or her perception of it (i.e., loss of control) or reaction to it (e.g., apprehension, avoidance). The interpretation that disfluent episodes are involuntary in nature further reflects the perception of the person who stutters. A few definitions make inferences concerning the underlying cause of the disorder (e.g., psychological reaction to disfluency, timing disruptions). In all, the definitions reflect the changing trends within the field that have emphasized aspects of the disorder at different times.

Consider how the components of these various definitions might apply to a particular case.

*Laura's* parents report that she has stuttered since she was 3 years old. At the time of her speech evaluation at age 7, she was found to repeat the first sounds and syllables of many words at the beginning of a phrase or sentence. At times, she seemed to posture her mouth and blink, and no sound could be heard. She made no attempt to avoid talking and had moments of normal fluency; suddenly the fluency would end, seemingly without warning. During her stuttering, she would often purse her lips, close her eyes, and appear as if she were trying to push out the word she was attempting to say. Laura's parents reported that she has expressed frustration at times over her inability to speak fluently.

In this brief case description, we recognize some of the common components of many definitions of stuttering:

- Repetition and prolongation of sounds and syllables
- Sudden or involuntary fluency interruptions
- Often accompanied by physical signs of struggle
- Often perceived negatively by the speaker

Therefore, despite the differences in definitions of stuttering, it is possible to observe the various components that these definitions present within a single case.

## THEORIES OF STUTTERING

There is probably no clinical area in speech-language pathology that has generated more controversy than our understanding of the cause and nature of stuttering. The number of causative theories is astonishing and reflects an evolution in thought over the last century. At any given time, one theoretical position becomes more popular as research advances and changing social mores shift the clinical perspective on this disorder. As Van Riper indicated in 1971, the pendulum of popular and clinical opinion tends to swing between physical and psychological causes. Despite these shifts in theoretical perspective over the years, we will clearly see the impact of these various theories reflected in approaches to intervention later in this chapter. Let us consider a few of the more prominent theoretical positions that have appeared over time.

Wendell Johnson is considered one of the founding fathers of the field of speech-language pathology. He spent his professional life studying the onset of stuttering. He concluded that the normal disfluencies experienced by many children were often labeled by their parents and other listeners as stuttering (Johnson, 1959). His **diagnosogenic theory of stuttering** was built on the belief that stuttering begins when normal disfluencies are labeled as stuttering. This theory recognized that normal children often pass through a period of nonfluent speech as they are in the process of language acquisition. Parents may hear their young children's normal episodes of disfluent speech and react negatively to them. They may call attention to their children's speech by telling them to "slow down" or to "take a deep breath and start over." Johnson suggested that these children are sensitive to their parents' reactions and become nervous or self-conscious about their speech. This leads them to become more disfluent in response, until stuttering becomes a learned behavior. Although there has never been any direct evidence in support of Johnson's theory, we continue to see its influence today. For example, some approaches to stuttering therapy involves indirect treatment methods that avoid calling attention to the stuttering behaviors themselves.

Johnson was also concerned with the psychological effects of disfluent speech. He believed the fear of stuttering could eventually become as great a problem as the actual stuttering episodes. As we saw earlier in this chapter, those who stutter can show physical signs of stress and anxiety (Blood et al., 1994; Weber & Smith, 1990) and may report higher levels of anxiety about possible speaking situations (Blood, Blood, Tellis, & Gabel, 2001). Signs of anxiety associated with speaking led to the idea that stuttering might be a manifestation of an underlying emotional conflict (Blanton, 1965; Glauber, 1958; Travis, 1971). In the mid-twentieth century, some recommended psychotherapy with the goal of uncovering hidden or repressed feelings that were thought to be at the root of stuttering. Today most speech-language pathologists reject the idea that stuttering is caused by a psychological disturbance. However, in some cases, sustained stuttering may cause significant psychological stress. Therapy approaches that include a component designed to address anxiety associated with stuttering episodes can produce long-term reductions in negative psychological consequences of stuttering (Blomgren, Roy, Callister, & Merrill, 2005). Likewise, many individuals derive benefit from participation in social support groups for persons who stutter (Yaruss et al., 2002).

In contrast to psychological explanations, some theories have proposed that stuttering has its roots in a form of neurological dysfunction. One early neurological theory was made popular by Orton in the 1920s. He proposed that a disturbance in the normal pattern of hemispheric specialization might account for disorders including stuttering (and also dyslexia). Early studies designed to examine cerebral functioning failed to identify any gross neurological deficit or robust differences between those who stutter and those who do not (see Andrews et al., 1983). However, advances in the techniques available to study brain structure and function have led to evidence of altered patterns of brain activation in adults who stutter. This includes overactivation in regions of the right hemisphere, typically the nondominant hemisphere for speech (e.g., De Nil, Kroll, Lafaille, & Houle, 2003; Fox, Ingham, Ingham, et al., 1996: Neumann et al., 2003). Furthermore, these anomalous patterns of activation may shift after successful participation in stuttering treatment (De Nil et al., 2003; Neumann et al., 2003), suggesting that altered speech is accompanied by altered patterns of brain activation in those who stutter.

To date, the neurological findings for stuttering do not explain why the speech of those who stutter is sometimes fluent and sometimes disfluent, even within the same conversation. Perkins and colleagues (1991) attempted to address this enigma by proposing that stuttering occurs as the consequence of dysynchrony among any of the neural systems that support communication, including phonology and language, in addition to the control of speech movements. There is support for the idea that the linguistic aspects of speech do indeed affect the occurrence of stuttering. Stuttering is often first reported at an age when children are starting to formulate complete sentences. When young children first begin to stutter, they rarely do so on single-word utterances and often do at the beginning of sentences, clauses, and phrases (Bloodstein, 2006). In addition, young children are more likely to stutter on utterances that are relatively long compared to what they typically produce (Zackheim & Conture, 2003). These patterns suggest that individuals who stutter may have difficulty coordinating speech movements when language formulation is also demanding. This idea is supported by the finding that the conversational language of young children who stuttered was more advanced than expected during pretreatment language testing. Their posttreatment speech was both more fluent and closer to the language level expected for their age (Bonelli et al., 2000). However, not all studies show this same pattern. Several have indicated that language skills of children are unchanged by success in treatment (see Lattermann, Shenker, & Thordardottir, 2005, for a review).

Aspects of language are known to influence stuttering in adults. Adults are more likely to stutter on content words (i.e., nouns and verbs) and long words than on words that serve grammatical function (e.g., articles). This may reflect subtle problems in the ability to rapidly access specific word forms while the overall message is being formulated. Support for this idea comes from Prins, Main, and Wampler (1997), who showed an effect for one's speed at naming pictures that reflected the frequency with which words appear in the language. When words are relatively infrequent, and therefore less familiar, it took longer to retrieve the name. This effect was magnified for individuals who stutter. Furthermore, disfluencies are more likely to occur on low-frequency words than on high-frequency words (Dayalu, Kalinowski, Stuart, Holbert, & Rastatter, 2002), further reinforcing the idea that subtle difficulty with word retrieval may provoke stuttering episodes. Similarly, adults have shown a reduction in speech articulation rate following treatment to enhance fluency (Andrews et al., 1983), suggesting that initial faster articulation rates were taxing the speech production system sufficiently to result in stuttering.

Whether these interactions between language and stuttering reflect a dyssynchrony between the neural systems that support speech and language is unknown. An alternate explanation is that speakers who are operating at the edge of their capacity for fluent speech may become disfluent when the demands for the speaking task exceed their capacity for producing the motor patterns for speech (Venkatagiri, 2005). Under this explanation, stuttering interacts with language, not because of mistakes in the coordination of the neural systems, but because use of more difficult language forms (e.g., complex sentences, less common vocabulary) is sufficiently demanding that language formulation interferes with automatic speech production. In contrast, speaking more slowly than usual, speaking in concert with other speakers, or singing forces the speaker to use a more deliberate rather than automatic means of programming speech, thus enhancing fluency. Therapy approaches that seek to reduce the demands on the speaker, so that his or her capacity for fluent speech is not exceeded, are consistent with this idea (e.g., Adams, 1990; Franken, Kielstra-Van der Schalk, & Bolens, 2005).

## EVALUATION OF DEVELOPMENTAL STUTTERING

The broad goals of a fluency evaluation are to determine whether clinically significant disfluencies are present, to understand (to the extent possible) the nature and potential cause of these disfluencies, and to understand the impact of these disfluencies within the context of the client's life. As we have discussed throughout the chapter, everyone experiences disfluent speech from time to time, and many young children typically pass through a period of normal disfluency as they acquire language skills. One of the first jobs of the clinician is to assess the likelihood that the client's disfluencies fall outside the range of normal. Typically, the clinician will consider the types of disfluencies observed, their frequency and duration, associated nonspeech behaviors (e.g., struggle, avoidance), and the client's (or parents') attitudes toward the disfluent episodes. The clinician may need to assess fluency in more than one context, because stuttering severity can change remarkably depending on the situation. School-based clinicians, for example, may observe a child in the classroom or out on the playground or even request a taped speech sample from home. Different task demands, such as making a phone call or providing an explanation, often alter the frequency of disfluent speech as well.

As we will see later in this chapter, there are other forms of disfluent speech besides stuttering. Disorders such as cluttering can produce disruptions in fluency that are qualitatively different from stuttering. The clinician must also differentiate between stuttering and the breakdowns in fluency that result from an expressive language disorder. A sudden disruption of fluency, particularly in later childhood, may be the first sign of a neurological disorder, which would prompt referral to a neurologist. Formal and informal measures of speech and language, as well as a detailed case history, are invaluable in distinguishing among disorders that affect fluency. Failure to do so can lead to inappropriate treatment choices.

Finally, the perceptions and attitudes of clients who stutter can have an enormous impact on the degree to which their lives are altered by stuttering and their readiness and motivation for change. Gaining this information is an ongoing process that starts with an initial interview and continues over the course of intervention. Clients and families may have very specific intervention goals ("I need to be able to conduct interviews for my job") or completely unrealistic ones ("I want my child to stop repeating himself all the time when he's excited"). A client's internal anxiety or lack of confidence about speaking may interfere with his or her ability to benefit from speech modifications. Unless we know what these attitudes and perceptions are, subsequent intervention may be fruitless or even offensive to the client.

## STUTTERING THERAPY

Stuttering can be successfully treated. There are now numerous reports in the literature that show that clients can develop and maintain fluency over time (e.g., Blood, Blood, Tellis, & Gabel, 2001; Hasbrouck, 1992; Hewat, Onslow, Packman, &

O'Brian, 2006; Onslow, Costa, Andrews, Harrison, & Packman, 1996; Packman, Onslow, & van Doorn, 1994). The primary questions in intervention are who should receive treatment, when it should begin, and what form it should take. For adults, the decision to seek treatment is a personal one. For children, a number of factors may influence parents' decisions to initiate treatment. Because many children who show early signs of stuttering will overcome this difficulty, some professionals have advocated vigilant waiting, with parent counseling and regular monitoring of the child's speech (Zebrowski, 1995). In contrast, Starkweather (1990) noted a growing emphasis on early intervention for stuttering. He also noted that a wait-and-see attitude is more risky than the cost of treatment for a child who would have recovered later on his or her own. In addition, he reported that recovery rates with treatment routinely exceed the rate of spontaneous recovery. Finally, there is some evidence to suggest that waiting to initiate treatment for the child who stutters is associated with more time in treatment. All these factors support the trend toward early intervention for children who show early signs of stuttering.

## Parental Involvement

There are a number of components of fluency therapy. For children, one critical component may be parent and family attitudes. Family involvement in the therapy process may be key to its success (e.g., Healy, Scott, & Ellis, 1995; Rustin & Cook, 1995). Kelly (1995) noted that mothers and fathers often differ in terms of how they interact with their children and may require different advice and guidance in order to best improve their child's fluency. We can see the need to understand the parents' perspectives in the following case:

> *Gerry* and *Anna* had very different reactions to their 4-year-old son's periods of disfluency. Anna told of her anxiety whenever Gerry Jr. would stutter: "It hurts me to see him struggle. I don't want other kids teasing him, either." She went out of her way to "not call his attention to it." As a result, she would allow her son to interrupt her conversations with others, and she often intervened when she thought his brothers and sisters might upset him and cause him to stutter. Gerry Sr. interpreted his wife's actions as "spoiling the boy." He didn't see his son's disfluencies as a problem. If anything, he thought that stuttering was one way that Gerry Jr. could get more attention in a household that included four other children. Needless to say, these differences in how each parent reacted to their son's disfluencies were a source of friction between them. It was apparent that intervention would have to include the parents' reactions to their child's disfluencies. This began with discussions to help the parents differentiate between the actual disfluent episodes and their reactions to it. The parents were provided with weekly "homework assignments" designed to help them develop workable and appropriate means of responding to specific situations that were problematic from either a fluency or a social-interaction perspective (e.g., should Gerry Jr. be allowed to interrupt at will?). For these parents, this approach allowed them to develop new perspectives on their son's disfluencies.

Parents may have many roles in the intervention process. They are often the first ones to seek help on behalf of their children and should be involved in setting long- and short-term goals for their child. As we saw in Gerry's case, parents may hold a range of attitudes and beliefs about stuttering. They may need information about what changes they can reasonably expect from therapy (Healey et al., 1995). They can also become invaluable assets in the intervention process. A number of therapy methods involve training parents to promote fluency in the child as the primary means of intervention (e.g., Jones, Onslow, Harrison, & Packman, 2000; Stephenson-Opsal & Bernstein Ratner, 1988; Yarus, Coleman, & Hammer, 2006). Parents may also be asked to reinforce treatment goals outside of therapy. Some intervention programs have used parents as the primary service provider with success (e.g., Craig et al., 1996; Franken et al., 2005).

## Treatment Approaches

Therapy approaches can be conceptualized as one of two types: indirect or direct. Indirect therapy methods are those that attempt to bring about fluent speech without direct instruction on how the client should modify his or her own speech. Indirect therapy may be selected because of the belief that calling attention to stuttering episodes only serves to raise the anxiety of the individual who stutters and may worsen stuttering as a consequence. This idea has its roots in Johnson's diagnosogenic theory, discussed earlier. In some cases, indirect therapy approaches may be preferred because the client is a young child. Young children may not have the skills to think about how they are speaking as a separate phenomenon from what they are speaking about. Therefore, it may be difficult for young children to monitor or modify their own speech. Direct therapy approaches train the client in specific techniques to modify or eliminate their stuttering. These techniques require clients to focus on how they are speaking as well as what they are speaking about.

## Indirect Methods

Indirect treatment methods have taken several forms over time. In some cases, a clinician may work to reduce the client's anxiety about stuttering without addressing the stuttering directly. For children, the clinician may advise the parents concerning changes they can make to increase fluency in their child. For example, parents can enhance fluency by slowing their own speaking rate in conversation with their child (Stephenson-Opsal & Bernstein-Ratner, 1988). Other indirect methods may call attention to the stuttering without offering explicit guidance in how to correct stuttering behaviors. One such example uses a time-out after a disfluent episode (e.g., Hewat et al., 2006; James, 1981; Martin, Kuhl, & Haroldson, 1972; Onslow, Packman, Stocker, van Doorn, & Siegel, 1997; Prins & Hubbard, 1988). For example, when a client stutters, he or she may immediately hear a tone (James, 1981) or some other signal (e.g., Martin et al., 1972) that requires the client to stop speaking. The time-out may even be self-administered by the client (Hewat et al., 2006; James, 1983). Why these time-out episodes are effective in reducing stuttering is unknown. However, they appear to reduce stuttering frequency in both children and adults.

One of the best-studied forms of indirect therapy is the Lidcombe Program (e.g., Bonelli, Dixon, Bernstein Ratner, & Onslow, 2000; Franken et al., 2005; Harris, Onslow, Packman, Harrison, & Menzies, 2002; Harrison, Onslow, & Menzies, 2004; Lattermann et al., 2005). This is a parent-delivered therapy program for children who stutter. Parents are trained to explicitly acknowledge or even praise the fluent speech of their child. In addition, parents call attention to disfluent speech by acknowledging its occurrence and asking the child to repeat his or her message fluently. Other than verbally differentiating between fluent and disfluent speech, no explicit instruction is used to teach the child how to produce stutter-free speech. Despite the fact that this program requires parents to explicitly draw attention to their child's stuttering, children seem to tolerate the program without ill psychological effects (Woods, Shearsby, Onslow, & Burnham, 2002). The treatment reduces stuttering in children during the treatment period (Harris et al., 2002), and the improved fluency persists after treatment has ended (Lincoln & Onslow, 1997).

A final class of indirect methods includes devices that are known to produce fluency. These devices involve earpieces that cause the person who stutters to hear his or her own speech in some altered fashion (Armson, Kiefte, Mason, & Croos, 2006; Howell, El-Yaniv, & Powell, 1987; Kalinowski, Armson, Roland-Mieszkowski, Stuart, & Gracco, 1993). Commercially available devices resemble a hearing aid that is worn in the ear canal or behind the ear. One class of devices presents the speaker's voice with a short time delay. The effect of this is that the speaker hears his or her own words just after they are produced. This effect, called **delayed auditory feedback**, is known to produce fluent speech, at least temporarily, in people who stutter. Other devices present speech that is altered in terms of its frequency or tone or that masks the speaker's voice with noise. These devices may be used as the sole method of intervention or in conjunction with instruction to the client on how to modify speech (a combination of indirect and direct therapy methods). The devices may enhance fluency for some individuals, but not all clients derive the same degree of benefit (Armson et al., 2006). There are various reasons why these devices may provide at least temporary relief from stuttering. It is well known that those who stutter can become temporarily fluent when singing, talking in unison with others (choral speech), talking to the beat of a metronome, talking with a sing-song cadence, and the like. It may be that altered auditory feedback causes speakers to adopt slower speech or speech that is otherwise altered from their normal pattern. In addition, speaking in the presence of altered auditory stimuli may cause the speaker to use more deliberate speaking methods that enhance fluency (see Venkatagirir, 2005). One concern is whether the effect of these devices on fluency will be maintained as those who use them become accustomed to their influence.

## Direct Methods

Direct therapy methods involve direct instruction to the client concerning speech production. Direct therapy methods can be divided into two basic approaches: those that modify stuttering to help the client stutter more fluently and those that modify speech to eliminate stuttering completely.

**Modifying Stuttering.**   Charles Van Riper, an early contributor to study and treatment of stuttering, concluded that "the stutterer already knows how to be fluent. What he doesn't know is how to stutter. He can be taught to stutter so easily and briefly that he can have very adequate communication skills. Moreover, when he discovers he can stutter without struggle or avoidance, most of his frustration and negative emotions will subside" (1990, p. 318). This statement implies that the primary goal of treatment is better communication skills; reduction of stuttering episodes is a secondary consideration. The philosophy behind stuttering modification approaches is that "the root of stuttering is in the struggle to be fluent" (Perkins, 1980). Consequently, therapy to modify stuttering often involves two components. The first involves improving the client's attitude toward speaking, so that the client is not apprehensive about the possibility of stuttering, and the actual stuttering episodes are no longer associated with anxiety. The second involves learning to stutter with less effort and fewer secondary stuttering behaviors, such as tension or avoidance behaviors. Techniques used by clients may involve intentionally extending the number of part-word repetitions produced on a stuttered word so that the client gains control over his behavior. Clients may be taught to cease a word attempt when their speech is blocked (known as "cancellation") or to ease out of blocked sounds by using intentional prolongations on stuttered words. Because the aim of this form of therapy is not to eliminate stuttering, it is not surprising that it is not necessarily effective in reducing the number of episodes of stuttering, even though patients may feel better about their overall ability to communicate (Blomgren et al., 2005). This type of stuttering modification may be the therapy approach of choice for clients who have stuttered for many years and consider true fluency to be an unrealistic goal.

**Modifying Speech.**   In the treatment of stuttering during the mid-1970s, there was a shift away from modification of stuttering toward the shaping of fluent speech. The fluency-shaping approach came directly out of learning theory, in which behavior was modified by degrees until it reached the target of natural sounding, fluent speech. Clients may use any of a variety of methods, such as slowing their speech, changing the prosody of speech, using light contacts of the tongue and lips when forming sounds, or prolonging the vowel sounds in words. For children, these techniques may be described in easy-to-understand terminology to assist their comprehension of the desired behaviors. For example, Druce, Debner, and Byrt (1997) taught young children a technique they referred to as "sleepy talk" to represent the slow, easy nature of the speech they wanted children to produce. The client, whether a child or adult, may apply the fluency-shaping techniques at first to very short utterances, on which they are highly likely to produce fluent speech, and then systematically increase the length of utterances (e.g., Druce et al., 1997; Riley & Ingham, 2000).

One problem with the techniques used to modify speech is that they can result in somewhat unnatural-sounding speech. For example, if clients are asked to slow or prolong their speech in order to attain fluency, the slow speech may be as disruptive to communication as the original stuttering was. Individuals who stutter may be reluctant to speak in an unnatural manner and may revert to stuttering (Martin, Haroldson, & Triden, 1984). Therapy may include a component that further shapes the clients' speech to be more natural sounding (Ingham, Sato, Finn, & Bekknap, 2001; Onslow, Costa, Andrews, Harrison, & Packman, 1996). Attention to speech naturalness, in addition to fluency, appears to improve overall outcomes for those who stutter.

A common component of programs designed to modify speech is transfer of the trained behaviors to settings outside the clinic or therapy setting. The clinician may use activities, such as telephone calls or field trips, during which the client is asked to use the fluent speech he or she has developed through treatment. This phase may be completed in the company of a clinician or through homework assignments. In either case, the client must eventually take responsibility for maintaining fluency outside of the therapeutic setting in order for fluency to be long lasting.

## OTHER DISORDERS OF FLUENCY

### Cluttering

Another clinical disorder associated with altered fluency is **cluttering**. Like those who stutter, children who are described as clutterers have abnormally high frequencies of word and phrase repetitions. In contrast to stuttering, however, cluttering involves fewer sound- or syllable-level disfluencies (e.g., prolongations, sound repetitions). In addition, cluttering usually occurs without the signs of struggle, tension, or avoidance that are common in stuttering (St. Louis, Hinzman, & Hull, 1985). However, there are reports of both cluttering and stuttering occurring in the same individual, indicating that signs of both disorders may coexist (Craig, 1996; Williams & Wener, 1997). Although the prevalence of cluttering is unknown, speech-language pathologists in the United States tend to report few cases of cluttering in their practices.

Wood (1971) defined cluttering as "rapid, nervous speech marked by omissions of sounds and syllables" (p. 10). This definition gives equal prominence to the symptoms of rapid rate and articulatory errors and is similar to that of Wingate (1978), who defined cluttering as "a fluency disorder of unknown origin characterized by sporadically excessive rate and incomplete and distorted articulation" (p. 268). In an early monograph written on the topic, Arnold (1966) reviewed literature from Europe that described cluttering as involving rapid rate, faulty articulation, and related reading and writing problems. Wall (1988) said that cluttering is characterized by rapid speed and disordered articulation but added this important part to the definition: "a lack of awareness of the problem on the part of the speaker" (p. 637). It would appear that most clutterers, unlike stutterers, are not upset by their continuing disfluency.

Clutterers speak much faster than stutterers; in fact, the word *tachyphemia*, which is sometimes used as a synonym for cluttering (although it is not), literally means "rapid speech." Clutterers may be differentiated from stutterers by the former's slurred and omitted phonemes, periods of unusually rapid rate of speech, lack of awareness of their poor speech, and the fact that they neither avoid nor feel tense about the act of speaking. In addition, clutterers are often observed to exhibit disorganized thought processes, some problems in language formulation and comprehension, and problems in reading and writing (St. Louis et al., 1985; Teigland, 1996). Such problems may require services for language and learning disabilities during the school years (St. Louis & Hinzman, 1986). By combining the views of several writers, let us define cluttering:

> *Cluttering* is speech characterized by rapid rate, disfluencies, and articulation errors, often accompanied by spoken and written language difficulties. These signs usually occur without the speaker's awareness or concern.

**Treatment of Cluttering.**    Although both stuttering and cluttering involve disfluencies, the differences between the two disorders dictate very different treatment approaches. St. Louis and Meyers (1995) offered a series of working principles to guide treatment of cluttering. St. Louis and Meyers begin with a recognition that stuttering and cluttering are, in fact, independent disorders. For the child who clutters, disfluencies are a direct combination of fast speaking rate combined with a weak ability to handle the phonologic, syntactic, or semantic aspects of spoken language.

Children who clutter can increase their fluency by slowing their rate. However, as anyone who has tried to change his or her speaking rate knows, sustaining a slower speaking rate while thinking about what to say is difficult. We can use direct methods to address speaking rate. The speaker might pace his or her speaking rate with a metronome to raise awareness about rate of speech. Later, a clinician might provide visual feedback, such as an arrow to signal whether speech is too fast, too slow, or just fine. The following case illustrates an indirect method of addressing rate, having the speaker alter loudness (which later can be reduced to normal levels when rate has been reduced). This 17-year-old was asked to listen to a recording of himself followed by one of a normal male speaker near the client's age:

CLINICIAN:   I bet you talk twice as fast as that other kid. Did you hear him?

CLIENT:   He donna wanna go fatter than me.

CLINICIAN:   Maybe if we just had you talk a little louder, like this: "I'm going to speak loudly for a bit." That sure makes me sound better, doesn't it?

CLIENT: Talin' loud is easy for me. I tal' loud at home and they all hear me.

CLINICIAN: Well, let's make a recording of you talking louder, and we'll see how that sounds.

Rather than working on the components of rate and articulation, both of which were far from normal in this case, the clinician elected to work holistically on making the patient aware that he could "speak better" by changing his speaking habits. Given a tangible method of changing his speech, that patient could monitor his loudness, which served to slow the rate of speech and improve his articulation.

Sometimes, indirect methods can be used to decrease rate by concentrating on another element of speech or language. For example, if a child's poor articulation contributes to cluttering, exercises designed to remediate articulation may have the side effect of reducing speaking rate. Likewise, if fluency breakdowns are occurring because of linguistic deficits such as word-finding problems or difficulty with syntactic constructions, then it makes sense to remediate these linguistic problems directly. In many cases, improved fluency is a side effect of a linguistic approach.

St. Louis and Meyers (1995) pointed out that a synergistic approach that focuses on improved communication may be best. Language formulation problems may be aided when rate is slowed, because the individual has more time to organize his ideas and give them linguistic structure. Improved self-monitoring may help the individual concentrate on correct articulation, which in turn will tend to slow speaking rate. Word-finding strategies may help prevent semantic breakdowns that reduce fluency. This dynamic approach may also include services coordinated with others (e.g., family members, teacher, psychologists) who can help to manage social and educational aspects associated with cluttering.

## Acquired Neurogenic Disfluency

Most adults who stutter have a history of childhood stuttering. There are, however, numerous cases of previously fluent adults who have an abrupt onset of stuttering (Market, Montague, Buffalo, & Drummond, 1990). In most instances, acquired stuttering is associated with neurological disease or exposure to toxins (Helm-Estabrooks, 1998; Ringo & Dietrich, 1995). Less frequently, acquired stuttering may have a psychological origin related to anxiety, depression, or other psychological disturbance (Baumgartner & Duffy, 1997). Although the symptoms of neurogenic and psychogenic stuttering may be difficult to distinguish from one another, a review of the patient's history is usually helpful in determining the cause of the disfluencies. We were asked recently to help interpret the disfluencies of a 69-year-old man.

*Mr. Nelson* was referred by his neurologist after a series of transient ischemic attacks or possibly small strokes. The most recent episode was followed by what appeared to be stuttering. The disruption of speech was a concern to Mr. Nelson, who was a highly educated, articulate man and a frequent public speaker as president of a volunteer organization. Despite his neurological history, the referral letter from the neurologist described Mr. Nelson's disfluency as "a functional acquired stuttering, possibly secondary to some sort of depression or anxiety."

Prior to his visit, Mr. Nelson was asked to write a narrative of his recent medical history and to describe any changes in his speech or language. His description clarified that he had experienced two episodes two years apart involving neurological signs. The first episode included persistent numbness and tingling on the left side of his body that lasted for about a week. The second included a more dramatic onset of right-sided weakness and some problems speaking. Mr. Nelson was hospitalized following the second episode and put on blood-thinning medication because of his risk for a stroke. He wrote that he was recovering fully from the second episode, but within a month he began to have increasing difficulty talking. He had some trouble coming up with the names of things, but his most vexing problem was stuttering, which he described as having "a lot of hesitation" in his speech.

An evaluation of Mr. Nelson's speech revealed many disfluencies. For example, as he read a 100-word passage aloud, he was disfluent on 10 words: 5 were tense pauses, 3 were sound prolongations, and 2 were sound repetitions. His conversational speech was similarly disrupted by pauses—although his articulators were postured correctly to produce a word, he seemed unable to proceed. No secondary stuttering characteristics such as facial grimacing, hand clenching, or head movements were observed. In fact, Mr. Nelson appeared to be annoyed by his disfluencies but not overly upset by them.

Mr. Nelson's disfluencies and his medical history suggested that he had acquired neurogenic stuttering. Although an MRI brain scan revealed some small areas of white matter changes, and it was not clear the Mr. Nelson had suffered a stroke, his medical history clearly indicated some compromise of his neurological functions. Neurogenic stuttering is not limited to damage to a particular region of the brain but has been related to left- and right-hemisphere and cortical and subcortical damage, as well as damage to the cerebellum and brainstem. About one-third of individuals with neurogenic stuttering also exhibit an aquired language impairment (Baumgartner & Duffy, 1997). In Mr. Nelson's case, he evidenced some mild word-finding problems **(anomia)**, but his overall performance was excellent for spoken and written language.

**Neurogenic versus Developmental Stuttering.**   Neurogenic stuttering refers to an acquired disruption of fluency that can be linked with an identifiable neurological event, such as a stroke or head injury. This is in contrast to developmental stuttering, which may also have an underlying neurological component, as described earlier. The disruptions in normal speech production that are observed in neurogenic disfluency are similar in some ways to developmental stuttering, but there are some differences. Whereas instances of disfluency in developmental stuttering occur more often on words that start with consonants than with vowels, neurogenic stuttering occurs equally often on words beginning with consonants and vowels (Ringo & Dietrich, 1995). Likewise, neurogenic stuttering occurs equally often on substantive and function words, whereas content words are more likely to be disfluent for adults who have stuttered since childhood. As was true with Mr.

Nelson, most individuals with neurogenic stuttering are notably free of anxiety about their speech and characteristics such as accessory behaviors and facial tension that are common in stuttering having a developmental origin.

**Neurogenic versus Psychogenic Stuttering.**   Mr. Nelson's disfluencies differed from psychogenic stuttering in several ways. Although psychogenic stuttering can be similar to neurogenic stuttering, Baumgartner and Duffy (1997) found several distinguishing features. Unlike neurogenic stuttering, psychogenic stuttering may be intermittent and associated with specific speaking situations. In addition, struggle behaviors and other signs of anxiety are not uncommon, and unusual or bizarre speech patterns not observed in other speech or language disorders, such as using "me" for the pronoun "I," are often present. Moreover, psychogenic stuttering usually responds quickly to behavioral treatment.

**Intervention.**   After we determined that Mr. Nelson's disfluencies were consistent with those of a neurogenic origin, we needed to decide whether treatment was warranted. Cases reviewed in the literature indicated that neurogenic stuttering often resolves on its own without treatment within a month or two of onset. Therefore, we assured Mr. Nelson that his stuttering appeared to be related to the neurological episodes he had experienced and told him that we suspected his fluency would improve on its own. He was scheduled for a follow-up visit six weeks later, at which time he showed considerable improvement in fluency. Some brief pauses were still observed as he spoke, but they were relatively subtle, and he reported that they were not as bothersome to him. In fact, he said that he was most annoyed by his occasional word-finding difficulty at that time, a problem he had minimized during his initial visit.

Had Mr. Nelson's stuttering persisted and had he wanted treatment, we might have treated it behaviorally in much the same way as developmental stuttering. Approaches that enhance fluency, such as slowed speaking rate and easy onset of voicing, have been used with success in neurogenic stuttering (Market et al., 1990). Fluency can also be facilitated by pacing speech production so that it is not disrupted by hesitations, prolongations, or repetitions (Helm-Estabrooks, 1998). In some cases, medications have been shown to improve neurogenic stuttering, although other cases of acquired disfluency appear to have been caused by medication (reviewed in Helm-Estabrooks, 1998). Thus, a careful review of a patient's history and medications are essential in instances of adult-onset disfluency.

## CLINICAL PROBLEM SOLVING

Annette first came to the attention of the school speech-language pathologist through a phone call from the district director of special education. Annette's parents had been phoning the director's office and home requesting that their daughter be treated for her stuttering. Annette's father was an adult stutterer, and both parents wanted Annette's speech to be "corrected before her stuttering became permanent." They also reported that Annette began speaking somewhat late, but they had no concerns about her speech or language other than the stuttering. Annette was enrolling in kindergarten that fall. After school began, the clinician was able to observe Annette on several occasions in the classroom, during which her speech was consistently fluent. The clinician reported her observations to the parents, advising them to allow Annette time to settle into the school routine. The parents were adamant that Annette stuttered frequently at home and were insistent that she be treated through the school. At the parents' urging, the clinician set up a classroom monitoring program to permit the classroom teacher to systematically document Annette's speech. From September to December, only two disfluent episodes were noted. After receiving this news, the parents sent the clinician a taped sample of Annette's speech at home. The tape revealed frequent episodes of disfluent speech, including part-word repetitions, sound prolongations, and silent episodes, which may well have reflected blocks.

1. Do you think that Annette does stutter? What makes you think so/not?
2. What risk factors for stuttering appear in Annette's history?
3. Select two theories and discuss how this case profile might relate to each theory.
4. Speculate on the reasons why Annette may stutter at home but not in her new kindergarten.
5. Do you think that Annette should receive therapy for stuttering? If so, what factors would you consider in developing a plan of intervention for Annette?

## REFERENCES

Adams, M. R. (1990). The demands and capacities model I: Theoretical elaborations. *Journal of Fluency Disorders, 15*, 135–141.

Andrews, C., Craig, A., Feyer, A., Haddinott, S., Neilson, M., & Howle, P. (1983). Stuttering: A review of research findings and theories circa 1982. *Journal of Speech and Hearing Disorders, 48*, 226–245.

Andrews, C., & Harris, M. (1964). *The syndrome of stuttering.* London: Heinemann Dynamic Medical Books.

Andrews, G., Howie, P., Dozsa, M., & Guitar, B. (1982). Stuttering: Speech pattern characteristics under fluency-inducing conditions. *Journal of Speech and Hearing Research, 25,* 208–216.

Armson, J., Kiefte, M., & Mason, J. (2006). The effect of SpeechEasy on stuttering frequency in laboratory conditions. *Journal of Fluency Disorders, 31*, 137–152.

Arnold, C. (1966). *Studies in tachyphemia: An investigation of cluttering and general language disability.* New York: Speech Rehabilitation Institute.

Baumgartner, J., & Duffy, J. R. (1997). Psychogenic stuttering in adults with and without neurologic disease. *Journal of Medical Speech Language Pathology, 5*, 75–95.

Blanton, S. (1965). Stuttering. In D. Barbara (Ed.), *New directions in stuttering.* Springfield, IL: Charles C. Thomas.

Blomgren, M., Roy, N., Callister, T., & Merrill, R.M. (2005). Intensive stuttering modification therapy: A multidimensional assessment of treatment outcomes. *Journal of Speech, Language, and Hearing Research, 48,* 509–523.

Blood, G. W., Blood, I. M., Bennett, S., Simpson, K. C., & Susman, E. J. (1994). Subjective anxiety measurements and cortisol responses in adults who stutter. *Journal of Speech and Hearing Research, 37,* 760–768.

Blood, G. W., Blood, I. M., Tellis, G., & Gabel, R. (2001). Communication apprehension and self-perceived communication competence in adolescents who stutter. *Journal of Fluency Disorders, 26,* 161–178.

Bloodstein, O. (2006). Some empirical observations about early stuttering: A possible link to language development. *Journal of Communication Disorders, 39,* 185–191.

Bonelli, P., Dixon, M., Bernstein Ratner, N., & Onslow, M. (2000). Child and parent speech and language and the Lidcombe Program of early stuttering intervention. *Clinical Linguistics and Phonetics, 14,* 427–446.

Conture, E. G. (1990). Childhood stuttering: What is it and who does it? *ASHA Report Series, 18,* 2–14.

Conture, E. G., & Kelly, E. M. (1991). Young stutterers' nonspeech behaviors during stuttering. *Journal of Speech and Hearing Research, 34,* 1041–1056.

Cooper, E. B., & Cooper, C. S. (1995). Treating fluency disordered adolescents. *Journal of Communication Disorders, 28,* 125–142.

Cooper, E. B., & Cooper, C. S. (1996). Clinicians' attitudes toward stuttering: Two decades of change. *Journal of Fluency Disorders, 21,* 119–135.

Craig, A. (1990). An investigation between anxiety and stuttering. *Journal of Speech and Hearing Disorders, 55,* 290–294.

Craig, A. (1996). Long-term effects of intensive treatment for a client with both a cluttering and stuttering disorder. *Journal of Fluency Disorders, 21,* 329–335.

Craig, A., Hancock, K., Chang, E., Mccreay, C., Shepley, A., Mccaul, A., Costello, D., Harding, S., Kehren, R., Masel, C., & Reilly, K. (1996). A controlled clinical trial for stuttering in persons age 9–14 years. *Journal of Speech and Hearing Research, 39,* 808–826.

Curlee, R. F. (1980). A case selection strategy for young disfluent children. *Seminars in Speech, Language, Hearing, 1,* 277–287.

Dayalu, V., Kalinowski, J., Stuart, A., Holbert, D., & Rastatter, M. P. (2002). Stuttering frequency on content and function words in adults who stutter: A concept revisited. *Journal of Speech, Language, and Hearing Research, 45,* 858–870.

De Nil, L. F., Kroll, R. M., Lafaille, S. J., Houle, S. (2003). A positron emission tomography study of short- and long-term treatment effects on functional brain activation in adults who stutter. *Journal of Fluency Disorders, 28,* 357–380.

Druce, T., Debner, S., & Byrt, T. (1997). Evaluation of an intensive treatment program for stuttering in young children. *Journal of Fluency Disorders, 22,* 169–186.

Fox, P. T., Ingham, R. J., Ingham, J. C., Hirsch, T., Downs, J. H., Martin, C., Jerabek, P., Glass, T., & Lancaster, J. L. (1996). A PET study of the neural systems of stuttering. *Nature, 382,* 158–162.

Franken, M-C. J., Kielstra-Van der Schalk, C. J., & Boelens, H. (2005). Experimental treatment of early stuttering: A preliminary study. *Journal of Fluency Disorders, 30,* 189–199.

Glauber, I. P. (1958). The psychoanalysis of stuttering. In J. Eisenson (Ed.), *Stuttering. A symposium.* New York: Harper and Row.

Harris, V., Onslow, M., Packman, A., Harrison, E., & Menzies, R. (2002). An experimental investigation of the impact of the Lidcombe Program on early stuttering. *Journal of Fluency Disorders, 27,* 203–213.

Harrison, E., Onslow, M., & Menzies, R. (2004). Dismantling the Lidcombe Program of early stuttering intervention: Verbal contingencies for stuttering and clinical measurement. *International Journal of Language and Communication Disorders, 39,* 257–267.

Hasbrouck, J. M. (1992). FAMC intensive stuttering treatment program: Ten years of implementation. *Military Medicine, 157,* 244–247.

Healey, E. C., Scott, L. A., & Ellis, G. (1995). Decision making in the treatment of school-age children who stutter. *Journal of Communication Disorders, 28,* 107–124.

Helm-Estabrooks, N. (1998). Stuttering associated with acquired neurological disorders. In R. F. Curlee (Ed.), *Stuttering and related disorders of fluency* (pp. 255–268). New York: Thieme Medical.

Hewat, S., Onslow, M., Packman, A., & O'Brian, S. (2006). A Phase II clinical trial of self-imposed time-out treatment for stuttering in adults and adolescents. *Disability and Rehabilitation, 28,* 33–42.

Howell, P., El-Yaniv, N., & Powell, D. J. (1987). Factors affecting fluency in stutterers. In H. F. M. Peters & W. Hulstijn (Eds.), *Speech motor dynamics in stuttering* (pp. 361–369). New York: Springer.

Howie, P. M. (1981). Concordance for stuttering in monozygotic and dizygotic twin pairs. *Journal of Speech and Hearing Research, 24,* 317–321.

Hull, F. M., Mielke, P. W., Willeford, J. A., & Timmons, R. J. (1976). *National speech and hearing survey.* Final Report, Project 50978. Washington, DC: Office of Education, Bureau of Education for the Handicapped, Department of Health, Education, and Welfare.

Ingham, R. J., Sato, W., Finn, P., & Belknap, H. (2001). The modification of speech naturalness during rhythmic stimulation treatment of stuttering. *Journal of Speech, Language, and Hearing Research, 44,* 841–952.

James, J. (1981). Behavioral self-control of stuttering using time-out from speaking. *Journal of Applied Behavioral Analysis, 14,* 25–37.

James, J. (1983). Parameters of the influence of self-initiated time-out from speaking on stuttering. *Journal of Communication Disorders, 16,* 123–132.

Janssen, P., Kraaimaat, F., & Brutten, G. (1990). Relationship between stutterers' genetic history and speech-associated variables. *Journal of Fluency Disorders, 15,* 39–48.

Johnson, W. (1955). A study of the onset and development of stuttering. In W. Johnson & R. R. Leutenegger (Eds.), *Stuttering in children and adults.* Minneapolis: University of Minnesota Press.

Johnson, W. (1959). *The onset of stuttering.* Minneapolis: University of Minnesota Press.

Jones, M., Onslow, M., Harrison, E., & Packman, A. (2000). Treating stuttering in young children: Predicting treatment time in the Lidcombe Program. *Journal of Speech, Language, and Hearing Research, 43,* 1440–1450.

Kalinowski, J., Armson, J., Roland-Mieszkowski, M., Stuart, A., & Gracco, V. L. (1993). Effects of alterations in auditory feedback and speech rate on stuttering frequency. *Language and Speech, 36,* 1–16.

Kalinowski, J., Lerman, J., & Watt, J. (1987). A preliminary examination of the perceptions of self and others in stutterers and nonstutterers. *Journal of Fluency Disorders, 12,* 317–331.

Kelly, E. M. (1995). Parents as partners: Including mothers and fathers in the treatment of children who stutter. *Journal of Communication Disorders, 28,* 93–106.

Kidd, K. K. (1980). Genetic models of stuttering. *Journal of Fluency Disorders, 5,* 187–202.

Lattermann, C., Shenker, R. C., & Thordardottir, E. (2005). Progression of language complexity during treatment with the Lidcombe Program for early stuttering intervention. *American Journal of Speech-Language Pathology, 14*, 242–253.

Lincoln, M. A., & Onslow, M. (1997). Long-term outcome of early intervention for stuttering. *American Journal of Speech-Language Pathology, 6*, 51–58.

Market, K. W., Montague, J. C., Buffalo, M. D., & Drummond, S. S. (1990). Acquired stuttering: Descriptive data and treatment outcome. *Journal of Fluency Disorders, 15*, 221–233.

Martin, R. R., Haroldson, S. K., & Triden, K. A. (1984). Stuttering and speech naturalness. *Journal of Speech and Hearing Disorders, 49*, 53–58.

Martin, R., Kuhl, P., & Haroldson, S. (1972). An experimental treatment with two preschool stuttering children. *Journal of Speech and Hearing Research, 15*, 743–52.

Miller, S., & Watson, B. C. (1992). The relationship between communication attitude, anxiety and depression in stutterers and nonstutterers. *Journal of Speech and Hearing Research, 34*, 789–798.

Morley, M. E. (1952). A ten-year survey of speech disorders among university students. *Journal of Speech and Hearing Disorders, 17*, 25–31.

Morley, M. F. (1972). *The development and disorders of speech in childhood.* Edinburgh: Churchill Livingstone.

National Institutes of Deafness and Other Communication Disorders (NIDCD). (1992). *Research in human communication.* (NIH Publication No. 93–3562.) Washington, DC: U.S. Government Printing Office.

Neumann, K., Euler, H.A., von Gudenberg, A. W., Giraud, A-L., Lanfermann, H., Gaul, V., & Preibisch, C. (2003). The nature and treatment of stuttering as revealed by fMRI: A within- and between-group comparison. *Journal of Fluency Disorders, 28*, 381–410.

Onslow, M., Costa, L., Andrews, C., Harrison, E., & Packman, A. (1996). Speech outcomes of a prolonged-speech treatment of stuttering. *Journal of Speech and Hearing Research, 39*, 734–749.

Onslow, M., Packman, A., Stocker, S., van Doorn, J., & Siegel, G. (1997). Control of children's stuttering with response-contingent time-out: Behavioral, perceptual, and acoustic data. *Journal of Speech, Language, and Hearing Research, 40*, 121–133.

Packman, A., Onslow, M., & van Doorn, J. (1994). Prolonged speech and modification of stuttering: Perceptual, acoustic, and electroglottographic data. *Journal of Speech and Hearing Research, 39*, 724–737.

Perkins, W. H. (1980). Prevention and treatment of stuttering. *The Annals of Otology, Rhinology, & Laryngology, Supplement, 89*, 150–152.

Perkins, W. H. (1980). Disorders of speech. In T. Hixon, L. Shriberg, & J. Saxman (Eds.), *Introduction to communication disorders.* Englewood Cliffs, NJ: Prentice Hall.

Perkins, W. H., Kent, R. D., & Curlee, R. F. (1991). A theory of neuropsycholinguistic function in stuttering. *Journal of Speech and Hearing Research, 34*, 734–752.

Prins, D., & Hubbard, C. (1988). Response contingent stimuli and stuttering: Issues and implications. *Journal of Speech and Hearing Research, 31*, 696–709.

Prins, D., Main, V., & Wampler, S. (1997). Lexicalization in adults who stutter. *Journal of Speech Language and Hearing Research, 40*, 373–384.

Riley, G. D., & Ingham, J. C. (2000). Acoustic duration changes associated with two types of treatment for children who stutter. *Journal of Speech Language and Hearing Research, 40*, 965–978.

Ringo, C. C., & Dietrich, S. (1995). Neurogenic stuttering: An analysis and critique. *Journal of Medical Speech-Language Pathology, 3*(2), 111–122.

Rustin, L., & Cook, F. (1995). Parental involvement in treatment of stuttering. *Language, Speech, and Hearing Services in Schools, 26,* 127–137.

Schwartz, H. D., Zebrowski, P. M., & Conture, E. G. (1990). Behaviors at the onset of stuttering. *Journal of Fluency Disorders, 15,* 77–86.

Shames, G. H., & Florence, C. L. (1980). *Stutter-free speech: A goal of therapy.* Columbus, OH: Charles E. Merrill.

Sheehan, J. G. (1970). *Stuttering: Research and therapy.* New York: Harper and Row.

Speech Foundation of America. (1987). *Self-therapy for the stutterer* (6th ed.). Publication 12. Memphis, TN: Author.

St. Louis, K. O., & Hinzman, A. R. (1986). Studies of cluttering: Perceptions of cluttering by speech-language pathologists and educators. *Journal of Fluency Disorders, 11,* 131–149.

St. Louis, K. O., Hinzman, A. R., & Hull, F. M. (1985). Studies of cluttering: Disfluency and language measures in young possible clutterers and stutterers. *Journal of Fluency Disorders, 10,* 151–172.

St. Louis, K. O., & Meyers, F. L. (1995). Clinical management of cluttering. *Language, Speech, and Hearing Services in Schools, 26,* 187–195.

Starkweather, C. W. (1990). Current trends in therapy for stuttering children and suggestions for future research. *ASHA Report Series, 18,* 82–90.

Stephenson-Opsal, D., & Bernstein Ratner, N. (1988). Maternal speech rate modification and childhood stuttering. *Journal of Fluency Disorders, 13,* 49–56.

Teigland, A. (1996). A study of pragmatic skills of clutterers and normal speakers. *Journal of Fluency Disorders, 21,* 201–214.

Travis, L. E. (1971). The unspeakable feelings of people with special reference to stuttering. In L. D. Travis (Ed.), *Handbook of speech pathology and audiology* (2nd ed.). Englewood Cliffs, NJ: Prentice Hall.

Van Riper, C. (1971). *The nature of stuttering.* Englewood Cliffs, NJ: Prentice Hall.

Van Riper, C. (1990). Final thoughts about stuttering. *Journal of Fluency Disorders, 15,* 317–318.

Venkatagiri, H. S. (2005). Recent advances in the treatment of stuttering: A theoretical perspective. *Journal of Communication Disorders, 38,* 375–393.

Wall, M. J. (1988). Disfluency in the child. In N. J. Lass, L. V. McReynolds, J. L. Northern, & D. E. Yoder (Eds.), *Handbook of speech-language pathology and audiology.* Philadelphia: B. C. Decker.

Weber, C. M., & Smith, A. (1990). Autonomic correlates of stuttering and speech assessed in a range of experimental tasks. *Journal of Speech and Hearing Research, 33,* 690–706.

Williams, D. F., & Wener, D. L. (1997). Cluttering and stuttering exhibited in a young professional. *Journal of Fluency Disorders, 21,* 261–269.

Wingate, M. E. (1962). Personality needs of stutterers. *Logos, 5,* 35–37.

Wingate, M. E. (1976). *Stuttering theory and treatment.* New York: Irvington.

Wingate, M. E. (1978). Disorders of fluency. In P. Skinner & R. Shelton (Eds.), *Speech, language, hearing: Normal processes and disorders.* Reading, MA: Addison-Wesley.

Wood, K. S. (1971). Definitions and terms. In L. D. Travis (Ed.), *Handbook of speech pathology and audiology* (2nd ed.). Englewood Cliffs, NJ: Prentice Hall.

Woods, S., Shearsby, J., Onslow, M., & Burnham, D. (2002). The psychological impact of the Lidcombe Program of early stuttering intervention: Eight case studies. *International Journal of Language and Communication Disorders, 37,* 31–40.

World Health Organization (WHO). (1977). *Manual of the international statistical classification of diseases, injuries, and causes of death* (Vol. I). Geneva: Author.

Yairi, E., & Ambrose, N. (1992). Onset of stuttering in preschool children: Selected factors. *Journal of Speech and Hearing Research, 35*, 782–788.

Yairi, E., Ambrose, N. G., & Cox, N. (1996). Genetics of stuttering: A critical review. *Journal of Speech and Hearing Research, 39*, 771–784.

Yairi, E., Ambrose, N. G., Paden, E. P., & Throneburg, R. N. (1996). Predictive factors of persistence and recovery: Pathways of childhood stuttering. *Journal of Communication Disorders, 29*, 51–77.

Yaruss, J. S., Coleman, C., & Hammer, D. (2006). Treating preschool children who stutter: Description and preliminary evaluation of a family-focused treatment approach. *Language, Speech, & Hearing Services in Schools, 37*, 118–136.

Yaruss, J. S., Quesal, R. W., Reeves, L., Molt, L. F., Kluetz, B., Caruso, A. J., Mclure, J. A., & Lewis, F. (2002). Speech treatment and support group experiences of people who participate in the National Stuttering Association. *Journal of Fluency Disorders 27*, 115–134.

Young, M. A. (1975). Onset, prevalence, and recovery from stuttering. *Journal of Speech and Hearing Disorders, 40*, 49–58.

Zackheim, C. T., & Conture, E. G. (2003). Childhood stuttering and speech disfluencies in relation to children's mean length of utterance: A preliminary study. *Journal of Fluency Disorders, 28*, 115–142.

Zebrowski, P. M. (1995). The topology of a beginning stutterer. *Journal of Communication Disorders, 28*, 75–92.

## READINGS FROM THE POPULAR LITERATURE

Bobrick, B. (1996). *Knotted tongues.* New York: Kodansha International.

Jezer, M. (1997). *Stuttering: A life bound up in words.* New York Nasic.

Shields, D. (1998). *Dead languages.* New York: Random House. (novel)

St. Louis, K. O. (2001). *Living with stuttering.* Morgantown, WV: Populore.

# CHAPTER SIX

# DISORDERS OF VOICE AND SWALLOWING

## JULIE BARKMEIER-KRAEMER

## PREVIEW

The larynx is the source of our voice for speaking, but it also serves to protect the airway during eating. Damage to the larynx or structures of the vocal tract may result in voice or swallowing problems. Most people experience problems with their voice due to improper voicing habits. Such voice disorders can usually be treated or improved by therapy that identifies and changes damaging voicing behaviors to healthy ways of voicing. Voice disorders related to physical damage to the laryngeal structure(s) may also be treated effectively with voice therapy; however, in some cases, medical intervention is needed. Swallowing problems can occur as a result of normal aging effects, neurological conditions, cancer, psychological problems, or structural abnormalities associated with birth defects or subsequent to surgery to the head and neck. Swallowing problems may be corrected by changing the consistency of food or making postural adjustments. Exercises are sometimes used to strengthen oral and pharyngeal structures for safe and effective eating. More recently, sensory stimulation and electrical stimulation have been studied for facilitating improved swallowing.

## VOICE DISORDERS

As described in Chapter 2, vocal fold vibrations produce sound, which is modified by the vocal tract. Individual differences in the vocal mechanism and its resonance characteristics contribute to the individual characteristics of each person's voice. Many temporary conditions, such as a stuffy nose or the effects of prolonged yelling, can change the voice. These types of problems tend to resolve on their own and typically do not require professional attention. However, permanent changes to the voice may occur with damage or disease. These conditions often require professional intervention.

The exact number of individuals who experience voice disorders in the population is not known. For children, the incidence of dysphonia has ranged from 6 percent (Nilson & Schneiderman, 1983) to 23.4 percent (Silverman & Zimmer, 1975). Duff, Proctor, and Yairi (2004) estimated the prevalence of dysphonia in preschool-aged African American and European American children to be 3.9 percent. In school-aged children, the prevalence of dysphonia is estimated at between 6 to 9 percent (McNamara & Perry, 1994). The prevalence of voice disorders in adults has been estimated at 7.2 percent for men and 5 percent for women, based on voice screenings (LaGuaite, 1972). Several occupations carry a high risk for developing voice problems due to the intense communication demands. Based on data from the University of Wisconsin, the most represented occupations in a voice disorder clinic included teachers (20%), singers (11%), salespeople (10%), clerks (9%), administrators and managers (7%), and factory workers (6%) (Titze, Lemke, & Montequin, 1997). Two other studies (Fritzell, 1995; Smith, Gray, Dove, Kirchner, & Heras, 1997) also reported that teachers have the highest incidence of voice disorders. A majority of voice patients report that their problem had a negative impact on their career options, social interactions, and other aspects of their daily lives (Smith et al., 1996).

Voice disorders can be described as problems related to pitch, loudness, voice quality, and resonance. These problems may stem from vocal misuse, disease, congenital defects, laryngeal trauma, aging effects, and neurological disorders. Emotional and psychological factors may also contribute to acquired voice disorders. Treatment usually requires the combined specialties of the ear-nose-throat doctor (otolaryngologist) and a speech-language pathologist with experience in assessing and treating voice disorders.

## VOICE DISORDERS RELATED TO VOCAL FOLD TISSUE CHANGES

Most voice disorders arise from overuse or frequent improper use of the voice, which can result in tissue changes that disrupt normal fold vibration.

*Susan*, age 17, was a cheerleader for her high school varsity football team for three years. During her first two years as a cheerleader, she experienced temporary bouts of hoarseness following each game. These usually subsided in a couple of days. During her third year as a cheerleader, however, she began to experience longer periods of hoarseness that did not fully resolve before the next game. By the end of the football season, her voice almost always sounded hoarse, and she had difficulty being heard in the football stands. Eventually, she was no longer able to cheer.

An otolaryngologist found bilateral nodules on her vocal folds (see Figure 6.1). Vocal nodules typically result from chronic vocal misuse that causes the vocal folds to repeatedly collide forcefully. The size of Susan's nodules prevented her vocal folds from coming together unless she increased her loudness. She was discouraged from participating in cheerleading until the vocal nodules diminished. She was also referred to a speech-language pathologist for voice therapy. The speech-language pathologist helped Susan identify other habits that were contributing to physical damage of the vocal folds, such as coughing, clearing her throat frequently, and yelling at her younger brother when he teased her. Susan reduced the frequency of these behaviors and learned better ways to produce her voice. After one month, the size of the vocal nodules had reduced dramatically, and Susan's voice was significantly improved.

### Traumatic Laryngitis

In the early stages of her voice disorder, Susan experienced repeated bouts of **traumatic laryngitis**. This condition is characterized by swollen and red vocal folds resulting from excessive yelling, screaming, or other traumatic uses of the voice (see Figure 6.2). Traumatic laryngitis is common and usually resolves within days of its onset. It often results from continuous vocal misuse such as yelling or cheering throughout an exciting athletic event. In such situations, yelling at high

**FIGURE 6.1** **The vocal folds viewed from above showing bilateral vocal nodules, indicated by arrows. Note that the larynx is oriented with the front of the structure at the bottom of the figure (i.e., the bottom is anterior and the top is posterior)**

intensity over loud environmental noise causes the vocal folds to slam together at high velocities. This results in trauma to the vocal fold tissue at the site of impact. As a result, the vocal folds become swollen and irritated (Brodnitz, 1971). Tissue swelling along the length of the vocal folds disrupts normal vocal fold vibration, causing changes in voice quality. In severe cases, there may be a complete loss of voice (**aphonia**). The best treatment for traumatic laryngitis is to rest the voice, allowing the vocal folds to heal. After two to five days, depending on the extent of damage, vocal fold swelling and irritation typically resolve, and the normal voice returns. In Susan's case, she experienced this cycle of trauma and recovery during her first two years of cheerleading.

If the vocal misuse continues, however, vocal fold irritation can become chronic. The tissue that covers the vibrating portion of the vocal folds may thicken. Chronic irritation may result from attempts to talk over environmental noise (e.g., machinery noise in a factory or the cheering and other crowd noise that occurs at an athletic event) or talking for long periods of time. Changes in daily voice use are needed to prevent further permanent damage and allow healing. Voice therapy may be necessary to identify poor vocal habits and teach improved techniques for using the voice.

## Vocal Nodules

**Vocal nodules** are small bumps that develop on the medial border of the vocal folds (see Figure 6.1). These bumps consist of fibrous tissue (Gray, Hammond, & Hanson, 1995), much like calluses that develop on the hands or feet. Nodules occur along the anterior one-third of the vocal folds as a result of persistent improper

**FIGURE 6.2    An example of the appearance of traumatic laryngitis, obtained using videoendoscopy. Notice the swollen and irregular borders of the vocal folds.**

voicing patterns, such as excessive yelling or sustained overuse of the voice. Although vocal nodules certainly are not life-threatening, they can result in significant voice problems. The symptoms of vocal nodules arise gradually and manifest as increasing hoarseness and difficulty projecting the voice. Vocal nodules can occur on one vocal fold but most frequency develop on both vocal folds at the site of impact. In early stages, nodules may appear as small swollen areas on the vocal folds. In later stages, the nodules become hard and impair normal vocal fold vibration. If the nodules become large enough, they can prevent the vocal folds from coming together completely, as occurred with Susan. She also demonstrated signs of traumatic laryngitis that preceded the development of nodules. She could have prevented the development of vocal nodules with modification of her voice use. Instead, Susan's vocal fold tissue adjusted to the continual irritation and traumatic impact by developing vocal nodules. This condition can be treated effectively with voice therapy that identifies voice misuse and teaches improved voicing habits (McCrory, 2001; McFarlane & Watterson, 1990; Yamaguchi et al., 1986) including better methods for producing and projecting the voice.

## Vocal Polyps

**Vocal polyps** are small, fluid-filled sacs that develop on the vocal folds as a result of yelling and other excessive uses of the voice (Johns, 2003; Kleinsasser, 1979, 1990). Compared to nodules, which are fibrous and usually bilateral, polyps are soft and compliant and typically occur on one side only. They may appear anywhere in the larynx, including on the vocal folds or ventricular folds or between the arytenoids. In contrast to the prolonged vocal misuse that leads to vocal nodules, it is believed that a single event of vocal misuse, such as screaming or even intense coughing, can lead to development of a polyp (McFarlane & Von Berg, 1998).

> *Mrs. Delvechio,* age 56, began to experience a gradual onset of hoarseness after an upper respiratory infection with severe coughing episodes. She was seen by an otolaryngologist who identified a polyp located near the posterior segment of the vibrating portion of the left vocal fold. The physician suspected the polyp had resulted from traumatic vocal fold impact during repeated episodes of severe coughing. The physician referred Mrs. Delvechio to a speech-language pathologist for counseling concerning excessive coughing and throat clearing. During counseling, Mrs. Delvechio also mentioned that her husband was hard of hearing and she often tried to talk to him over the television or from another room in the house. She was encouraged to speak at comfortable loudness and not to speak over noise. In addition, she was instructed to talk to her husband only when they were in the same room. After six weeks, her polyp was reduced in size, and her voice was almost completely normal.

A vocal polyp may result in significant voice problems, including breathiness or hoarseness. The polyp may also cause each vocal fold to vibrate at a different rate, causing a double voice, or **diplophonia**. Treatment for a vocal polyp frequently entails identification of the behaviors that led to the problem (e.g., yelling, throat clearing, coughing). In Mrs. Delvechio's case, once she became aware of the behaviors that were contributing to the voice problem, she could eliminate those habits. Subsequently, the polyp reduced in size as the laryngeal tissue healed. In some cases, the individuals may need specific therapeutic instruction by a speech-language pathologist to improve use of the voice. In still other cases, surgical removal of a polyp by an otolaryngologist is necessary (Johns, 2003; Kleinsasser, 1979, 1990).

## Laryngeal Papilloma

Papillomas are wartlike growths found along the vocal tract and respiratory system. They are caused by the human papilloma virus, and they occur predominantly in preschool children, 60 to 80 percent of all cases (Derkay & Darrow, 2006). Although a rare disorder, infants, children, and adults can all be affected by papilloma. The onset of this condition may be characterized by breathiness and hoarseness. If the papilloma grows large enough, it can impede or obstruct the airway. In such cases, a whistling sound may be heard during breathing. Papilloma may be treated with laser surgery, but it grows back quickly, and multiple surgeries may be necessary. Unfortunately, frequent laser surgeries may result in vocal fold scarring that cannot be repaired. In extreme cases, the vocal folds may become so scarred that the voice cannot be produced due to the stiffness of the vocal fold tissue. Voice therapy can sometimes help these individuals make the best of their voices after surgery. Other forms of treatment include chemotherapy and antibiotic treatments.

## Laryngeal Cancer

Cancer, or **carcinoma**, of the larynx can be a life-threatening disease if not identified during its early stages. Persistent hoarseness is the most common symptom associated with laryngeal cancer. Other warning signs include swallowing problems, swelling in the throat and neck regions, and persistent throat pain.

> *Mr. Mahr*, age 45, smoked a pack of cigarettes per day for twenty-five years. He also enjoyed a cigarette along with several drinks during cocktail hour every night before dinner. Over a period of six months, his voice became increasingly hoarse. He did not report any illness during this time, although he noticed that he experienced more fatigue than usual and sometimes felt as though he could not breathe in enough air. Mr. Mahr loved his work as an attorney and usually had a lot of energy. He finally went to see an otolaryngologist, who discovered that his vocal folds were covered with a whitish mass that impaired their normal movement. The physician scheduled surgery to remove a piece of the mass and determine its pathology. The biopsy revealed that it was cancer. Mr. Mahr was told that the cancer had invaded much of the laryngeal region and that the entire larynx would need to be removed. After surgery, Mr. Mahr also needed to undergo a series of radiation treatments to reduce the risk that the cancer would recur. Fortunately, Mr. Mahr's laryngeal cancer was caught early enough that survival was likely. However, the treatment cost him his voice. Mr. Mahr was referred to a speech-language pathologist to explore alternatives for creating a new voice after the laryngectomy.

As in Mr. Mahr's case, those who develop laryngeal cancer usually smoke and drink alcohol (McKenna, Fornataro-Clerici, McMenamin, & Leonard, 1991; Rafferty, Fenton, & Jones, 2001). When caught in its early stages, laryngeal cancer frequently can be treated using conservative medical approaches. These include radiation, chemotherapy, and surgery to remove the cancer, leaving the larynx as intact as possible (Mendenhall, Parsons, Stringer, Cassisi, & Million, 1988). In its later stages, laryngeal cancer is typically treated by surgical removal of the entire larynx.

When the larynx is removed, the trachea is attached to a permanent opening in the neck called a **tracheostoma** (or stoma, for short). After his laryngectomy, Mr. Mahr will be able to breathe normally except that the air will enter and exit the body through an opening in his neck rather than the nose and mouth (see Figure 6.3). Food and drink are still taken by mouth, although the sense of taste is diminished because airborne odors are no longer breathed through the nose.

After laryngectomy surgery, a speech-language pathologist will work with the individual to develop alternative ways of generating a sound source for speech. One method is esophageal speech. To use this method, an individual must learn to trap air in the mouth and push it into the esophagus (McKenna et al., 1991). Once the air is trapped in the esophagus, it is belched back up, creating a sound source by vibration of the esophageal tissues. This sound source is trans-

FIGURE 6.3   This woman is showing the location of the airway opening in her neck called a tracheostoma. Since undergoing a laryngectomy, she now breathes through the tracheostoma. The white tab attached to the skin outside the tracheostoma secures a one-way valve. This valve shunts airs into the esophagus to create voice by vibrating esophageal tissue in a similar but less predictable way than the vocal folds.

formed into words by the articulatory movements of the teeth, tongue, and lips, as with normal speech.

A second method of speech production involves an electronic device called an **electrolarynx**, or artificial larynx (Casper & Colton, 1993). The electrolarynx is a handheld device that makes a buzzing sound that substitutes for vocal fold vibration. The device is placed against the neck so that the sound travels through the skin into the vocal tract, providing a "voice" that is then modified into speech by mouthing words (see Figure 6.4). The speech-language pathologist provides therapy to help improve speech intelligibility using the electrolarynx.

A popular method to provide voice is a tracheo-esophageal puncture. This surgical procedure creates a hole for the placement of a small tube into the tissue that divides the trachea from the esophagus (see Figure 6.3). The tube has a one-way valve that shunts air from the trachea into the esophagus when the tracheostoma is covered by the individual's thumb or finger. The shunted air vibrates the esophageal tissue in the same way as the belching does in esophageal speech, resulting in voice.

**FIGURE 6.4** This gentleman is holding an electrolarynx securely against the front of his neck to provide his "voice" for speech.

Whichever method Mr. Mahr uses to communicate, he will need training and practice to maximize speech intelligibility. Many individuals like Mr. Mahr are grateful that they have another chance at life and resume their activities with great enthusiasm. Others may fall into depression and need professional counseling to help them deal with the psychological and social issues that arise.

## NEUROLOGICAL VOICE DISORDERS

*Mrs. Finley,* age 45, developed a voice problem after undergoing surgery to remove her thyroid gland. After the surgery, her voice was breathy, and she choked whenever she drank liquids too quickly. She was evaluated by an otolaryngologist, who diagnosed paralysis of the right vocal fold. The doctor suggested that the nerve serving the vocal fold had probably been injured during thyroid surgery. Because this nerve may recover from such damage, the physician decided to wait six months before considering surgical intervention. In the meantime, Mrs. Finley was referred to a speech-language pathologist to learn techniques for stimulating the left vocal fold to vibrate against the paralyzed right vocal fold. In addition, the speech-language pathologist provided Mrs. Finley with strategies for swallowing that would reduce her choking episodes.

Through voice exercises, Mrs. Finley learned to produce a soft voice instead of a breathy one. She was able to avoid choking by taking small sips of liquid while tilting her chin toward her chest. At five months postsurgery, her voice had become stronger and closer to normal, indicating that nerve innervation was returning. By six months, her voice was clear and strong. The otolaryngologist reexamined her larynx at that time and determined that her right vocal fold had regained near-normal function.

## Vocal Fold Paralysis

The recurrent laryngeal nerve is a branch of cranial nerve X (the vagus nerve). It provides neural input to muscles that move the vocal folds during voicing and swallowing (see Chapter 2). Vocal fold paralysis may result from damage to one or both recurrent laryngeal nerves on either side of the larynx. Unilateral vocal fold paralysis is most common. As in Mrs. Finley's case, damage to the nerve can occur when it is cut or compressed during surgery. Nerve damage can also result from a tumor or viral infection. In some cases, there is no known cause for nerve damage. Once the nerve to the laryngeal muscles is damaged, the vocal fold on the same side as the nerve is immobilized. Because the vocal folds cannot close completely, the voice is breathy, and patients often choke on liquids. In many cases, the impaired nerve recovers or regenerates within six months, resulting in recovery of the voice (Hockauf & Sailer, 1982; Mu & Yang, 1991).

To compensate for the paralyzed vocal fold, patients are taught to use greater effort to increase the movement of the unaffected vocal fold. With increased exertion, the healthy vocal fold may be able to vibrate against the paralyzed vocal fold to produce voicing. If the impaired nerve does not recover within six months, several surgical procedures are available to improve voice production. The surgical procedures move the immobile vocal fold medially so that the working vocal fold can vibrate against it. This was not necessary in Mrs. Finley's case because her vocal fold function recovered over time.

Paralysis of both vocal folds is a more serious problem than one-sided vocal fold paralysis. This disorder is typically caused by an impairment to the central nervous system, such as a tumor or stroke that interferes with the generation of the neural signals that control movement of the vocal folds. Bilateral paralysis may result in difficulty breathing if the vocal folds are paralyzed in the closed (or nearly closed) position. Surgical intervention is usually necessary to create an open airway adequate for breathing.

## Spasmodic Dysphonia

Spasmodic **dysphonia** is a rare voice disorder often characterized by a strained-strangled voice quality. The cause of this disorder was once believed to be related to psychological dysfunction (Arnold, 1959). It is currently thought to result from a dysfunction of the neural signals that control the vocal folds during speaking (Ludlow, 1995b). There are two types of spasmodic dysphonia: *adductor* and *abductor*. The adductor type occurs when the vocal folds close together too tightly during voiced speech sounds, resulting in a strained-strangled voice quality. The abductor type occurs when the vocal folds spasm apart during production of unvoiced speech sounds, resulting in excessive breathiness. Thus, the difference between the two types of spasmodic dysphonia can be remembered by these two rules:

1. The "AD" part of *adductor* means that the vocal folds spasm together.
2. The "AB" part of *abductor* means that the vocal folds spasm apart.

Adductor spasmodic dysphonia is characterized by intermittent onset of the strained-strangled voice quality, or voice stoppage. Additional muscular force is needed to move the folds from the midline, resulting in effortful voice production. The abductor type of spasmodic dysphonia occurs less frequently than the adductor type and is characterized by intermittent bursts of breathy voice quality. The breathiness results from spasms that keep the vocal folds apart during speech. Thus, these individuals may complain that they cannot make their voice loud enough to be heard.

> *Mr. Sparks,* age 42, began to experience a catch in his voice while giving business reports to his employer. When this first began, he thought it was related to being nervous. However, he noticed the catches in his throat occurred more frequently over time. They also occurred at times when he was not nervous, such as after a church service or at home. Over the course of a year, the condition worsened. He put such effort into forcing his voice to function that he often became exhausted after a short period of talking. As the voice problem increased, his employer became displeased with Mr. Sparks's productivity and inability to provide regular business presentations. In desperation and frustration, Mr. Sparks went to see his doctor.
>
> Mr. Sparks's primary care physician thought the problem was related to stress but agreed to refer him to a speech-language pathologist specializing in voice disorders. The speech-language pathologist recognized Mr. Sparks's problem as spasmodic dysphonia. Voice therapy was initiated to modify some of the problematic voice patterns he had developed as compensation for his uncooperative larynx. The speech-language pathologist also recommended consultation with an otolaryngologist for further evaluation. The otolaryngologist diagnosed Mr. Sparks with adductor spasmodic dysphonia and recommended medical treatment that consisted of injections of a toxin (Botox®) into the muscles of the vocal folds to reduce spasms during talking.

The injection of toxin into the vocal folds is the current treatment of choice for adductor-type spasmodic dysphonia. The toxin is botulinum type A, most often referred to as Botox. Botox impairs the ability of nerved endings to cause contraction of the vocal fold muscles. This results in weakened vocal fold muscles that can no longer spasm closed during talking. However, the vocal folds may be so weak that they cannot come together to create a strong voice or protect the airway during swallowing. After a few weeks the Botox is absorbed by the body, and new nerve endings grow. At this point, the vocal folds begin to move normally, resulting in an improved voice quality. After three to six months, the Botox wears off, and the symptoms of spasmodic dysphonia typically return, requiring reinjection of Botox to maintain an improved voice.

In some individuals, Botox does not effectively weaken the vocal fold muscles. In those cases, an alternative is surgery to cut one of the laryngeal nerves, creating unilateral vocal fold paralysis (Dedo & Behlau, 1991; Dedo & Izdebski, 1983; Weed et al., 1996). Although the resulting voice is slightly breathy, it allows the individual to function more normally in daily communication. In approximately 20 percent of individuals who undergo surgical cutting of the laryngeal nerve, the nerve regrows, and symptoms of adductor spasmodic dysphonia return within one to three years after the surgery (Dedo & Behlau, 1991). Although cutting the nerve is a treatment of last resort, newer methods show promise for more successful long-term benefits for those who do not respond well to Botox treatment (Weed et al., 1996).

Despite its successes in the treatment of adductor-type spasmodic dysphonia, Botox injections are not as effective with abductor spasmodic dysphonia. Botox treatment is typically attempted with abductor spasmodic dysphonia to see if it will effectively weaken the laryngeal muscles that pull the vocal folds apart during a spasm. However, the improvement is usually minimal and lasts only two to four weeks. In addition, these individuals often experience an extremely breathy voice for several weeks after treatment before their voice improves (Ludlow, 1995a). Presently, there is no known effective way to treat abductor spasmodic dysphonia.

## VOICE ASSESSMENT

The goal of a voice evaluation is to determine the nature of the problem, its probable cause, and the options available to treat the problems. Some people go to their primary care physician first, who then refers them to an otolaryngologist or speech-language pathologist. Others seek help on their own and go directly to the otolaryngologist. Otolaryngologists with specialized interest in voice disorders often work with a speech-language pathologist with similar interests. Thus, medical evaluation and treatment may be augmented by voice therapy from a speech-language pathologist. Depending on the setting and equipment available for assessing the voice problem, various methods of evaluation may be used.

Voice evaluations begin with gathering information about the history of the problem and the symptoms present at the time of the examination. This information influences the evaluation procedures as well as the treatment.

> *Ms. Norwood* worked as a real estate agent for the past six years and was one of the top salespeople in her company. Her company relocated to a new building two

years ago. Since the relocation, numerous renovation projects were necessary, such as putting in new carpeting and painting. She noticed that whenever she worked in her new office, her voice became increasingly hoarse over the course of the day. When her productivity dropped significantly and she felt increasingly anxious about her work, she sought medical help from an otolaryngologist.

The otolaryngologist looked at Ms. Norwood's larynx and noted that both vocal folds were swollen and red and did not vibrate normally during voicing. Thinking that she probably developed improper voicing patterns that led to changes in the vocal folds, the otolaryngologist referred her to a speech-language pathologist for voice therapy. The speech-language pathologist documented events leading to Ms. Norwood's voice disorder and discovered her problems began after her office was relocated to the new building. More specifically, her voice problems coincided with the new carpet and paint in her office. The speech-language pathologist suspected that Ms. Norwood was sensitive to chemicals in the air from the renovations. Ms. Norwood also had begun to cough frequently and clear her throat because it felt like something was in her throat. Furthermore, she reported drinking a lot of coffee and only small amounts of water each day. The caffeine from the coffee and the low amount of other fluids may have caused dehydration that exacerbated her voice disorder. The speech-language pathologist helped Ms. Norwood monitor and eliminate the daily habits that were irritating her voice and taught her techniques to improve the sound of her voice. In addition, she was instructed to avoid the office for two weeks to determine if the chemicals from the new carpet and paint were irritating her vocal folds.

Ms. Norwood's voice improved dramatically over the two weeks she was away from her office. Upon her return, the voice problem returned despite her efforts to use the techniques she learned from the speech-language pathologist. Thus, it appeared that Ms. Norwood's voice problem was caused by her sensitivity to the chemicals in her office. She decided to work from home to avoid exposure to the chemical fumes until the renovation was completed.

In the example above, the true source of Ms. Norwood's voice problem was uncovered after all the information related to the onset of her voice disorder was obtained. The physical appearance of her larynx was similar to that associated with chronic improper and effortful use of the voice. However, use of the following case history guidelines helped to determine the probable causes of a voice problem and, consequently, influenced the course of treatment:

1. Obtain the client's description of the voice problem.
2. Determine whether the onset of the voice problem was associated with an illness, accident, or other significant circumstance.
3. Note the duration and consistency of the symptoms of the voice problem.
4. Note patterns or variability in the reported symptoms or severity of the voice problem on a daily, weekly, monthly, and seasonal basis.
5. Obtain a description of the client's daily voice use.
6. Obtain a description of the client's work, home, and social activities.
7. Note whether the client's voice changes across different environments, speaking situations, or times of the day.

The case history provides information concerning development and impact of the voice disorder on the client's life. It also provides an opportunity for the speech-language pathologist to get to know the client as an individual, which is important for designing successful behavioral therapy. In Ms. Norwood's case, an examination of the circumstances leading to the voice problem helped reveal the true cause of the voice problem, resulting in an effective voice treatment plan.

In addition to the case history, a voice evaluation also includes examination of the vocal mechanism. In Ms. Norwood's case, the otolaryngologist examined the larynx to determine whether vocal pathology was present. To observe the pharynx and larynx, the physician may use a tongue depressor, a light to illuminate the structures, and a laryngeal mirror to reflect their image. Other ways of viewing the soft palate and throat utilize fiberoptic equipment to obtain a video recording of the soft palate or throat. This procedure is called videoendoscopy. Videoendoscopy can be performed using a scope placed through the mouth or nose. The scope inserted through the nose (i.e., **nasoendoscope**) is a small tube with fiberoptic cables that illuminate and allow viewing of the nasal passages, soft palate, pharynx, and larynx. The type of scope inserted through the mouth is a rigid scope that looks like a steel rod with a lens on the end. It acts like a periscope in that it is placed over the tongue and provides a view of the larynx from just beyond the back of the tongue (see Figure 6.5). The image obtained by either scope is displayed on a television monitor and can be recorded on videotape. The rigid scope obtains a closer view of the vocal folds than the flexible scope, but the client cannot talk with the rigid scope in his or her mouth. The flexible scope is a good way to obtain a recording of the structures in the throat during speech. The lighting used for both

FIGURE 6.5   **The vocal folds are viewed from above using a rigid scope placed at the back of the mouth. Note the image of the healthy vocal folds on the video monitor.**

scopes can be changed into a strobe light while the client sustains a vowel sound such as "ee." The strobe light illuminates only a fraction of the vocal fold vibrations so that they appear to occur in slow motion and are easier to evaluate.

The voice evaluation should include assessment of the facial muscles, lips, teeth, soft and hard palate, tonsils, and pharynx, because these structures may be affected when a voice disorder is present. Other components of a voice evaluation include respiration testing, acoustic measurements of the voice (e.g., frequency and intensity), and descriptions of the voice quality (e.g., breathy, hoarse) as perceived during different speaking tasks. The combined information from observation and measurements helps the speech-language pathologist determine the best approach for treating the client's voice problem. They can also be compared to findings after therapy.

> *Ms. Alvarez* worked as a kindergarten teacher. During the first six months of her job, she began experiencing increased hoarseness that worsened from morning to night. By the end of each week, she could barely make herself heard in the classroom. Ms. Alvarez became frightened that she might have laryngeal cancer, so she went to see an otolaryngologist. The otolaryngologist looked at Ms. Alvarez's larynx and noted the presence of two vocal nodules. In addition, her vocal folds were red and swollen. Ms. Alvarez was referred to a speech-language pathologist for further evaluation of her voice and voice therapy.
>
> To assess vocal fold vibration, the speech-language pathologist performed videoendoscopy on Ms. Alvarez using the rigid scope and a strobe light. The speech-language pathologist also tape-recorded Ms. Alvarez's voice during sustained phonation of "ah" and "ee" and while reading. The speech-language pathologist asked Ms. Alvarez about her work, family, and social life to obtain a better idea of how she uses her voice in different environments. From this information, the speech-language pathologist determined that Ms. Alvarez's problems were primarily related to how she used her voice at work. She often needed to shout above noise to get the children's attention. The speech-language pathologist suggested using a microphone system so that Ms. Alvarez could project her voice above the noise without much effort. In addition, they discussed instructional strategies such as using a whistle to get attention and using more visual aids to help preserve her voice. Finally, the speech-language pathologist taught Ms. Alvarez how to project her voice without straining. After one month, Ms. Alvarez's voice had improved noticeably. On reexamination, the vocal nodules appeared smaller than they had been initially.

In Ms. Alvarez's case, the strain on her voice at work led to the development of vocal nodules. The speech-language pathologist knew that vocal nodules usually occurred with chronic misuse of the voice. The type of therapy done with Ms. Alvarez could be described in two ways:

1. Elimination of harmful daily vocal habits
2. Learning new techniques to effectively use the voice without strain

As discussed earlier, these are the two primary approaches used to treat voice disorders resulting from harmful vocal habits. In severe cases, surgical removal of a growth may be necessary; however, more frequently, voice therapy is successful in treating clients such as Ms. Alvarez and Ms. Norwood.

# DYSPHAGIA

Eating is vital to maintaining life and providing the energy for basic bodily functions. The process of ingestion begins with chewing and swallowing food, a complex process that we do not often think about. However, when swallowing is impaired, we become more aware of how large a role eating plays in our lives. In addition to providing nutrition, eating serves as the focus of many social functions. Impaired eating, called **dysphagia** (pronounced dis-fay-jah), may create such difficulties that eating becomes an unpleasant activity and social occasions are avoided.

Although individuals diagnosed with dysphagia can be of any age, most are over 55 years old. In that age group, the prevalence is estimated at between 16 to 22 percent (Bloem et al., 1990; Kjellen & Tibbling, 1981). This includes a wide range of problems with eating that are related to stroke, neuromuscular problems, traumatic brain injury, progressive neurological diseases, surgery to structures involved in ingestion, head and neck cancer, and cognitive problems such as dementia. In young people, dysphagia primarily relates to illness, trauma, surgeries of the head and neck, severe reflux, or congenital malformations.

In order to understand dysphagia, one must appreciate the components of normal eating. There are four phases involved, any of which may be impaired in someone with dysphagia. Figure 6.6 illustrates the sequence of the phases of swallowing.

## The Normal Swallow

**Phase One.**    The first phase of eating is referred to as the *oral preparatory phase* (see Figure 6.6A). This phase is important for preparing food in the mouth for transport to the stomach. During this phase, the lips, tongue, and soft palate play a major role in holding the food within the oral cavity. The tongue moves the food around so that it can be chewed and then gathered into a central groove formed by the tongue prior to swallowing. The collection of food held together by the tongue is referred to as a food **bolus**. Saliva produced by glands in the mouth begins the digestion process. Saliva coats the food so that it is moist, and the digestive chemicals soften the food prior to swallowing. Problems with the oral preparatory phase may arise because of congenital malformations of the oral structures or changes related to age, surgery, trauma, or neurological problems.

> *Mrs. Baker*, age 71, had lost all of her teeth and had not replaced them with dentures. As a consequence, she was unable to eat any food that required chewing, such as meat, popcorn, salad, or fruit. Her self-imposed diet was restricted to soups, applesauce, oatmeal, and fluids. Over time, Mrs. Baker lost considerable weight and became malnourished. She sought help from her doctor, who recognized that her health issues were related to her diet and chewing problems. Mrs. Baker was

A          B          C          D

FIGURE 6.6   The four phases of eating are shown: (A) the oral preparatory stage, (B) the oral transport stage, (C) the pharyngeal stage, (D) and the esophageal stage. The black shape represents the food bolus as it travels from the oral cavity to the esophagus.

admitted to the hospital, where she received intravenous fluids to rehydrate and rebalance her body chemistry. She was seen by a dietician, who recommended that Mrs. Baker obtain dentures to allow her to eat more normally. Once Mrs. Baker regained weight and was healthy, she was released from the hospital and instructed to check back with her doctor and dietician periodically for monitoring of her health and diet.

In this example, Mrs. Baker's lack of teeth resulted in difficulty chewing, which limited her food options. She did not make wise food choices to ensure adequate nutritional and caloric intake. As a consequence, she lost weight and jeopardized her health due to poor nourishment. Mrs. Baker's situation could be easily remedied by obtaining dentures. However, if dentures were not an option for her, Mrs. Baker would need to consider using nutritional supplements to balance her diet and ensure adequate caloric intake.

**Phase Two.**   Once food is chewed and ready to be swallowed, the tongue gathers it into a cohesive bolus held between the tongue and hard and soft palate. The tongue propels the bolus into the pharynx by pressing up against the hard palate and pushing the bolus backward. This phase of transporting the bolus from the oral cavity into the pharynx is called the *oral transport phase* of the swallow (see Figure 6.6B).

*Mr. Roswell,* age 85, suffered a stroke that impaired his ability to control tongue and lip movements. As a consequence, it was difficult to control the food in his mouth while chewing. Food and fluids often spilled out of his mouth because his lips were too weak to keep them in his oral cavity. Mr. Roswell also had difficulty collecting the food in his mouth into a cohesive bolus for swallowing. After swallowing, some food remained in his mouth.

The speech-language pathologist assessed Mr. Roswell while he ate and determined that his primary difficulty was controlling food in the mouth. A procedure called *flexible endoscopic examination of swallowing* (FEES) was performed to visualize the pharynx while he swallowed measured amounts of milk and then applesauce. FEES involves the placement of a fiberoptic tube in the nose to allow viewing of the pharynx from above. This exam showed that after a teaspoon of milk was placed in Mr. Roswell's mouth the milk ran back into the pharynx before he initiated a swallow. Milk also spilled through his lips. Mr. Roswell was able to control the applesauce so that it did not spill into the pharynx or out through his lips. He was able to swallow all of the applesauce so that none remained in his mouth.

The speech-language pathologist recommended that Mr. Roswell's wife try thickening liquids and soups using cornstarch or a food-thickening product. This allowed Mr. Roswell to place a spoonful of food with a consistency similar to applesauce on his tongue and immediately swallow without having to chew first. Adding thickener to liquids also allowed Mr. Roswell improved oral control so that liquids did not spill out of his mouth or into his throat before initiating a swallow. Treatment included exercises to strengthen his tongue, lips, and jaw and to increase the range of their motion in order to control food in his mouth. The combination of strengthening exercises and the use of foods with preferred consistencies helped Mr. Roswell recover most of his oral control so that he could enjoy a wider variety of foods.

As seen in the example of Mr. Roswell, difficulty with the oral transport phase can prevent an individual from moving food out of the oral cavity to be swallowed. However, simple measures can be taken to help compensate for this problem by restricting foods to those the client can manage best. In addition, weakness of the oral musculature may be improved by strengthening and range-of-motion exercises for the tongue, lips, and jaw (Logemann, 1983).

**Phase Three.**    The *pharyngeal phase* of swallowing is characterized by movement of the bolus of food through the pharynx and into the esophagus (see Figure 6.6C). The bolus is propelled into the pharynx, and, as it passes the back of the tongue, muscles of the pharynx contract to continue the propulsive action initiated by the tongue. As the superior portion of the pharynx contracts, the airway closes and the larynx elevates. This raised position during the swallow maximizes protection from *aspiration* of food into the airway. After the bolus enters the esophagus, the pharyngeal structures return to their resting positions. This phase is less than one second in duration.

*Mrs. Lasser*, age 65, began having difficulty swallowing. She felt as though there was something caught in her throat, and she needed to drink extra fluid to clear the food that was stuck. In addition, she experienced choking on the fluids she drank as she tried to clear her throat. Her swallowing difficulties required so much time and effort that she stopped enjoying meals and was embarrassed to eat in front her friends. As a result, she reduced the amount of food eaten and declined invitations to join friends for meals. After losing weight and becoming malnourished, Mrs. Lasser went to see her doctor.

Mrs. Lasser's doctor referred her for a swallowing examination, which was performed jointly by a radiologist and speech-language pathologist. During the test, Mrs. Lasser experienced all of the swallowing difficulties described earlier. The examination revealed that Mrs. Lasser's pharyngeal muscles appeared weak and her larynx was not elevating as it should during swallowing. The food she swallowed was not cleared completely from her throat. The speech-language pathologist showed Mrs. Lasser a way to swallow while tilting her chin downward. Mrs. Lasser used this posture while eating and found swallowing less difficult. However, she still needed to follow each bite of food with water or juice to clear her throat completely.

As shown in this case, impairment of the pharyngeal phase of the swallow can often be compensated for by simple posture changes. If food does not clear the throat during this phase of the swallow, the individual risks aspiration of food into the airway. This can lead to inflammation of the lungs, which is a potentially serious illness called aspiration pneumonia.

A team assessment by the radiologist and speech-language pathologist is the best way to assess the pharyngeal phase of swallowing. Using a procedure called a modified barium swallow, the patient is given food or liquid mixed with a radiocontrast material, barium, which is detected using an X-ray procedure called **videofluoroscopy**. Videofluoroscopy allows visualization of the pharyngeal structures and their movement during swallowing. It also allows identification and estimation of the amount of food aspirated into the airway before, during, and after the swallow. In addition, videofluoroscopy permits determination of whether changes in posture or food consistency improve the clearance of food from the mouth and throat.

**Phase Four.**    The final, *esophageal phase* of swallowing involves transportation of the bolus to the stomach by the esophagus (see Figure 6.6D). The esophagus pushes the bolus toward the stomach using muscle contractions, called **peristaltic contractions**, that squeeze each portion of the esophagus from the top to the bottom. This muscle action is similar to that used by a worm as it moves along the ground. That is, each muscle segment surrounding the esophagus contracts in sequence from the upper esophagus to the stomach so that the bolus is moved into the stomach.

*Rocco*, age 6 months, began spitting up copious amounts after drinking a bottle of formula. When he spits up, he tends to exhibit gagging behaviors and difficulty breathing. More recently he has developed a wet cough and appears to have stopped gaining weight. His crying voice and cooing voice appear hoarse. Rocco's mother also reports frequent occurrence of hiccups and frequent burping. However, there was no sign of a fever or loss of hunger or thirst. Rocco's mother sought help from a pediatrician. The pediatrician suspected that Rocco exhibited a severe form of gastrointestinal **reflux**. The severity of Rocco's reflux warranted referral to a pediatric gastroenterology specialist. The gastroenterologist confirmed the diagnosis of reflux using a barium swallow examination to assess Rocco's esophagus and digestive tract. This radiologic test entailed swallowing a liquid barium contrast while videofluoroscopy was used to monitor the path of the barium. The test revealed that any food swallowed by Rocco was propelled back into the esophagus from the stomach within minutes of being swallowed. The gastroenterologist prescribed a medication to increase the rate at which the stomach empties. He also recommended a different formula that did not contain lactose, in case Rocco had a food sensitivity. Strategies for positioning Rocco during eating were offered by the occupational therapist and speech-language pathologist. The occupational therapist also recommended using a special bottle that reduced the amount of air swallowed during feeding sessions. The combined strategies were successful in reducing the degree and frequency of Rocco's reflux. In fact, within one month, Rocco was happily feeding, with minimal regurgitation, and had gained three pounds.

As all of these cases demonstrate, dysphagia occurs when there is a problem with any or all of the four phases of swallowing. Common signs of dysphagia include the following:

- Difficulty initiating a swallow
- Difficulty chewing food due to poor dentition (as in Mrs. Baker's case)
- Difficulty controlling food in the oral cavity, such that it spills out of the mouth or into the airway before the larynx closes to protect the airway (as in Mr. Roswell's case)
- Choking when swallowing food, and food sticking in the throat (as Mr. Lasser experienced)
- Reflux of food from the esophagus or stomach back up to the throat or mouth (as in Rocco's case)

Various methods exist for assessing the swallow, as described in the above examples. Imaging techniques such as the FEES method (Langmore, Schatz, & Olsen, 1988) and the modified barium swallow (Logemann, 1993) are most frequently used to visualize the oral, pharyngeal, and esophageal structures. Although the speech-language pathologist can perform the FEES method if properly trained, an otolaryngologist may obtain FEES images while the speech-language pathologist administers the test food substances. During a modified barium swallow, the radiologist or radiology technician performs the videofluorographic imaging while the speech-language pathologist administers the barium contrast substances and determines which postures or consistencies appear to be successfully swallowed during testing. The gastroenterologist and radiologist are best trained to assess esophageal and other digestive organs during the barium swallow.

Assessing and providing care to someone with dysphagia may involve many professionals, including a speech-language pathologist, radiologist, gastroenterologist, otolaryngologist, neurologist, dentist, nurse, social worker, dietician, occupational therapist, and psychologist. The speech-language pathologist plays a major role in the assessment procedures, making recommendations to compensate for the dysphagia and referring the individual for further assessment by other dysphagia team members. Treatment of dysphagia most frequently entails simple measures such as changing the posture of the head and body during eating and swallowing, altering the consistency of the foods eaten, changing the temperature of foods to improve initiation of the swallow, and performing exercises to increase strength and range of motion of oral structures. Other treatment methods provided by medical specialists include the use of drugs to improve smooth muscle contraction, non-oral feeding using a nasogastric or gastric tube, and surgical intervention.

## CLINICAL PROBLEM SOLVING

Mrs. Hepple, age 65, underwent surgery to remove a portion of her esophagus that was cancerous. After surgery, her voice was breathy, and she choked every time she drank water. In addition, the food she swallowed came back up. She was sent to an otolaryngologist who examined her vocal folds and noted that the left vocal fold was not moving during voicing. She was referred to a speech-language pathologist, who used rigid videoendoscopy with a strobe light to further evaluate her voice. Mrs. Hepple's vocal folds did not come together completely when vibrating. The speech-language pathologist was concerned about Mrs. Hepple's difficulties with swallowing and suggested a modified barium swallow. During this test, the speech-language pathologist noted that liquids entered Mrs. Hepple's trachea during the pharyngeal phase of the swallow. Subsequently, she choked and coughed to clear the liquid from her airway.

1. Why does Mrs. Hepple have a breathy voice quality?
2. What do you think caused her left vocal fold to stop moving?
3. How might the speech-language pathologist try to help improve her voice quality?
4. Might the voice problem go away with voice therapy?
5. What phase of the swallow is impaired?

## REFERENCES

Arnold, G. E. (1959). Spastic dysphonia: I. Changing interpretations of a persistent affliction. *Logos, 2,* 3–14.

Bloem, B. R., Lagaay, A. M., van Beek, W., Haan, J., Roos, R. A. C., & Wintzen, A. R. (1990). Prevalence of subjective dysphagia in community residents aged over 87. *British Medical Journal, 300,* 721–722.

Brodnitz, F. S. (1971). *Vocal rehabilitation.* Rochester, MN: Whiting Press.

Casper, J. K., & Colton, R. H. (1993). *Clinical manual for laryngectomy and head and neck cancer rehabilitation.* San Diego: Singular Publishing Group.

Dedo, H. H., & Behlau, M. S. (1991). Recurrent laryngeal nerve section for spastic dysphonia: 5- to 14-year preliminary results in the first 300 patients. *Annals of Otology, Rhinology, and Laryngology, 100*(4), 274–279.

Dedo, H. H., & Izdebski, K. (1983). Intermediate results of 306 recurrent laryngeal nerve sections for spastic dysphonia. *Laryngoscope, 93,* 9–16.

Derkay, C. S., & Darrow, D. H. (2006). Recurrent respiratory papillomatosis. *Annals of Otology, Rhinology, & Laryngology, 115*(1), 1–11.

Duff, M. C., Proctor, A., & Yairi, E. (2004). Prevalence of voice disorders in African American and European American preschoolers. *Journal of Voice, 18*(3), 348–353.

Fritzell, B. (1995). *Occupation and voice problems.* Paper presented at the Proceedings from XXIII World Congress of IALP [abstract].

Gray, S. D., Hammond, E., & Hanson, D. F. (1995). Benign pathologic responses of the larynx. *Annals of Otology, Rhinology, and Laryngology, 104*(1), 13–18.

Hockauf, H., & Sailer, R. (1982). Postoperative recurrent nerve palsy. *Head and Neck Surgery, 4,* 380–384.

Johns, M. M. (2003). Update on the etiology, diagnosis, and treatment of vocal fold nodules, polyps, and cysts. *Current Opinion in Otolaryngology Head and Neck Surgery, 11*(6), 456–461.

Kjellen, G., & Tibbling, L. (1981). Manometric oesophageal function, acid perfusion test and symptomatology in a 55-year-old general population. *Clinical Physiology, 1,* 405–415.

Kleinsasser, O. (1979). *Microlaryngoscopy and endolaryngeal microsurgery: Technique and typical findings.* Baltimore: University Park Press.

Kleinsasser, O. (1990). Restoration of voice in benign lesions of the vocal fold by endolaryngeal microsurgery. In R. T. Sataloff (Ed.), *Voice perspectives.* San Diego: Singular Publishing.

LaGuaite, J. (1972). Adult voice screening. *Journal of Speech and Hearing Disorders, 37,* 147–151.

Langmore, S. E., Schatz, K., & Olsen, N. (1988). Fiberoptic endoscopic examination of swallowing safety: A new procedure. *Dysphagia, 2,* 216–219.

Logemann, J. A. (1983). *Evaluation and treatment of swallowing disorders.* Austin, TX: Pro-Ed.

Logemann, J. A. (1993). *Manual for the videofluorographic study of swallowing* (2nd ed.). Austin, TX: Pro-Ed.

Ludlow, C. (1995a). Treating the spasmodic dysphonias with botulinum toxin: A comparison of results with adductor and abductor spasmodic dysphonia and vocal tremor. In J. Tsui, & D. Calne (Eds.), *The dystonias.* New York: Dekker.

Ludlow, C. L. (1995b). Management of the spasmodic dysphonias. In J. S. Rubin, R. T. Sataloff, & G. S. Korovin (Eds.), *Diagnosis and treatment of voice disorders* (pp. 436–434). New York: Igaku-Shoin.

McCrory, E. (2001). Voice therapy outcomes in vocal fold nodules: A retrospective audit. *International Journal of Language and Communication Disorders, 36*(Suppl.), 19–24.

McFarlane, S. C., & Von Berg, S. (1998). Facilitative techniques in intervention for dysphonia. *Current Opinion in Otolaryngology and Head and Neck Surgery, 6,* 161–165.

McFarlane, S. C., & Watterson, T. L. (1990). Vocal nodules: Endoscopic study of their variations and treatment. *Seminars in Speech and Language, 11,* 47–59.

McKenna, J. P., Fornataro-Clerici, L. M., McMenamin, P. G., & Leonard, R. J. (1991). Laryngeal cancer: Diagnosis, treatment and speech rehabilitation. *American Family Physician, 44*(1), 123–129.

McNamara, A. P., & Perry, C. K. (1994). Vocal abuse prevention practices: A national survey of school-based speech-language pathologists. *Language, Speech, and Hearing Services in Schools, 25,* 105–111.

Mendenhall, W. M., Parsons, J. T., Stringer, S. P., Cassisi, N. J., & Million, R. R. (1988). T1-T2 vocal cord carcinoma: A basis for comparing the results of radiotherapy and surgery. *Head and Neck Surgery, 12,* 204–209.

Mu, L., & Yang, S. (1991). An experimental study on the laryngeal electromyography and visual observations in varying types of surgical injuries to the unilateral recurrent laryngeal nerve in the neck. *Laryngoscope, 101,* 699–708.

Nilson, H., & Schneiderman, C. R. (1983). Classroom program for the prevention of vocal abuse and hoarseness in elementary school children. *Language, Speech, and Hearing Services in Schools, 14,* 121–127.

Rafferty, M. A., Fenton, J. E., & Jones, A. S. (2001). The history, aetoiology and epidemiology of laryngeal carcinoma. *Clinical Otolaryngology, 26*(6), 442–446.

Silverman, E., & Zimmer, C. (1975). Incidence of chronic hoarseness among school-age children. *Journal of Speech and Hearing Disorders, 40,* 211–215.

Smith, E., Gray, S., Dove, H., Kirchner, L., & Heras, H. (1997). Frequency and effects of voice problems in teachers. *Journal of Voice, 11,* 81–87.

Smith, E., Verdolini, K., Gray, S., Nichols, S., Lemke, J., Barkmeier, J., Dove, H., & Hoffman, H. (1996). Effect of voice disorders on quality of life. *Journal of Medical Speech-Language Pathology, 4*(4), 223–244.

Titze, I. R., Lemke, J., & Montequin, D. (1997). Populations in the U.S. workforce who rely on voice as a primary tool of trade: A preliminary report. *Journal of Voice, 11*(3), 254–259.

Weed, D. T., Jewett, B. S., Rainey, C., Zealear, D. L., Stone, R. E., Ossoff, R. H., & Netterville, J. L. (1996). Long-term follow-up of recurrent laryngeal nerve avulsion for the treatment of spasmodic dysphonia. *Annals of Otology, Rhinology, Laryngology, 105*(8), 592–601.

Yamaguchi, H., Yotsukura, Y., Kondo, R., Horiguchi, S., Imaizumi, S., & Hirose, H. (1986). Nonsurgical therapy for vocal nodules. *Folia Phoniatrica, 38,* 372–373.

## READINGS FROM THE POPULAR LITERATURE

Fox, M. J. (2002). *Lucky man.* New York: Hyperion. (Parkinson disease)

Rehm, D. (1999). *Finding my voice.* New York: Alfred A. Knopf. (spasmodic dysphonia)

# CHAPTER SEVEN

# LANGUAGE

## PREVIEW

Human communication includes a wide range of activities. Much of it is nonverbal: A pointed stare or a strategic clearing of the throat is often sufficient to convey an emotion or prompt the recipient to respond. A speaker's body posture and hand gestures convey aspects of attitude, emphasis, and emotion. Often, these nonverbal forms of communication are unintentional and nonspecific. When a specific message must be conveyed, people typically employ language. Language, whether spoken, written, or signed, uses a system of symbols to convey meaning. Language involves the interaction of many skills that combine for effective communication. A speaker must know the rules for combining sounds into words and words into sentences. The speaker uses both sentence structure and word meanings to convey the content of the message. Finally, the speaker must appreciate the rules of social discourse to use language effectively for communication. We will present some approaches used to study language acquisition that highlight various aspects of language in children. To illustrate normal acquisition, we will follow the progression of language skills in a typically developing preschool child.

Human communication provides an opportunity for the exchange of feelings, knowledge, and wants between two or more people. In the first year of life, the baby communicates primarily through changes in the voice with accompanying facial expressions and gestures. These nonverbal vocalizations in the early part of life, primarily expressions of internal biological states, are affective in nature, and are interpreted by those around the baby as communicating emotion. The vocalizations soon begin to take on the melody of speech. When we left our discussion of infant vocalization in Chapter 3, Abraham, a child whose development we have been following, was just beginning to say his first words.

## THE COMPONENTS OF LANGUAGE

As effortless as language appears to be for most people, effective use involves the interaction of many skills. To understand the nature of language better, it is sometimes useful to examine the skills that contribute to overall language functioning. Bloom (1988) suggested that language skills can be described in terms of form, content, and use. **Form** includes phonology, syntax, and morphology. **Content** includes the meaning, or **semantics**, of words and utterances. **Use** includes pragmatic skills such as the rules of social discourse and the speaker's purpose for communication.

### Form

**Phonology.**   **Phonology** is the study of the sounds of speech. Linguists have been studying the phonological development of children since the early 1900s (Ingram,

1981). Much of current phonological investigation focuses on uncovering the rules required for combining speech sounds (or phonemes) to form syllables and words. As we saw in Chapter 1, any given language contains only a subset of the possible sound combinations that can be produced. For example, the phonology of English permits the /st/ blend at either the beginning or end of words, but /str/ can only appear at word beginnings. Likewise, there are specific rules for voicing or unvoicing in pluralization. If we were to pluralize the words *hat* and *hit,* we would add the unvoiced consonant /s/. Pluralization of a noun ending in a voiced consonant requires the use of the voiced cognate of /s/, the phoneme /z/. So, if we were to pluralize the word *bed,* we would add the /z/ phoneme, writing the word in phonetics as [bɛdz]. Such rules for how sound is used are part of the phonology of the language.

**Syntax.**   **Syntax** refers to the structure of sentences. The structure can be described in terms of hierarchically ordered components, as illustrated in Figure 7.1. A syntactic theory describes the rules by which words may be combined into grammatically acceptable sentences. For example, in English, the subject of a declarative sentence (a noun or noun phrase) must precede the predicate (a verb or verb phrase). Therefore, a sentence such as "He is swinging" is acceptable, whereas "Is swinging he" is not. Syntactic rules also describe the constraints in combining words and phrases of particular types. For example, for the predicate "is swinging," there are a limited number of phrases that might follow it in a sentence. We might say, "He is swinging wildly," or "He is swinging on the porch swing," or "He is swinging the baby." The predicate "is swinging" belongs to a class of verbs that can be followed by an adverbial phrase, prepositional phrase, or noun phrase. For most people, the rules for combining words into sentences are unconscious and automatic. Knowledge of these syntactic rules allows a speaker to produce

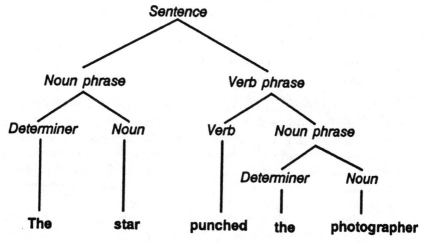

**FIGURE 7.1**   **The syntactic structure of a sentence.**

grammatical utterances effortlessly. In any language there is a limited number of acceptable syntactic structures. Therefore, knowledge of these structures allows listeners to anticipate the words they will hear and draw conclusions about how the words relate to one another to convey meaning. For example, in "Jamie asked Adelida . . ." there is a high probability that the sentence will continue with either a prepositional phrase (e.g., "about . . .") or a verb infinitive (for example, "to go . . ." or "to call . . ."). The listener, from the conversational context, may even be able to anticipate the precise phrase. Given the complete sentence "Jamie asked Adelida to go," the syntactic rules tell the listener that Jamie is doing the asking and that Adelida is being asked to go. In this way, the syntax has represented the general meaning of the utterance in a structured, rule-governed way. This phenomenon is referred to as mapping a deep structure (meaning) to a surface structure (syntax).

We will talk more about syntax in the next section of this chapter when we discuss language acquisition. Problems in syntactic comprehension and production in language-impaired children and adults will be presented in Chapters 8 and 9.

**Morphology.**   **Morphology** refers to how meaning is represented by the use of words, affixes, various grammar tenses (such as past tense), and plurality. A **morpheme** is the smallest unit of a language that has meaning. It can be a whole word, one of several parts of a word, the beginning of a word (i.e., a prefix, such as *un-*), or a word ending (i.e., a suffix, such as *-ing*). The following words contain one morpheme; they cannot be divided into any smaller units and still carry meaning:

|          |                  |
|----------|------------------|
| quick    | (one morpheme)   |
| build    | (one morpheme)   |
| structure| (one morpheme)   |

Words that can stand alone are called *free morphemes*. A second class of morphemes is called *bound morphemes* because they must be attached to other words. Bound morphemes include the suffixes *-ly, -er,* and *-ed* in:

|           |                  |
|-----------|------------------|
| quickly   | (two morphemes)  |
| builder   | (two morphemes)  |
| structured| (two morphemes)  |

Each of these words contains two morphemes, one free and one bound. Notice that the bound morpheme changes the meaning of the word in each case. In some cases the addition of a morpheme actually changes the syntactic classification of the word. The addition of *-ly* changes *quick* from an adjective to an adverb. The addition of *-er* changes *build* from a verb to a noun. The addition of *-ed* to *structure* can change it from a noun to an adjective. In other cases, morphemes add meaning without changing the class of the word (e.g., *dog* versus *dogs*).

Children's acquisition of morphology seems to follow predictable stages. After analyzing the utterances of children over time, Brown (1973) developed five stages of sentence construction that seem to parallel (or mirror) overall language development. The five stages correspond to the average of number of morphemes a child says per utterance, known as the MLU, or mean length of utterance, in morphemes:

> Stage I (1.75 morphemes).  The child is using single words and is starting to put noun-verb sequences together, such as "Car go."
>
> Stage II (2.25 morphemes).  The child starts to change word endings to portray grammar, as in "Cars going."
>
> Stage III (2.75 morphemes).  The child begins to use questions and imperatives, for instance, "That a car?"
>
> Stage IV (3.5 morphemes).  The child begins to use complex sentences, for example, "Where's car going?"
>
> Stage V (4 morphemes).  The child may use connectors and more functions, as in "Mom and Dad can come."

Although there is obvious overlap between successive stages, Brown and his colleagues conducted a number of studies over time that showed a progression from saying a single word to the two-word utterance to the telegraphic sentence, with the gradual refinement of grammar leading to complete sentences compatible with the adult model.

## Content

Content includes the meanings of individual words and words in combination. The study of word meanings is sometimes referred to as semantics. Our basic use of language as a tool for communication is to transmit meaning to someone else. Hubbell (1985) noted, "Meaning is the bridge between the thoughts and experiences of individuals and the sequences of sounds they produce to symbolize those thoughts and experiences. Words symbolize concepts, and concepts represent experiences or reality" (p. 33).

Of interest here is how young children attach meaning to a particular phonological sequence they have been hearing and how their meaning for a word develops into the adultlike meaning. As children hear words associated with particular actions and behaviors in social contexts, they begin to assign meaning to those words. Eventually, a word stands for those actions and feelings, without the need for the original context. As the child develops cognitively through various experiences, there is a greater coupling of words with meaning. The child begins to use "words to refer to or represent external objects and events" (Clark, 1979, p. 193).

Two kinds of meaning may develop for words, denotative and connotative. Denotative meaning is the literal meaning of the word. For example, for the word *milk,* we can use the dictionary definition of "a whitish fluid that is secreted by the mammary glands of female mammals for the nourishment of their young" as a literal, denotative meaning. (Few of us have thought of this meaning very often.)

Besides the literal, denotative meanings, words carry connotative meanings, which include the subtle overtones that distinguish words of very similar meanings. Thus, we would probably prefer to be called "unique" or even "unusual" rather than "atypical" or "abnormal." Connotative meanings often set the emotional tone of what is said. For example, "She requested it" has a more formal tone than "She asked for it." Connotative meanings also reflect concepts associated with particular words. For example, if we associate the concept of physical nourishment with milk, we can make the connection to spiritual nourishment to understand an alternate meaning of milk in the metaphorical "milk of human kindness." Speakers learn the rules of the semantic system by hearing and using words in ways appropriate to both their connotative and denotative meanings.

The sentence context influences the specific meanings that we attach to individual words. The meanings of nouns and verbs are modified by the use of adjectives and adverbs. The listener's expectations about the meaning of a sentence may change as later words cause its meaning to shift. For example, the noun *shoe* typically produces in the mind of the listener a picture of a leather covering of the foot mounted on a thicker sole. We can see how the sentence context is used to produce many different meanings for this word:

| | |
|---|---|
| If the shoe fits, wear it. | (a nonliteral, proverbial meaning) |
| It fits like an old shoe. | (from experience, old shoes feel good on the foot) |
| Make a ringer with a horseshoe. | (*horse* morpheme changes the meaning of *shoe*, and *ringer* requires specialized knowledge of horseshoe game) |
| You can't stop with worn shoes. | (a brake shoe is ineffective when worn) |

In the preceding examples, we see that the noun *shoe* (which we may first think of as the object we wear on a foot) can have many other meanings. We understand the particular meaning in the context in which the utterance was made. Disagreements in interpreting what someone intended to say may sometimes relate to different interpretations of word meaning.

## Use

How we use words, and in what situations, is the focus of language use, or pragmatics. Bates (1976) and Bruner (1975) pointed out that the human interaction a baby experiences in the first year of life establishes various pragmatic roles long before the baby is using language. The preverbal behaviors described in Chapter 3 are basically employed to control and manipulate the environment. After the first six months of life, spontaneous vocalization begins to be replaced with intentional vocalization accompanied by expression and gesture (Oller, 1980). From about the age of 9 months, the baby enjoys interaction with the caregiver, using vocalization appropriately for such games as pat-a-cake and peek-a-boo. In these early games, the child is using vocalizations, to interact with others. Bates (1976) calls these "preverbal performatives," (p. 426). Even between 12 and 18 months, the baby uses single-word responses like "bye-bye" more as part of a physical interaction with the caregiver than as true words that represent concepts. These utterances are called "performative acts" by Bates. The performative act serves a communicative purpose for the child, such as declaring, promising, asking questions, and so forth (Bates, Benigni, Bretherton, Camaioni, & Volterra, 1977).

The speech acts theory, developed by Searle (1969), focuses on the speaker's intention rather than on the words used. Searle described three types of intents: *asserting, requesting,* and *ordering.* These categories focus on how the speaker is using language rather than on the specifics of what was said. Assertions are almost as varied as topics of communication, whereas requests are usually for some kind of action or information. Others have elaborated on this focus with additional functions that language serves. Lahey (1988) provided a description of many functions that children's language serves. Some examples follow:

1. Comment (I did it!)
2. Rejection (No anchovies!)
3. Pretend (Barbie goes in her dream house . . .)
4. Obtain information (What's that?)
5. Routine (I pledge allegiance to the flag . . .)

As young children grow, so does their verbal repertoire, enabling the use of language forms that meet the demands of particular situations. Children learn to communicate (verbally and nonverbally) one way to their peers, another way to their parents, and another way to the teacher or the doctor. The child learns that the situation or context of the communication has much to do with how things are phrased. The specific decision about what to say and how and when to say it is shaped by the success the child experiences in conversation. For example, the child soon learns that he can call his cousins by their first names but he'd better use "Aunt" or "Uncle" with their parents, even though the adults address each other by first name alone. Furthermore, the child soon understands that Grandmother likes to use baby talk and that Grandfather uses a very adult language form. In Chapter 3, we saw the use of "child-directed speech" by Abraham's parents when addressing their infant son. However, it is unlikely that these parents speak to their bosses or coworkers in this style of speech. Instead, they adjust their speech to match the age and social status of their listener.

## APPROACHES TO THE STUDY OF LANGUAGE ACQUISITION

During the first year of life, infants all over the world hear the languages spoken around them and eventually organize what they hear into some kind of meaning. Toward the end of the first year, babies respond to their name. They are also able to respond to simple verbal commands and make simple motor responses using the objects in their immediate environment. As we saw in Chapter 3, their vocalizations toward the end of the first year have become a complex vocal pattern that resembles the patterns of the spoken languages they have been hearing. The first spoken words are followed by the orderly acquisition of one- and two-word utterances; these first words such as *ma* and *mi(lk)*, have primary value to the baby. These first words are also relatively easy to say and phonetically simple. As language is acquired during the second year, children are able to produce (and understand) longer and increasingly complex language constructions. Children acquire a grammar (rules of structure and sequence) of the language through everyday use. As children put two or three words together, they use the rules of the grammar to keep the words in the form and sequence needed to facilitate comprehension by the listener. Children learn that, to be understood by the listener, the verbal message must be said in a way that is reasonably similar to the language code of the listener.

There are many similarities across cultures regarding the sequence and timing of language acquisition. In contrast, there is great diversity in theories of language acquisition. In addition to speech-language pathologists and audiologists, many scholars from different backgrounds have studied language over the years. The philosopher and the psychologist have examined the relationship between language and thought. The linguist has studied the origins and forms of language. The psychologist and biologist have viewed language from its neurogenic origins. The neurologist and psychologist have studied the neurological foundations of both normal and disordered language. The child development specialist, the linguist, and psychologist have looked at cognition and language. Although some of the diversity of opinion about language is related to the particular discipline, some of it is related to the chronology or history of studying language. Over the years there have been major shifts in focus and viewpoint. The historical time at which language acquisition was studied (such as in 1950 as opposed to 1970 or 1990) has a influential role in one's approach to the topic. It would be convenient and encouraging to identify a sequential and progressive theme in the study of language over the years, but it appears that there is some randomness, perhaps even circularity in our study of normal language. Among the many theoretical approaches to the acquisition of language that are available, let us select four and cite a few of the theorists who have advocated each point of view.

It must be recognized that any selection or listing of theoretical approaches to language acquisition is an oversimplification. Further, there is considerable overlap of view between particular approaches, and there are single proponents advocating several theories. Cruttenden (1979) advocated a "balanced viewpoint" in consideration of various approaches to language acquisition, recognizing that there is some truth in each. In this introductory work, our intent is to present each approach briefly, with no attempt to advocate any one theory of language acquisition.

## The Behavioral Approach

According to the behavioral approach, language is a learned, conditioned behavior. This approach to language acquisition stresses the influence of environment rather than any innate abilities of the child. The origins of behavioral therapy perhaps started with the classical conditioning study of Pavlov, who conditioned dogs to salivate (Watson, 1970). Observing that dogs salivated when looking at meat, Pavlov presented a tuning-fork sound when the meat was presented. The dogs were soon *conditioned* to salivate when they heard the tuning fork (whether the meat was present or not). Like most automatic reflexes (such as salivation), many forms of human behavior can be conditioned (Skinner, 1957).

Behavioralists assert that language can be taught as well. For example, the 9-month-old baby learns to attend to the voice of her caregivers; when she hears these voices and looks closely at these people, she discovers that she finds comfort. She then repeats the comfort-producing behavior. The 12-month-old baby says "ma" when his mother is about to feed him. His *ma* production is followed by feeding, accompanied by many animated expressions of love from his mother. The positive response he received makes *ma* an attractive word to say. Every time he sees his mother (if there is enough positive reinforcement), he is likely to repeat it. He may also generalize the use of *ma* for all feeding situations regardless of who the caregiver may be. Such inappropriate stimulus generalization will eventually be extinguished through the reactions and feeding situations the baby experiences.

Skinner (1957) developed a behavioral theory of verbal learning. Language is conditioned when a child's early vocal behaviors receive positive reinforcement. As the child develops, correctly pronounced words and combinations of words are rewarded by approval or sometimes by the basic pleasure of verbalization (Cruttenden, 1979). Incorrect utterances are met with no approval and are subsequently replaced by correct (good) verbalizations. In this way, the caregiver becomes the teacher, providing reinforcements for the child's utterances, in effect *shaping* the child's productions to approximate those of the adult language model.

A behavioral approach to language learning strongly emphasizes shaping and reinforcement of speech attempts in the child's acquisition of language. In the first two years of life, when the child is in close proximity to a caregiver, one can appreciate that the latter has a primary role in reinforcing the child's utterances. However, the caregiver role may involve modeling and interacting as much as reinforcing. Once the child reaches the age of 2, it is difficult to see how a heterogeneous society can provide a consistent model for shaping verbalizations. Young children encounter a great variety of linguistic models (baby talk, fragmented sentences, and sentences spoken in a way they do not understand) and varied reactions to their utterances (anger, annoyance, laughter, ignoring, and friendliness). Moreover, children are capable of generating sentences they have never heard.

Despite its limitations for fully explaining normal language acquisition, the behavioral theory has been applied to teaching language in cases of language disorders. The behavioral approach to language acquisition was much utilized in the 1960s and 1970s as a clinical training model for children with deficient language. These approaches often involved repeated practice, with reinforcement for correct productions. Although therapy approaches have become more naturalistic over the years, Skinner's learning principles continue to be used for stimulating language in children with language disabilities of various kinds.

## The Nativist (Innateness) Approach

In some respects, the nativist approach was a reaction to the behavioral theory of language acquisition. Proponents of the nativist approach (e.g., Chomsky, 1988; Pinker, 1984) noted that children rarely receive explicit feedback about the grammatical correctness of their speech (e.g., "That's not right. You say it this way"). The "learning by shaping" tenet of the behaviorist approach seemed unrealistic in the absence of evidence of explicit teaching by adults. In fact, nativists felt that children's relatively rapid and seemingly effortless acquisition of language suggests that knowledge of the rules of language is part of their biological endowment. Children are presumed to have an innate knowledge of how words are organized into sentences, even before hearing all the types of sentences possible in their native language.

Early proponents of the nativist approach (e.g., Chomsky, 1965; McNeill, 1970) argued that children come equipped with a *language acquisition device* (LAD). All the language a child hears (the language "corpus") passes through the LAD, and this mechanism processes the structure of language so that the child becomes competent in his native language. McNeill provided a simple diagram of the LAD model as

Language Corpus → LAD → Grammatical Competence

The inner workings of how the LAD produces grammatical competence are not understood well, leading some to refer to it as a "black box" model. Explaining exactly what this black box does has occupied linguists for the past fifty years. Chomsky (1988) suggested that the LAD imparts knowledge of invariant features that characterize all languages (e.g., all languages use sentences that are constructed in rule-governed ways). These are referred to as language "universals." According to the theory, the child need only be exposed to his or her native language to recognize the specific rules that govern that particular language.

The nativist approach makes certain claims that set it apart from other theoretical approaches. The first is that language is not explicitly taught to children; rather, they acquire it because they are biologically predisposed to do so. Second, the child possesses a biological mechanism that is responsible for acquisition. This mechanism is thought to be independent of brain systems that handle other aspects of cognition. This theory has focused on language form and has not addressed aspects of communication that involve language content or use. The narrow scope of the nativist approach has prompted the development of other theoretical positions that encompass aspects of communication in addition to language form.

## The Cognitive Approach

The cognitive approach assumes that language skills represent the application of general cognitive skills for the purpose of communication. This theoretical approach has its early roots in the work of Piaget (1963) who proposed that children's developing facility with language is a reflection of their progression through hier-archical stages of cognitive development. The acquisition of words and sentences is thought to reflect the child's increasing ability to represent thoughts and experi-ences in the abstract form of language.

Like the nativist approach, the cognitive approach assumes that language acquisition is mediated by the brain. In contrast to the nativist approach, the brain systems that support language are not independent of those that support other as-pects of cognitive development. The cognitive approach also contrasts with the be-haviorist approach because it emphasizes the contribution of the child's abilities rather than the external feedback the child may receive. The types of abilities that cognitivist researchers have explored are perceptual skills that allow children to distinguish the sounds of speech, and cognitive skills such as pattern recognition that allow them to discern the ways sounds are arranged into words and words into sentences. Note that basic cognitive skills, such as perceptual capabilities and pattern recognition, are used not only for language but also for nonlinguistic skills (e.g., recognizing faces, learning sequenced activities).

According to the cognitive approach, language acquisition is dependent on the child's experiences with communication. The child learns about his or her lan-guage from the patterns available in the environment. For example, let us suppose a child hears words associated with actions, like *jump* and *jumped*, *cry* and *cried*. He or she might learn the association between *-ed* and the ends of verbs. This child may even overextend this association to verbs that do not take the *-ed* ending (e.g., *runned, sitted*) for a period of time (as some children do). However, after he or she hears enough examples of the irregular forms (e.g., *ran, sat*), the child will use these forms correctly as well. If these irregular words occur frequently in the speech he or she hears, the child might learn these "exceptions to the rule" quite quickly. And in fact, irregular verbs are quite common in conversational speech.

This line of thinking led to the development of the cue-competition theory of language acquisition (Bates & MacWhinney, 1987). This theory is based on the premise that all native languages provide the child with cues as to their underly-ing structure. The effectiveness, or strength, of these cues is related to how fre-quently they occur in the language and how reliably they lead the child to the correct conclusion about communication. For example, English-speaking children hear subject-verb-object sentences quite frequently. Therefore, interpreting the ini-tial noun of a sentence as the subject is quite reliable for understanding the sen-tence. This makes the first-noun-as-subject cue strong for English-speaking children. However, this same rule would not have high cue strength in all other languages. This language-to-language variation in cues accounts for the fact that there are differences in when specific linguistic elements are aquired across languages.

A recent evolution in the cognitivist tradition has been the application of computer models to the problem of language acquisition (e.g., Cartwright & Brent, 1997; Huiskens, Coppen, & Jagtman, 1991; McClelland & Rumelhart, 1986). In some ways, the computer models are a reaction to nativist claims that specialized, language-specific mechanisms (such as the LAD) underlie language acquisition.

Instead, these models use general associative processes that are not language specific. Few researchers would claim that a successful computer model proves how children acquire language. Instead, these models serve to broaden thinking about the possibilities that could account for acquisition. Simply put, the fact that a computer can mimic aspects of acquisition indicates that it is possible that those skills could be acquired without a language-specific mechanism.

Cognitive approaches have the advantage of being broad enough to account for not only language form but also its content and use. Because cognitive theories acknowledge the role of a child's experiences in shaping language acquisition, it is easy to see how the environment can dictate the types of words a child acquires and the social conventions the child uses when communicating. In fact, some theorists have suggested that the social function of language (why the child wants to say something) drives much of early language acquisition. This focus on the communication interaction also separates the cognitive approach from the other theoretical approaches discussed so far.

## The Biological Approach

The modern biological approach to language actually has its roots in nineteenth-century Europe. At a time that preceded direct methods to study brain-behavior relations, physicians and anatomists developed theories that have persisted centuries later. The concept of localization of function (see Chapter 2) was championed by Francis Gall. Gall was an anatomist who dedicated his career to study of the human brain. He received both international fame and later considerable derision for his ideas that variation in brain structure could account for individual differences in behavior. He developed maps that assigned different skills, attitudes, and personality traits to small regions of the brain. Given that there were no methods for directly measuring variations in these areas in the living brain, he inferred brain differences by mapping the topography of the skull. Although time has refuted his methods and brain maps, his concept of localization of function has proved to be an important and powerful concept even today.

The localizationist perspective was further reinforced by the work of Paul Broca and Carl Wernicke, whose case studies of specific types of language loss led to assignment of particular language functions to the left hemisphere of the brain. Broca and Wernicke began a tradition that continues today of examining the language deficits that occur after stroke, disease, or injury in order to infer function of the damaged area. With the advent of neuroimaging techniques in the mid-twentieth century, researchers were able to locate the area of damage in living patients. This has allowed greater specificity in the ability to localize function.

Others have used both the time-tested methods of autopsy work and modern brain-imaging techniques to discover if structural variations in the intact brain might explain the propensity of the left hemisphere to support language. Geschwind and Levitsky (1968) were the first to discover that the one area serving language was larger in the left hemisphere than in the right. Later work established that these asymmetries are present at birth (Chi, Dooling, & Gilles, 1977), supporting the idea that these structural differences provide an anatomical substrate for developing left hemisphere language representation. These twentieth-century discoveries in many ways were the legacy of Gall's ideas two centuries earlier.

Today, researchers are fortunate to have a variety of tools to study the living brain's structure and function in amazing detail. These tools are being applied to the study of language acquisition during childhood (e.g., Molfese, 1990 Plante, Schmithorst, Holland, & Byars, 2006), normal language in adults (e.g., Bookheimer, 2002; Kutas & Hillard, 1983), and the language deficits and recovery patterns in those with neurological disorders (e.g., Hertz-Pannier et al., 2002; Rosen et al., 2000). New discoveries are modifying our view of language in the brain. We now know that language is better described as lateralized (more on the left than the right) rather than strictly localized to the left hemisphere (see Figure 7.2). There are indications that the language areas of the right hemisphere might be one mechanism of recovery in some cases of left hemisphere brain damage. We are also developing a better appreciation of how the language systems interact with other regions that support memory and attention (e.g., Plante, Ramage, & Maglöire 2006; Shaywitz et al., 2001). These investigations are guided by the three-hundred-year legacy of brain-language discoveries and by modern theories on the nature of language. Ultimately, the biological approach may provide evidence to support or refute the tenets of other approaches to language acquisition discussed in this text.

## Summary

In many ways, the approaches described differ more in their focus than in their substantive claims. Indeed, writers frequently combine aspects of various positions or switch between them over time. Cognitive approaches tend to emphasize

**FIGURE 7.2   Activation (areas in white) found when normal adults listened to stories. Note that multiple areas of the brain are engaged in this task and more activation is seen in the left hemisphere than the right. This pattern is consistent with the left hemisphere lateralization of language.**

Data from Plante, Ramage, & Maglöire (2006), used by permission of the first author.

the importance of the communicative function of language. Nativist approaches are frequently designed to account for language form. Cognitive and behavioral approaches often address language content as it is mapped to the child's experiences. Biological approaches concentrate on anatomical and physiologic correlates of language. The differences in focus reflect, in part, the different disciplines that have contributed to the field of language. As the study of language becomes increasingly interdisciplinary, we can look forward to a greater integration of such approaches.

Several of these perspectives on language acquisition reflect a nature-versus-nurture argument. For example, nativist theories have historically emphasized the child's innate endowment (nature) for language. In contrast, behavioral theories have emphasized the role of the environment (nurture). Recent advances in the neurosciences demonstrate that strict nature–nurture dichotomies are unrealistic. We now know that experience shapes the structure and function of the brain at very basic levels. The pattern of neuron activation is shaped and changed by sensory input and experiences. Activation, in turn, promotes neuronal survival and outgrowth. These changes in the brain's basic organization make the brain a ready and increasingly efficient processor of experience, including experience with language.

This type of dynamic interaction between children's biological nature and their experiences forces a redefinition of innate versus experience-based skills. The word *innate* typically means "present from birth," although this definition no longer means that experience has no effect. Many brain systems rely heavily on sensory input to develop normally, and such input may begin prenatally. For example, the auditory system becomes functional during the third prenatal trimester. Some aspects of spoken language, such as prosodic patterns and certain sound contrasts, are audible in the womb. As we saw in Chapter 3, infants hear and respond differentially to sounds they were exposed to while in the womb (e.g., DeCasper & Spence, 1986). Thus, infants are born with some knowledge of acoustic characteristics of their language community, and this knowledge appears to be experience based. These types of discoveries force a reevaluation of the assumptions that underlie traditional approaches to language acquisition. As Locke (1990) suggested, language may be both innate and learned, because certain biological characteristics may predispose a child to attend to language-relevant information, prompting the child to learn more about it. From this perspective, it is more productive to explore the interactions between the child and his or her experiences than to divide them artificially.

## LANGUAGE DEVELOPMENT FROM SOUNDS TO SENTENCES

In Chapter 3, we followed the development of a young boy named Abraham. We saw his communicative development progress from his first exposure to the sounds of language to the point where he was able to produce sound sequences recognizable as single words. This is a truly remarkable accomplishment. It signals coordination of the range of biological systems (respiratory, vocal, articulatory, auditory, and cognitive) to support spoken language. Once the first words appear, others soon follow. A child learns words that characterize his environment. The family dog's name is learned, and the word *dog* itself will follow. If there is no neighborhood cat, however, that word will take longer to appear. Sometimes these first words are highly context specific. For example, Abraham could name animals from his Noah's ark book that he did not name at the zoo. Nonetheless, with each day and every new experience, there were opportunities to learn new words and refine his understanding of words recently acquired. Let us continue to look at Abraham's communication from the perspective of his emerging language skills.

## 21 Months

Abraham visited us at the language clinic at 21 months of age. When he entered the large playroom, he was immediately attracted to the crayons and paper that we had set out on a child-size picnic table. He loved to color, which at this point consisted of light marks scribbled mostly on the page and occasionally on the table. At

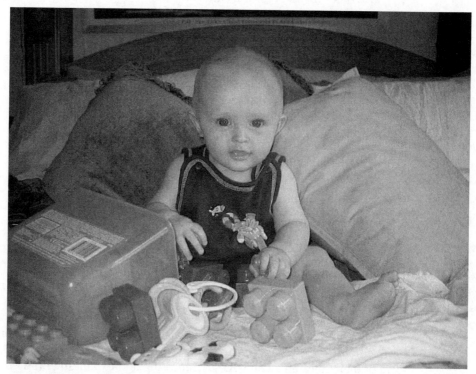

**Infants build vocabulary through their experiences. Play and exploration are important in this process.**

this age, Abraham's attention span for any one activity was fairly short. When he began to color, his mother had the following conversation with him:

MOTHER:   You like to color, huh?

ABRAHAM:   Gah!

MOTHER:   Yeah, you like to color, huh?

ABRAHAM:   Ah deh. Out.

MOTHER:   Want to get out? (She lifts him out from between the table and bench.) You want to go look in that bag? Bring your bag. Bring the bag over here. (Abraham brings the bag.) All right! (Laughs) What's in there?

(Abraham and Mother look into the bag.)

ABRAHAM:   Bribee [baby].

MOTHER:   Yeah.

ABRAHAM:   Beebee [baby].

MOTHER:   That's your baby. (Takes it out)

ABRAHAM:   Night night. Deh coo.

MOTHER:   Blanket for the baby.

ABRAHAM:   Deh yi gah.

MOTHER:   Yeah, that's your grrrr bear. (Takes it out)

(Abraham wanders off . . .)

MOTHER:   Where are you going, hun?

ABRAHAM:   Ow meh.

MOTHER:   You're coming here?

ABRAHAM:   Eeehhh [yes].

MOTHER:   What else is in the bag?

ABRAHAM:   Ehhh off. (Abraham pulls at the vest he is wearing.)

MOTHER:   Oh, we're gonna leave it on. Look how nice you look.

ABRAHAM:   Ah hah.

MOTHER:   Very handsome.

This short conversation illustrates many aspects of Abraham's current stage of language acquisition. The first thing we notice is that, although he is now using words, we don't always understand what he is saying. Even his parents do not always understand everything he says. However, when the context gives clues to the meaning of the words (e.g., pulling objects out of a bag), his mother can translate his attempts into actual words. In fact, parents provide indirect feedback about the form of their children's language by repeating and expanding on their children's utterances (Demetras, Post, & Snow, 1986).

At this age, Abraham's language consists mostly of single words. He is just beginning to use two-word combinations and an occasional three-word utterance. Abraham's production of single words, with few multi-word combinations, is reflected by an overall MLU (mean length of utterance in morphemes) of 1.49. These utterances consist almost exclusively of content-rich words (e.g., nouns, verbs). Completely absent are any of the grammatical morphemes (e.g., articles, plurals, verb tense markers). In contrast, Abraham can comprehend much longer utterances than he is able to produce. For example, his mother's direction to him ("Oh, we're gonna leave it on") is longer than what he produced.

Abraham has between fifty and hundred different words in his language repertoire. However, his understanding of the meanings of words may be different from those of an adult. This is the age when toddlers point to strange men in grocery stores and exclaim, "Daddy!" For them, the word *Daddy* may be broadly defined as including all adult males. The narrower meaning of, *Daddy* as "my male parent" will develop later. Conversely, other words may have too narrow a definition. *Doggie* may be used only with the household pet, and not for other dogs. Still other words are actually social routines (e.g., *Night night*) or parts of songs, which may not be used outside of that specific context. As children grow in both experience and cognitive maturity, their understanding of the meaning of words will become more refined and adultlike.

Despite the fact that most of his language consists of single words, Abraham gets a lot of "mileage" out of those single words. He is actually able to convey a range of meanings with similar utterances, depending on the situational context and his intonation. When we look at his utterances from the perspective of language content and use, we can see this flexibility of expression.

> **MOTHER:**  We got a bunch of different books here.
>
> **ABRAHAM:**  Elmo book! Elmo book! (Content: item name) (Use: requests an action [reading])
>
> **MOTHER:**  You want to read the Elmo book?
>
> **ABRAHAM:**  Elmo book. (Content: item name) (Use: confirmation)
>
> (They read.)
>
> **MOTHER:**  Who's that?
>
> **ABRAHAM:**  Gower. (Content: character name) (Use: labeling; reply to mother)
>
> **MOTHER:**  Grover.
>
> **ABRAHAM:**  Gower coffee. (Content: possession) (Use: comment)

## 28 Months

At 2 years of age, Abraham is quite the conversationalist. At this point, Abraham can be understood well by both family members and those who hear him speak less frequently. We can see an example when Abraham talks about his toddler gymnastics class.

MOTHER:   What did you get to do at class?

ABRAHAM:   Jump!

MOTHER:   You get to jump. On what?

ABRAHAM:   Trampoline.

AUTHOR:   Did Mommy get to jump on the trampoline?

ABRAHAM:   Yeah.

MOTHER:   Did I jump on that trampoline?

ABRAHAM:   No.

MOTHER:   No.

AUTHOR:   No? Why not?

ABRAHAM:   She want to get off.

MOTHER:   Who else got to jump on it?

ABRAHAM:   Other boy turn.

MOTHER:   Yeah. You guys shared, didn't you?

ABRAHAM:   Yeah. (Abraham crouches and makes a funny face.) Went nnnnnggggggggg.

MOTHER:   Is that what he said?

ABRAHAM:   Yeah. I say that.

As this conversation illustrates, Abraham is talking in single words and short sentences. We hear the major content words (e.g., nouns, main verbs). We also hear the earliest-acquired grammatical morphemes (e.g., "com*ing* our house!" "Flower*s*"). However, most other grammatical units tend to be missing. In this early stage of language development, it is common to hear such "telegraphic speech" (Brown, 1976). Abraham's MLU on the day this conversation took place was 2.03, which is about average for children at this age.

We sometimes have difficulty understanding what Abraham says, not because the words themselves are mispronounced, but because he does not always provide enough information or background to convey the general context. For example, the word "jump" does not necessarily bring to mind bouncing on a trampoline when it is first said. In this case, Abraham's mother was filling in the background information and structure of the conversation by cueing him as to what information should be given next. In addition, children at this stage are likely to agree with what adults say, regardless of its actual truth, as we see here. Pragmatically, they understand that a positive response will continue the conversation, without appreciating that the listener's understanding has diverged from their own. Although Abraham's mother gets the conversation back on track, we can see that this tendency in young children can also lead to miscommunications.

Despite these limitations in form and content, Abraham is exhibiting a range of language use. During a play visit to the author at the clinic, we observed various pragmatic functions. The following is a small sample of these:

| | |
|---|---|
| What that? | (request for information) |
| Mommy do it! | (request for action) |
| A doll. | (labeling) |
| Now him sad. | (commenting) |
| No! No! | (negating) |

## 39 Months

Children's speech changes rapidly between the ages of 2 and 4. In twelve months, we can already see changes in the form of Abraham's language. We recorded this interaction between Abraham and his mother when Abraham was 39 months.

MOTHER:  Oh, you know what? I should have brought your pictures of you and Christopher to show. They were so pretty. Remember?

ABRAHAM:  You forgot?

MOTHER:  I forgot to bring them. They were really neat.

ABRAHAM:  The pictures that I made and colored?

MOTHER:  Yep.

AUTHOR:  You colored them by yourself?

ABRAHAM:  Mmmhmm. I made 'em mixed with for the sky.

MOTHER:  Yep, you mixed the color of the sky.

ABRAHAM:  And I made the clouds inside.

MOTHER:  You sure did.

ABRAHAM:  But the 'nuther one was messed up.

MOTHER:  Well, yeah. You did make one that you didn't like much.

ABRAHAM:  It was messed up.

MOTHER:  It was. But you really liked it because you put legs and feet and arms and hands.

ABRAHAM:  There wasn't enough room for the legs.

Although we still see a few form errors (e.g., "the 'nuther one" for "another one") we see noteworthy gains as well. Abraham increased the length of his utterances. His MLU on this day was 5.28. This is actually above average for his age. MLUs for children at this age typically range between 2.71 and 4.23 (Miller, 1981). Abraham's MLU fluctuates from day to day as well. In a sample collected one month later, his MLU was 4.03. Other aspects of language form are entirely appropriate for Abraham's age. Most of his utterances now are complete sentences with nouns and verbs serving as subjects and predicates. Notice that Abraham now uses both content words and a number of grammatical morphemes (e.g., past tense *-ed*, plural *s*, articles *the* and *a*). Occasionally, we see complex sentences (e.g., "The pictures that I made and colored?").

Compared with the conversation we saw at age 28 months, Abraham's contributions carry much more content. Instead of just providing input when prompted, he is now contributing new information spontaneously. There are still instances in which his meaning is not entirely clear (e.g., "And I made the clouds inside"), but most of the time others can follow his conversations with little effort.

We can clearly see how form, content, and use have developed and interact by revisiting some of the pragmatic functions we saw at 28 months and looking at the form and content now being used to code those functions at 39 months.

| | |
|---|---|
| What does mine do? | (request for information) |
| Buy some at the store. | (request for action) |
| It is a tool. | (labeling) |
| That looks like a robot. | (commenting) |
| Mickey doesn't have shoes. | (negating) |

At this age, Abraham is using language not just for communication with others but for imaginative uses as well. He talks about what he is doing even when there is no one to hear or respond to him. The following excerpt was recorded while Abraham played alone with a large doll house and a family of dolls. What we hear is a verbal monologue of his ongoing thoughts as he plays. In this case, he is using language as a tool to organize and encode his thoughts and experiences in a pretend situation.

> Oh, wow, oh man, I need all these guys. There's a bunch of people. I don't want the bunch of people, just a little bit. A little bit means, this is a little bit. Yeah, this is a little bit. (Looks at one figure.) Gross. I don't want you. Well, get your mom and dad. I'll get the mom. I'll get the dad. (Talks for the boy doll.) Mom, could we go to the park? Dad, could we go to the park? This is the park already. Okay, I want to sit right . . . Let's go over. . . let's take. . . take a nap. Our bed. Oh wow. Your bed is. . . my bed is right down. . . your bed is right down there. That's right. These are not the big people's. No, these are ours. The baby's is right there where his is. Mommy and Daddy are busy down there. You guys, you can't wait to go to the nap like that. You need someone to help you get into bed. You guys already got back into bed and get the baby.

## 44 Months

At age 4, children's language is adultlike in many respects. We rarely hear violations of language form, although we do hear false starts and revisions (even adults produce these periodically). At 44 months, Abraham's MLU is now 5.35, which indicates no increase in utterance length compared to five months before. In fact, Abraham has now passed the age where MLU is sensitive to gains in language acquisition. This is because his sentences are becoming more complex rather than simply becoming longer. We hear complex verb phrases ("He *wants to get* in there") and conjoined sentences ("But not the boy, *'cause* he's hiding in a hiding place up there").

The content of language continues to be dictated by experience. Children must hear new words to learn them (later, reading will contribute significantly to vocabulary growth). When children read a new book, play with others, go new places, or watch television programs, they are exposed to new words. Therefore, the words that children know depend, in large part, on their range of experience, which provides a context for new words to be learned. Once words are acquired, they are available to the child to help frame his or her future experiences and to support further learning. We can see the role of experience in building vocabulary when Abraham's preschool class made a trip to a local fire station. Although Abraham had never been there before, it was clear that he already had some very specific concepts about what a fire station is like and vocabulary to go along with the experience. In his case, a likely source of this vocabulary was a book that had been read to him many times. A home video of the field trip captured the following conversation:

(The children enter the fire station.)

ABRAHAM:   What is. . . What's that? A fire truck. An old fire truck.

(The children go through the living areas.)

ABRAHAM:   We don't have one right here? We don't have a pole here?

FIREFIGHTER:   We don't have a pole. There's only one or two left in the country that still has a pole and we don't. . .

ABRAHAM:   Whoa! Look at this. This is where the firefighter sleeps.

(The children look at the ambulance.)

ABRAHAM:   I have a question.

FIREFIGHTER:   I have an answer. What can I do for you?

ABRAHAM:   These are the people that drive the ambulance?

FIREFIGHTER:   That's right. Do you know I can drive this ambulance? That's my job.

In this conversation, we can see that Abraham is quite confident talking to others, although other children at this age may be shy. He is also beginning to show some of the subtleties of language use. For example, he uses the indirect "I have a question" before asking the actual question. We also see that his use of conversational conventions is still not perfect. Earlier, he asked a question and interrupted the adult before receiving the full answer. He will continue to refine skills within the domain of language use as he grows.

In four short years, Abraham has gone from an infant, whose only means of expression was crying, to a preschooler, whose language contains many of the features one would see in an adult speaker. In this chapter, we have seen the development of language *form* as he progressed from word attempts that were only approximations of the adult phonological form to fully intelligible speech. We saw single words progress to multiword phrases to sentences containing clauses and complex verbs. We saw increased use of morphology as phrases and sentences emerged. We saw language *content* grow from the restricted meanings of the first few words to the multitude of words whose meanings approximate adult versions. Finally, we saw improvement in the *use* of language for a variety of communication functions. Although certain aspects of language form, content, and use will continue to expand as he grows, Abraham's language is, by age 4, already a remarkable tool for communication.

## THE DEVELOPMENT OF LITERACY

In addition to spoken language skills, children develop skills with reading and writing language. Like spoken language, the foundations for reading and writing may begin in early infancy and emerge over time. If the child is read to frequently, the development of early literacy skills may be as natural to the child as the development of spoken language. Let us look at Abraham's development of literacy skills.

*Abraham* was born to parents who value and enjoy reading. They purchased baby books and began reading to him shortly after his birth. This was part of their daily routine and provided an opportunity for baby and parents to interact. A typical book session involved his mother or father holding Abraham so that both could see the book. After reading a page, they would point out and name the things pictured on the pages before turning to the next page. By 12 months, Abraham was actively joining in this activity. We saw him waiting for his father to read the words before pointing to the picture and babbling. Then he helped to turn to the next page. When the book was closed, he babbled two syllables remarkably like "the end" would have sounded if he had said real words. By 2 years, Abraham wanted the same few books read over and over again. He would bring books to his mother during play times and was always read one of these stories before going to sleep. If his mother paused when reading the text, Abraham would fill in the final words. By 3, his mother started to point not only to pictures on the page but also to each word as she read. Some time after that, Abraham started to recognize words that occurred frequently in his favorite books. He was also given an alphabet book at this point and began to learn the names of the letters. Although his alphabet book associated letters with words ("A" with *apple, ants*), he showed no sign of recognizing that the letters made specific sounds that went with the items pictured on the page. However, he can recognize a handful of words in his favorite books. These tend to be those words that occur most frequently in the story, like *the,* a, or the name of the main character.

As we see from Abraham's experience, literacy experiences often arise well before a child is formally taught to read and write. Abraham's early literacy experiences are typical of many children who are raised in households where reading is a common activity and where parents consider it their role to introduce their children to books (Weigel, Martin, & Bennett, 2006). Before such children even enter kindergarten, they have many preliteracy skills that will facilitate learning to read and write. Children who are read to develop social routine for books. They know how to hold them, know that the reader says some words, everyone looks at the picture, the page is turned, and the routine repeats until the end. Their experience with books teaches them that individual letters have names and that the groups of letters the reader points to correspond to the words said, and the words correspond to the pictures on the page. Perhaps most important, these children see book reading as an enjoyable activity. These children have a strong advantage when they enter school because they already know much about the process of reading. In contrast, children who lack experience with books at home may still be gaining the skills other children mastered as preschoolers when their classmates are learning to sound out words. These children may also be less motivated to learn to read because they never had the experience of enjoying the stories that books contain.

The path to normal reading involves not only the practical skills involved with handling and appreciating books but also a growing awareness of the function of print. Even children who are not read to encounter print in their daily lives. Road signs, billboards, children's television programming, and toy boxes all offer exposure to print in the environment. One model for the progression from pre-reading to true reading (Frith, 1985) suggests that children first develop an awareness of whole printed words through repeated environmental exposure. For example, Abraham would point to a stop sign and say "stop" long before he had any notion that the word was made of individual letters that, when pronounced in combination, made up the word "stop." In some regards, the "stop" on a stop sign or the "Lego" label on a toy box functions more like a picture that has a specific name than a written word.

In order to differentiate between words like *stop* and *step* or *stop* and *top*, children must recognize that there is a difference in the individual letters that make up these words, and these letters make a difference. Children's increasing familiarity with the alphabet assists them in this process. However, alphabetic knowledge does not come through environmental exposure alone but must be taught. Many children learn to sing the alphabet song or are given alphabet books as preschoolers. Others may have limited opportunities to learn the alphabet and the corresponding sounds each letter can represent before they begin formal schooling. Regardless of when awareness of the alphabet arises, children must eventually learn that printed words are made up of individual letters, and changing these letters changes the words. The ability to pair sounds with letters is a key skill necessary for "sounding out" words in print. This requires children to associate sounds with the printed letter symbols, a skill known as **sound–symbol correspondence**.

As Abraham enters school, he learns that he can tell what a word is by "sounding it out." As he is taught to read, Abraham will learn that certain combinations of letters are not sounded out individually (e.g., "th" in "these") and that a vowel in one word can sound different than the same vowel in another word. These skills are critical for decoding words he has not encountered before. If Abraham knows the story being read, he finds he often just needs to sound out the first one or two sounds before he can guess what the word is. Most of the time, he guesses correctly. This demonstrates that he is using his comprehension of the prior text to predict what a new word should be. He also relies on the pictures that accompany the text to help his comprehension and to anticipate the text to come.

The child who is developing reading normally may sound out words the first few times they are encountered. However, if the same word is encountered repeatedly, the child will quickly begin to recognize the whole word. At this point, the word is said to be in their "sight vocabulary." Books geared to young children facilitate this process by presenting the same vocabulary items repeatedly within the context of the story. The more books the child reads, the more sight words he or she will accumulate, further speeding the reading process.

The early stages of reading demonstrate the importance of two skills for reading development: phonological decoding and language comprehension. For early readers, phonological decoding may be the most important skill. This allows readers to turn letters into sound sequences and sound sequences into words with meaning. Until the reader builds a corpus of words that are known by sight, he or she must rely on decoding as a primary strategy for accessing meaning. For later readers, comprehension becomes more critical. Readers have to not only track the meaning of the individual words, but also make sense of the sentences and the overall narrative of the text being read. As readers become more proficient, and are sounding out fewer words per page, their ability to follow the overall meaning of a story is more predictive of their success as a reader than their ability to decode individual words. This is also the point at which children are expected to use reading as a means for learning in school. Children transition from reading as an instructional objective to reading textbooks to gain information around third grade. After this point, children who have not mastered reading sufficiently to learn class material are at risk for academic failure. We will consider two such individuals in Chapter 8.

Literacy skills develop in parallel with spoken language skills. Abraham's earliest literacy skills emerged even before his first words were spoken. Early literacy experiences also provide a mechanism for language growth. The pictures in the book provide a context for learning new words. For example, words like *pair*, *zebra*, and *ark* may have little opportunity to arise in conversational language, but a child will be repeatedly exposed to these words if he or she is given a book on Noah's ark. The pictures and text provide a means of teaching the meaning of these words, as does the opportunity for the child and the reader to talk about these concepts. Books also contain language forms that may not occur frequently in conversational language as well. Books for young children may include rhyming text or use alliteration liberally. These literary devices cue children into similarities and differences in the sound sequences of words. Books for older children may include sentence structures that do not occur in oral language (e.g., "'Get the dog!' he said"). The stories read to children provide a framework for how information may be organized when they tell stories of their own. For these reasons, language and reading are considered reciprocal skills (e.g., Raikes et al., 2006). Reading builds a variety of language skills. In turn, children with stronger language skills are better able to understand the books they read.

> By age 4, Abraham is interested in writing on his own. He can recognize his own name when his mother writes it. He also likes to copy his name onto the pictures that he draws. The letters are uneven in size, and often he needs to continue part of his name below the initial few letters if he runs out of room. Sometimes he misses a few of the letters despite having a model. By 5, he is interested in writing captions to pictures he draws. He will sometimes make up words by stringing random letters together. Other times, he asks his parents what letters he should use. He can form both uppercase and lowercase letters. However, he does not understand when each type of letter is used, so sometimes uppercase letters appear in the middle of words rather than just at the start of sentences. He commonly reverses letters as well. Often there is no space between words, or letters are spaced randomly on the page. However, he "reads" his written captions with pride to his parents.

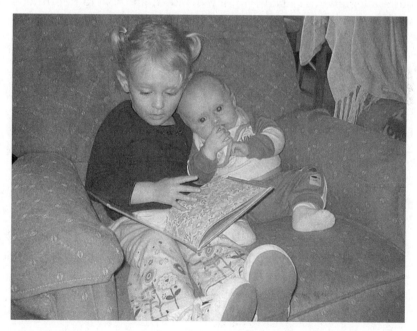

**Literacy skills have their earliest roots in children's first experiences with books.**

By the time a child like Abraham begins school, he or she already has rudimentary writing skills. This may include being able to copy letter forms or even write letters that are named for him. Other children may lack the experience or even the basic motor skills to control a pencil or crayon to form letters. Early home or school experiences may include practice in forming letters. By kindergarten or first grade, children will be taught the sounds that go with each letter as a prerequisite to spelling words. Some words, like those the child recognizes consistently from stories or his environment, may be spelled correctly even before he or she can sound out the individual letters of the word.

Just as reading occurs in a variety of contexts, from environmental print to books, writing also develops in a variety of contexts. A child may see a parent noting appointments on a calendar or typing emails on the computer. Many children will produce scribbles for words before they can form individual letters. A child might begin developing more functional writing skills with simple activities like copying his or her name onto a birthday card or putting a label on a hand-drawn picture. School assignments may include more formal activities like practice with letter formation, written spelling practice, and writing worksheets. Many teachers may allow young children to spell words phonetically in order to facilitate the child's experience of expressing him- or herself through print without the added burden of using the correct spelling conventions. However, as children become more proficient with the physical demands of writing, the expectations for correct spelling and grammar also increase. Advanced writing skills will eventually require integration of language form, content, and use to inform or persuade a reader.

## CLINICAL PROBLEM SOLVING

Here are two language samples obtained from Abraham at two different ages.

**28 months:**

MOTHER:    Is that a taco that you're making?

ABRAHAM:    Yeah.

MOTHER:    Where do you eat tacos?

ABRAHAM:    With a mat.

MOTHER:    On a placemat?

ABRAHAM:    (Pours beans into a bowl) Put all in.

(They start to fall on the floor.)

MOTHER:    Hey, honey, honey. . .

ABRAHAM:    Oh no, mommy!

MOTHER:    Do you want help with the beans?

ABRAHAM:    It's a cooking beans!

**44 months:**

ABRAHAM: I ate eggs for breakfast.

AUTHOR: Did mommy make it?

ABRAHAM: I got a gargoyle and I got a Casper today.

AUTHOR: What was the gargoyle on?

ABRAHAM: They're just on my underwear.

AUTHOR: Oh, you have gargoyle underwear on.

ABRAHAM: I have them not on today!

AUTHOR: You have Caspers on today?

ABRAHAM: Yeah.

Look at the transcripts above and consider them from the perspective of language form, content, and use:

1. How has Abraham's language changed from 28 to 44 months?
2. Do you think that his content is typical of other children at each age? Why or why not?
3. What evidence can you find that Abraham has not yet reached adultlike competence in form, content, and use at each age?

# REFERENCES

Bates, E. (1976). Pragmatics and sociolinguistics in child language. In D. Morehead & A. Morehead (Eds.), *Normal and deficient child language.* Baltimore: University Park Press.

Bates, E., & MacWhinney, B. (1987). Competition, variation, and language learning. In B. MacWhinney (Ed.), *Mechanisms of language acquisition* (pp. 157–193). Hillsdale, NJ: Lawrence Erlbaum Associates.

Bates, E., Benigni, L., Bretherton, I., Camaioni, L., & Volterra, V. (1977). From gesture to the first word: On cognitive and social prerequisites. In M. Lewis & L. Rosenblum (Eds.), *Interaction, conversation, and the development of language.* New York: Wiley.

Bloom, L. (1988). What is language? In M. Lahey (Ed.), *Language disorders and language development.* New York: Macmillan.

Bookheimer, S. (2002). Functional MRI of language: New approaches to understanding the cortical organization of semantic processing. *Annual Review of Neuroscience, 25,* 151–188.

Brown, R. (1973). *A first language: The early stages.* Cambridge, MA: Harvard University Press.

Brown, R. (1976). *A first language.* New York: Penguin.

Bruner, J. S. (1975). The ontogenesis of speech acts. *Journal of Child Language, 2,* 1–19.

Cartwright, T. A., & Brent, M. R. (1997). Syntactic categorization in early language acquisition: Formalizing the role of distributional analysis. *Cognition, 63,* 121–170.

Chi, J. C., Dooling, F. C., & Gilles, F. H. (1977). Gyral development of the human brain. *Annals of Neurology, 1,* 86–93.

Chomsky, N. (1965). *Aspects of the theory of syntax.* Cambridge, MA: MIT Press.

Chomsky, N. (1988). *Language and problems of knowledge: The Managua lectures.* Cambridge, MA: MIT Press.

Clark, E. (1979). What's in a word? On the child's acquisition of semantics in his first language. In V. Lee (Ed.), *Language development.* New York: Wiley.

Cruttenden, A. (1979). *Language in infancy and childhood.* New York: St. Martin's.

DeCasper, A. B., & Spence, M. B. (1986). Prenatal maternal speech influences newborns' perception of speech sounds. *Infant Behavior and Development, 9,* 133–150.

Demetras, M. J., Post, K. N., & Snow, C. E. (1986). Feedback to first language learners: The role of repetitions and clarification questions. *Journal of Child Language, 13,* 275–292.

Frith, U. (1985). Beneath the surface of developmental dyslexia. In K. E. Patterson, J. C. Marshall, & M. Coltheart (Eds.), *Surface dyslexia* (pp. 301–330). Mahwah, NJ: Lawrence Erlbaum Associates.

Geschwind, N., & Levitsky, W. (1968). Human brain: Asymmetries in temporal speech region. *Science, 7,* 5097–5100.

Hertz-Pannier, L., Chiron, C., Jambaque, I., Renaux-Kieffer, V., Van de Moortele, P. F., Delalande, O., Fohlen, M., Brunelle, F., & Le Bihan, D. (2002). Late plasticity for language in a child's nondominant hemisphere: A pre- and postsurgery fMRI study. *Brain, 125,* 361–372.

Hubbell, R. (1985). Language and linguistics. In P. Skinner & R. Shelton (Eds.), *Speech, language, and hearing* (2nd ed.). New York: Wiley.

Huiskens, L., Coppen, P. A., & Jagtman, M. (1991). Developing a tool for the description of language acquisition. *Linguistics, 29,* 451–479.

Ingram, D. (1981). Transitivity in child language. *Language, 47,* 888–910.

Kutas, M., & Hillyard, S. A. (1983). Event related brain potentials to grammatical errors and semantic anomalies. *Memory and Cognition, 11,* 539–550.

Lahey, M. (1988). *Language disorders and language development.* New York: Macmillan.

Locke, J. (1990). Structure and stimulation in the ontogeny of spoken language. *Developmental Psychobiology, 23,* 621–643.

McClelland, J., & Rumelhart, D. (1986). A PDP model of the acquisition of morphology. In B. MacWhinney (Ed.), *Mechanisms of language acquisition.* Hillsdale, NJ: Lawrence Erlbaum.

McNeill, D. (1970). *The acquisition of language.* New York: Harper & Row.

Miller, J. (1981). *Experimental procedures: Assessing language production in children.* Baltimore: University Park Press.

Molfese, D. L. (1990). Auditory evoked responses recorded from 16-month-old infants to words they did and did not know. *Brain and Language, 38,* 345–363.

Oller, D. (1980). The emergence of speech sounds in infancy. In G. Yeni-Komshian, J. Kavanaugh, & C. Ferguson (Eds.), *Child phonology. Vol. 1: Production.* New York: Academic Press.

Piaget, J. (1963). *The origins of intelligence in children.* New York: Norton.

Pinker, S. (1984). *Language learnability and language development.* Cambridge, MA: Harvard University Press.

Plante, E., Ramage, A., Maglöire, J. (2006). Processing narratives for verbatim and gist information by adults with language learning disabilities: A functional neuroimaging study. *Learning Disabilities Research and Practice, 21,* 61–76.

Plante, E., Schmithorst, V. J., Holland, S. K., & Byars, A. W. (2006). Sex differences in the activation of language cortex during childhood. *Neuropsychologia, 44,* 1210–1221.

Raikes, H., Luze, G., Brooks-Gunn, J., Raikes, A. H., Pan, B. A., Tamis-LeMonda, C. S., Constantine, J., Tarullo, L. B., Rodriguez, E. T. (2006). Mother-child bookreading in low-income families: Correlates and outcomes during the first three years of life. *Child Development, 77,* 924–953.

Rosen, H. J., Petersen, S. E., Linenweber, M. R., Snyder, A. Z., White, D. A., Chapman, L., Dromerick, A. W., Fiez, J. A., & Corbetta, M. D. (2000). Neural correlates of recovery from aphasia after damage to left inferior frontal cortex. *Neurology, 55,* 1883–1894.

Searle, B. (1969). *Speech acts.* London: Cambridge University Press.

Shaywitz, B. A., Shaywitz, S. E., Pugh, K. R., Fulbright, R. K., Skudlarski, P., Mencl, W. E., Constable, T., Marchione, K. E., Fletcher, J. M., Klorman, R., Lacadie, C., & Gore, J. C. (2001). The functional neural architecture of components of attention in language-processing tasks. *NeuroImage, 13,* 601–612.

Skinner, B. F. (1957). *Verbal behavior.* New York: Appleton-Century-Crofts.

Watson, B. B. (1970). *Behaviorism.* New York: Norton.

Weigel, D. J., Martin, S. S., & Bennett, K. K. (2006). Mothers' literacy beliefs: Connections with the home literacy environment and pre-school children's literacy development. *Journal of Early Childhood Literacy, 6,* 191–211.

# CHAPTER EIGHT

# DISORDERS OF LANGUAGE
# IN CHILDREN

## PREVIEW

When normal language acquisition is impeded because of a developmental disorder or childhood illness, language may become impaired. Language disorders in children may occur secondary to illness or injury, but they often arise without an identifiable cause. For the young child, impaired oral language may interfere with the ability to express needs or understand what others say. As children progress through school, weak language skills may also impact reading, writing, and academic success. Because developmental language disorders result from a variety of causes and are associated with diverse skill profiles, assessment and intervention methods are tailored to the needs of the individual child.

As we discussed in Chapters 3 and 7, the development of language follows a fairly predictable sequence. Infants begin with an awareness of sound and quickly develop a preference for the sounds and patterns of their native language(s). Sounds, first produced reflexively, are soon produced intentionally and take on the characteristics of speech. Across cultures and languages, first words appear around the child's first birthday. By age 2, most children know many words and are combining them into short phrases. By age 4, children sound remarkably adultlike in their spoken language.

Not all children experience normal language acquisition. Language disorders may affect up to 13 percent of children (Tomblin, Records, & Zhang, 1996). A variety of conditions may lead to a language disorder. Genetic conditions may disturb the development of the brain and alter its capacity for normal language development. The presence of a hearing impairment can have a profound effect on language development. Injury or illness can arrest language development after a period of normal development. Finally, there is a wide variety of developmental syndromes that include impaired language as part of the presenting signs.

Although many conditions can lead to a language disorder, the types of skills affected may vary considerably. A language disorder includes any impairment of the ability to understand or use language—when compared to same-age peers of the same community. Severity can vary widely among types of language disorders and even among children who are identified as having the same type of language disorder. Language disorders can affect language in any modality, spoken, written, or signed. In fact, it is often the case (although there are exceptions) that multiple modalities are affected when language is impaired. A language disorder is often first suspected because the child's language development lags behind the expected norms for children of the same age. Because age-expected language skills expand as the child grows, the nature of the language disorder may change too. For example, language impairment will not affect reading until the child has reached an age at which reading skills would be expected. Finally, language form, content, and use all vary from region to region and culture to culture. Therefore, language disorders must be distinguished from these regional and culturally derived language differences.

## LANGUAGE DIFFERENCES

There are children from particular cultural and social groups whose speech may differ in some respect from standard English. However, these differences do not, in themselves, constitute a language disorder. Such children have learned the language code of their community and may be quite competent in their use of the native language.

Some linguistic variation reflects regional differences in language, known as dialects. We recognize dialectal differences in the way certain sounds are produced in the Northeast and the Deep South and the Midwest. Other differences may affect the choices of words that are used within a region. Carbonated drinks may be "soda" in one region and "pop" in another. Large-scale sandwiches on long rolls are "submarines," "hoagies," or "po' boys" depending on the region. Dialects can vary with social or cultural groups within a particular region. Communities with strong Hispanic roots may use a variant of English that includes influences from Spanish. Residents of both inner cities and rural districts may speak one or more versions of a dialect known as Black English (sometimes called Ebonics). Although these dialects are culturally influenced, speakers do not necessarily have to be members of the particular minority group to speak the dialect. Furthermore, any given speaker of a dialect may not use it at all times. Social rules may dictate when a dialect, or even which variant of a dialect, is appropriate to the situation. Thus, an individual who uses one version of Black English among friends may use another with parents and switch to Standard American English when addressing a teacher. This situational shifting of speech and language patterns is referred to as **code switching**.

The variations in language *form* observed in dialects are rule governed, meaning that there are strict conventions that dictate correct use of these forms. However, for the listener who is unfamiliar with the conventions of a dialect, it may seem as if the speaker is making linguistic errors. For example, residents of Maryland may "go down the shore for the weekend," omitting the preposition "to" that speakers in other parts of the country would typically use in that sentence. Forms of Black English may include omissions of certain grammatical forms (e.g., the contracted "is" or "are"; the infinitive "to") and changes in grammatical form (e.g., "hisself" for "himself"; "be" for "has been [continually]") in certain sentence contexts. These are normal forms within some versions of this dialect. However, not all speakers of Black English and other dialects use all the linguistic or pragmatic elements associated with the dialect. For example, Washington and Craig (1994) reported that young children within the same region may vary in their frequency and types of Black English forms in their speech. Speech-language pathologists must be able to distinguish between linguistic variation that reflects a dialect and variation that signals a disorder and to treat those aspects that are attributable to the disorder alone. However, if a dialect speaker who shows no sign of a language disorder wishes to improve his or her use of Standard American English, a speech-language pathologist may provide such assistance (ASHA, 1983).

Children who speak more than one language may also show language content differences that may be mistaken for a disorder. For example, the Navajo child in northeastern Arizona may be bilingual, using Navajo at home and English at school. Vocabulary development in each language may be restricted to the environment in which it is used. For example, the child may know the Navajo word for *grasshopper* but not the English word. Likewise, the child may know the English word but not the Navajo word for it. These children may appear to have limited lexical knowledge, when tested in only one of their languages, but often have a large and rich vocabulary when both languages are considered. Furthermore, if a Navajo child moves to Los Angeles, his or her language use might be judged faulty by the non-Navajo listeners in the new city. Children in many parts of the world are multilingual, using a particular language for a specific situation. For most children, learning two or more languages (or dialects) in the preschool years is relatively easy, given adequate experience with those languages. Some children, however, are unable to use any of the languages of their community proficiently.

## EARLY SIGNS OF A LANGUAGE DISORDER

### Infants at Risk

Some infants are born with genetic conditions, illnesses, or disabilities that interfere with their development (Clark, 1994; Sparks, 1984). In Chapter 11, we will see that a great many genetic and acquired conditions may affect hearing and consequently alter the course of language development. Many other conditions, such as drug exposure (Johnson, Seikel, Madison, Foose, & Rinard, 1997), infection (Bent & Beck, 1994), low birth weight, and premature birth (Byrne, Ellsworth, Bowering, & Vincer, 1993), increase the risk that a child will experience language and learning difficulties. In some cases, prolonged serious illness itself may interfere with language development. Infants who require hospitalization will not receive the same stimulation from their parents as healthy babies. Infants who are confined to a hospital nursery will have limited opportunities to explore and interact with the people and objects around them. Other infants have physical disabilities that interfere with normal development, including speech and language development.

A speech-language pathologist may work with an infant's family and the hospital staff to provide experiences that facilitate language development. In these cases, speech and language intervention often must be integrated with medical treatments, physical therapy, and occupational therapy. The speech-language pathologist and audiologist are members of a multidisciplinary team, which may also include medical staff, rehabilitation staff, and social services. The team works closely with the infant's family to ensure understanding of the child's needs and the best ways to address them. When a child is born with an obvious disability, parent counseling and intervention for the child can begin right away. However, the impact pact of prematurity on language and academic disorders can appear years later as the child develops (e.g., Halsey, Collin, & Anderson, 1996). Therefore, parents and professionals may need to monitor progress throughout childhood.

## Late Talkers

One group of children at risk for language disorders is toddlers who lag behind their peers in the ability to understand or produce words. These children have been referred to as "late talkers." In the research literature, late talkers are typically defined as young children (between approximately 16 and 30 months) whose language skills fall below 90 percent of their same-age peers. These children are slow to acquire their first 50 words and slow to combine words into phrases. For example, Rescorla, Roberts, and Dahlsgaard (1997) reported their group of late talkers had an average of 20 words at age 26 months, compared with their normal peers who had an average of 226 words. Furthermore, only one of thirty-four late talkers was combining words into phrases. The parents of late-talking toddlers may also report that their children seem to understand fewer words than would be expected for their age. These children lack a history of hearing loss, cognitive impairment, or medical factors that would otherwise place them at risk for poor language development.

Investigators who have followed the development of late-talking children have demonstrated that these children are at risk for continued language problems. Toddlers who are identified as late talkers tend to remain behind their peers over time (Rescorla et al., 1997; Thal, Bates, Goodman, & Jahn-Samilo, 1997). However, what is true for the group is not necessarily true for all its members. In fact, some late talkers do "catch up" with their peers (Ellis Weismer, Murray-Branch, & Miller, 1994; Rescorla et al., 1997; Thal et al., 1997). Some studies have suggested factors that may predict language outcome, including poor comprehension skills (Thal & Tobias, 1992), limited use of gestures for communication (Thal et al., 1997; Thal & Tobias, 1992), limited vocabulary (Fischel, Whitehurst, Caulfield, & Debaryshe, 1979; Thal et al., 1997), and initial overall severity (Rescorla et al., 1997; Rescorla & Schwartz, 1990). In addition, the age at which a child is identified as a late talker also appears to be predictive, with the young late talkers faring better than older ones (Paul, 1993; Rescorla & Schwartz, 1990; Thal et al., 1997). However, there is currently no clear consensus concerning what early factors or signs might predict which children prove to be "late bloomers" and which ones will continue to experience language difficulty.

Late-talking toddlers are typically first identified by their impoverished vocabularies. For those late talkers who do not move into the normal range, a variety of signs of a language disorder emerge over time. Even those who do catch up with their peers in terms of vocabulary may continue to be at risk for other, later-appearing language impairments. As we saw in Chapter 7, normally developing children acquire a corpus of single-word utterances that they then begin to combine into two-word utterances. From this point, children lengthen their phrases and eventually begin to produce more complex sentences. By age 3 or 4, many children who were late-talking toddlers moved into the normal range for vocabulary skills (Rescorla et al., 1997). However, these same children produced much shorter and morphologically and syntactically simpler phrases than their normally developing peers (Paul & Alforde, 1993; Rescorla et al., 1997). Kindergarten children who were late talkers were less proficient in relating a story in logical order than their normally developing peers (Paul, Hernandez, Taylor, & Johnson, 1996). By second grade, these children appeared to have caught up in terms of narrative ability. However, there were still other differences in expressive language skills between this late-talking group and their peers (Paul, Murray, Clancy, & Andrews, 1997).

These studies demonstrate that long-term difficulty with language can be associated with late-talking status as a toddler. We also saw that not all late-talking toddlers have a poor language outcome. However, despite our imperfect ability to predict outcome, status as a "late talker" is sufficient to indicate risk for language disorder. The long-term risk warrants close monitoring of late-talking children so that those who go on to show clear signs of a language disorder may receive the earliest possible intervention (Thal et al., 1997).

## DEVELOPMENTAL LANGUAGE DISORDERS

For many children with language problems, there is no obvious cause for the impairment. They do not have the physical characteristics that would signal the presence of a developmental syndrome. They hear normally and lack any sign of brain damage or disease that might lead to impaired language, but their language skills lag behind those of their peers. These children are said to have a **developmental language disorder**.

*Developmental language disorder* is actually an umbrella term that encompasses children with a wide range of language-related problems. Although the exact cause of these disorders is unknown, parents are often relieved to know that it does not appear to be related to child-rearing practices or the way they have talked to their child. Instead, the underlying cause appears to be biological. Current information suggests that the brains of language-disordered children develop differently than those of most people (Cohen, Campbell, & Yaghmai, 1989; Gauger, Lombardino, & Leonard, 1997; Plante, Swisher, Vance, & Rapcsak, 1991). This altered brain development may underlie altered language development. Evidence of altered brain anatomy can also be found among the parents and siblings of these children (Jackson & Plante, 1997; Plante, 1991). Likewise, when one member of the family has a developmental language disorder, it is common that others do also (Tallal, Ross, & Curtiss, 1989; Tomblin, 1989). The fact that both the biological and behavioral aspects of this disorder tend to cluster in families is consistent with a genetic contribution to the disorder (Bishop, Laws, Adams, & Norbury, 2006; O'Brien, Zhang, Nishimura, & Tomblin, 2003; SLI Consortium, 2002).

Children may have developmental problems with receptive language, expressive language, or both. Language deficits may encompass any or all of the components of language *form, content,* or *use* (see Chapter 7 for a review), and an individual child's language difficulties may change over time. When language deficits occur in the absence of other handicapping conditions (e.g., cognitive, motor, sensory, emotional), the child is said to have a **specific language impairment**. To understand this disorder, let us look at the development of one child diagnosed with specific language impairment.

> *Troy* had difficulty with communication from a very early age. He was reportedly about 20 months of age before he used his first word. His parents became concerned when, at age 2, he used few words, communicating instead largely by grunting and pointing. Despite his limited expression, both parents felt that he understood speech well for his age. Troy's pediatrician also noticed his slow language development and arranged for him to be evaluated by a speech-language pathologist.
>
> During his initial evaluation, Troy passed a hearing screening. His parents completed a questionnaire that surveyed cognitive, motor, self-help, and social skills. Their responses placed him well within normal limits for each of these areas. Troy was then given a formal evaluation of language skills that involved a series of simple activities to test receptive and expressive skills. He correctly pointed to pictures and followed simple commands appropriate for his age. Test scores for receptive language confirmed relatively normal skills for his age. In contrast, his expressive score placed him in the first percentile, or below 99 percent of other children his age. He had great difficulty naming pictures and imitating words on request. He often used the same "word," /da/, to refer to a variety of pictures and objects. In addition, Troy had a limited number of sounds that he used spontaneously, relying mostly on stop consonant-vowel combinations in the words he attempted.

In Troy's case, early deficits involved vocabulary and phonology. These delayed communication skills were present despite the fact that he was developing normally in other areas. As we saw in our discussion of late talkers, such delay is a risk factor for a developmental language disorder. However, not all children with a developmental language disorder are noticeably different from other children at this young age. For some, the first words emerge right on schedule for normal development, and the disorder only becomes apparent as the child fails to progress from words to sentences.

> Troy was enrolled in a preschool program for children with specific language impairment at age 3. His parents reported remarkable improvement from that time forward. In addition to his preschool class, his parents implemented a home program of language stimulation. This involved techniques for introducing new vocabulary and encouraging him to produce longer utterances. Troy's vocabulary expanded rapidly from 14 words to well over 100 words in five months. His phonological repertoire also expanded, so that he was producing many more of the sounds appropriate for his age. At age 3, he was occasionally combining words to

form two-word utterances as well. His mother reported that Troy was showing fewer signs of frustration in his attempts to communicate and that people outside of the family were having much less difficulty understanding his speech.

At age 4, Troy was using many two- and three-word phrases, with an occasional four-word phrase in spontaneous speech. However, he used few grammatical morphemes (e.g., verb tense markers, prepositions), which is unusual for a child his age. At age 4 years, 7 months, the following conversation was recorded while he played with a toy fire station:

TROY:  This the fireperson. This the bell. (Indicating the fire alarm)

MOTHER:  Does the bell ring in an emergency?

TROY:  No. The bell, it has . . . the car come out.

MOTHER:  The cars come out when the bell rings?

TROY:  (Nods) The telephone do that too!

Not surprisingly, formal tests documented below-normal expressive language skills at this time, including morphology and syntax. Although language form was still delayed, Troy showed marked improvement in language content and use. He spoke readily in a variety of contexts and was able to use language for a variety of purposes (e.g., requesting, explaining, directing).

This pattern of differential impairment across language domains is fairly common for children with specific language impairment during the preschool years. In Troy's case, we observed a shift from the initial vocabulary deficit, which was apparent at age 2, to morphosyntactic deficits at age 4. This phenomenon is known as "growing into a deficit." We did not see morphosyntactic deficits early on, simply because English-speaking children do not use syntax or morphology until words are combined into phrases. Therefore, we had to wait until Troy reached a developmental stage where these skills could be expected before determining whether they were impaired.

Children with early language disorders may ultimately achieve parity with their normally developing peers. For some, this marks the end of their language difficulties. However, for others, this period of normal language is temporary and is referred to as a period of "illusory recovery" (Scarborough & Dobrich, 1990). Children who appear to recover may once again fall behind their peers as they progress through grade school. Still other children with early language problems continue to show signs of language deficits as they enter the school years. We saw this pattern with Troy.

Troy's speech and language skills were reevaluated by the school speech-language pathologist when he entered first grade at 5 years, 9 months. At that time, his early problems with phonology were almost completely resolved. His speech could be easily understood. The only remaining speech errors were occasional mispronunciations in conversation, and these involved only the late-acquired sounds of speech (see Chapter 3). However, his conversations consisted primarily of short, simple sentences. He continued to have difficulty with grammatical morphemes, making substitutions like "the paint guy" for "pain*ter*" and "the more big one" for "big*ger*" or omissions like "He run" for "He run*s*." Once again, formal testing documented poor language expression despite good overall comprehension. Both receptive and expressive vocabulary remained strong.

The school speech-language pathologist continued to see Troy twice a week to work on morphology. She also coordinated activities with the classroom teacher and Troy's parents to reinforce correct use of the morphological items that Troy was learning. This intervention was quite successful, and by the middle of second grade Troy's conversational speech no longer contained obvious morphological errors. He was retested at this time because the school was considering his dismissal from therapy. His standardized test scores continued to indicate that his expressive language skills lagged behind his peers. However, because he was keeping up in the classroom and was doing well socially, it appeared that his weak expressive language skills were not a handicapping factor at this time. The school decided to monitor his progress but discontinue direct services.

The school staff's decision to discontinue services for Troy is consistent with their mandate to provide services to children with *educationally handicapping conditions.* The public law (P.L. 94–142) that first mandated services in 1975 guaranteed a free and appropriate education for all children with educationally handicapping conditions. Speech and language disorders are among the disorders covered under this law, and subsequent legislation (e.g., P.L. 99–457 IDEA; Individuals With Disabilities Education Improvement Act of 2004; see also Chapter 11). Because Troy was functioning well in the educational system, the school staff decided he was best served in the regular classroom with monitoring and consultative support by the speech-language pathologist. For Troy, this educational plan places him in the *least restrictive environment* in which he is capable of functioning.

Other children with more serious handicaps may require greater educational support. This may include "pullout" services, in which the child leaves the classroom for brief periods of direct therapy, placement in special classrooms within the regular school, or even placement in specialized schools for severely handicapped children. Each of these modes of intervention involves increasing restrictions on the child's environment, because less time is spent with normally developing peers. The type and frequency of service each child receives may change over the years as the degree to which the child's disorder impacts educational progress changes. Where and how the child receives services is determined by a multidisciplinary team that includes parents, teachers, therapists, and others who can provide insight into a particular child's learning difficulties. This team develops an *individualized educational plan* (IEP) that specifies the level of services, who will provide the services, and what the goals will be.

Three years later, at age 10, Troy's skills were reevaluated. This testing session revealed a further evolution in his language profile. Up to this time, his comprehension test scores had always been a relative strength compared with his expressive scores. However, at age 10, his comprehension scores now fell below average. The appearance of comprehension deficits during the school years can be accounted for in part by the fact expectations for understanding language change between the ages of 7 and 10 years of age. For example, older children are expected to be able to follow complex and multistage directions and to be able to follow the plot of a story that may have multiple subplots. In school, children are expected to perform multiple language tasks simultaneously: listening to a lecture, extracting the principle concepts, and encoding them as written notes. Comprehension becomes a learning tool, not just in listening but also in reading. It is sometimes the case that a child's limitations in the receptive domain become apparent only when the demands increase to the point where the deficits emerge.

Troy's poor language comprehension was still apparent during his teen years. In fact, by age 14, his expressive language skills were slightly better than his receptive skills. However, he continued to show problems with expressive language as well. We no longer see the same types of expressive problems that characterized his spoken language at earlier ages. Troy no longer omits grammatical morphemes, for example. The effectiveness of his oral communication remains compromised. Consider Troy's attempt to relate the plot of a movie during a conversation, recorded when he was 12 years old:

> It was hilarious. He didn't put the . . . um . . . "owies." He only put the best "owie." No, that was the second best "owie." The first was when the rope that he went down was soaked in some kind of thing . . . that it makes fire go on . . . makes it go faster and they were on the rope and say "Hey Harry, are you there?" No, that's Clorox, or something like that. (Speaks for a movie character.) "Oh guys." (Sound effect of guys falling). "Get up! Get up!" (Sound effect of guys yelling and hand gestures.) Then there's like a bridge and they fall right through and they get covered with all kinds of . . . sticky stuff.

We can see a number of problems in this short sample. First, the story he is telling lacks the structure of a identifiable beginning, middle, and end. Characters are referred to without first being introduced to the listener (e.g., He didn't put the . . . um . . . "owies"). We hear pauses and revisions throughout. In addition, the use of sound effects and gestures suggests that Troy may have been having difficulty retrieving specific words to communicate his thoughts.

The ability to organize and sequence verbal information becomes increasingly important as a child progresses through school. In fact, Troy's written work showed many of the same characteristics that we saw in the verbal sample above. In addition, he often made the same morphological errors in written language that we saw in his spoken language at age 5. For example, at age 12 he wrote:

> Mom caned the riped vejedetables.
>
> I don't wan't any.
>
> But the two dog eat it.

At this point, Troy's language difficulties were still interfering with his academic progress. His reading was slow, and he did not always glean as much meaning from reading as he should. His writing was messy, with many spelling errors,

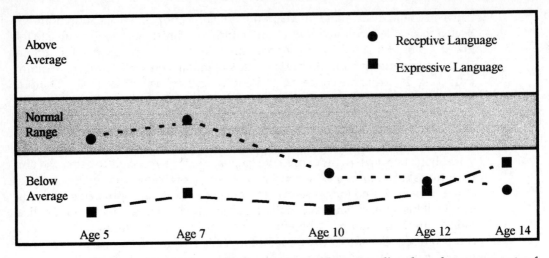

**FIGURE 8.1    For children with developmental language disorders, the components of language can change over time. Here we can see receptive and expressive language skills shift over time in a single child (Troy) relative to typically developing peers.**

and the flow of thoughts did not always follow a logical sequence. Because his weak language skills were having the greatest impact on educational skills, the school staff considered providing services for a **learning disability**. Children with learning disabilities often have difficulties in listening, speaking, reading, or writing. Their poor language skills can hold them back in any academic subject in which language is used as a tool for learning or problem solving.

The long-term outcome of children with developmental language disorders is quite variable (see Figure 8.1). Some will overcome the handicap of an early language disorder. Others may struggle with language in either the oral or written modalities for years. Even as adults, individuals with a history of language therapy may still show subtle, residual deficits on standardized measures (Tomblin, Records, & Freese, 1992). However, these language difficulties may or may not prove handicapping in the individual's everyday life. In fact, adults with a childhood history of language disorders appear no less satisfied with their quality of life than those without such a childhood history (Records, Tomblin, & Freese, 1992).

## READING IMPAIRMENTS

Reading and writing require a child to transfer what he or she already understands about oral language to visual and manual modalities. In Chapter 7, we saw the importance of two skills, phonological decoding and language comprehension, for developing reading competence. Here we consider two boys, both in second grade, who are having difficulty learning to read.

*Jimmy* had been receiving services targeting language and phonology since he was 4 years of age. He was now in second grade, and his mother had concerns about his reading ability. She had approached the school about her concerns when Jimmy was in first grade but had been assured that different children learn to read at different times and Jimmy would catch on in his own time. The speech-language pathologist, Therese, agreed to listen to Jimmy read. She selected some short stories at different reading levels. When Jimmy came into her room, she passed the easiest story to him. He looked quickly at it and immediately announced he didn't want that one. He picked up another and put it down again, saying maybe they should read later. Jimmy's attempt to get the third story was abandoned when Therese pointed out that it was even longer, and had no pictures besides. Jimmy reluctantly took the easiest story and then announced he "didn't know any of those words." Therese offered to read the story with him. In the title, he read the word "the" without sounding it out, but then stopped completely. Therese asked what the next word started with and Jimmy responded "B." Therese then asked what sound that made, and Jimmy responded that he didn't know. When Therese made the /b/ sound, Jimmy responded "oh yeah!" Therese then pointed to the picture to see if Jimmy could find something that might correspond to that sound. Jimmy guessed "dog." As they progressed through the title and first sentence, Jimmy never got past the first sound of any word. Furthermore, by the time he got to the last word, he had forgotten so much that he couldn't repeat the sentence they had "read together."

Jimmy demonstrates several traits that predict the occurrence of reading problems. First is his history of speech and language difficulties. Children with early language impairment are at an increased risk for later reading problems (Botting, Simkin, & Conti-Ramsden, 2006; Snowling, Bishop, & Stothard, 2000). Next, Jimmy appears to know the names of letters, but has a weak grasp on what sounds the letters make. This undermines his ability to use phonological decoding as a reading strategy. Not only is he not sounding out the letters that make up words, but he is unable to link letter sounds to corresponding pictures (e.g., /b/ with the picture of a boy). Therefore, he is not able to use the pictures to support his decoding of the text. Furthermore, his reading is so labored because of his lack of decoding skills and the very few words he knows by sight, he does not build up any comprehension of the text already read. This breakdown of comprehension, a major predictor of reading proficiency along with decoding, is a consequence of poor decoding. In fact, his comprehension of conversational language is much better than he displayed when attempting to read. However, his overall weak language skills may eventually interfere with reading comprehension when he encounters more complex reading matter. Finally, we see in Jimmy a boy who is already actively trying to avoid reading. He is well aware of his problems at this point, and also knows that others in his class are not struggling as he is. Furthermore, he is only a year away of having to start reading to gain knowledge in classes like social studies or to solve word problems in math. Because of this, the speech-language pathologist recommended that reading goals be added to his education plan. She will work with the school's reading specialist and the classroom teacher to strengthen his decoding skills beginning with linking letters to the sounds they make rather than just to their letter names. This skill is referred to as knowledge of **sound–symbol correspondence**. Along with this skill, intervention will include sounding out and blending the sounds in printed words along with building a core of sight words that occur frequently in text. These sight words provide a means of offering quick success for reading without having to sound out every word. Finally, Jimmy will be encouraged to use story pictures to help his comprehension of printed text.

> *Carlos* was another child who was on Therese's caseload. He had been diagnosed with specific language impairment. Therese was working in Carlos's class one day when he was asked to read aloud to his reading group. He proceeded to read the story from the title to "the end." The only things Therese noted was that he read relatively fast, and his intonation was somewhat flat, possibly because of his rapid reading rate. He mispronounced only two words (*gray* was pronounced as "grew," *try* was prounounced as "tie"), and he pronounced two words as if he was working out the sound at first (e.g., ssllled). Otherwise, his oral reading was error free. But when Therese asked questions about the story, which involved a boy who found a way to sneak out of the house to go sledding, Carlos recalled a plot that involved a boy who didn't want to go sledding and other major deviations from the actual meaning of the text. It was almost as if Carlos remembered key vocabulary words (e.g., boy, sledding) and then reconstructed a story that worked for those words.

Carlos showed indications that he was actively decoding words because he paused to sound out words on occasion. His strong decoding skills allowed him to build an impressive sight vocabulary over time. However, Carlos's reading illustrates a case where phonological decoding is strong, but reading comprehension is poor nonetheless. Such children are referred to as "poor comprehenders." The speech-language pathologist's job then becomes to discover why comprehension is poor. Some children may have a poor understanding of word meanings such that they do not build comprehension as a story is read. Others may have more complex comprehension problems that involve multiple components of language content and form. Reading intervention will address the specific reasons for an individual child's comprehension difficulty. Intervention for a child like Carlos, therefore, would take an entirely different form than that for a child like Jimmy.

Reading disorders in children can take a variety of forms. Perhaps the most well known reading disorder is **dyslexia**, sometimes also called *specific reading disability*. Dyslexia is diagnosed when children's poor word reading appears to be caused by especially poor phonological decoding. As with Jimmy, reading comprehension can also be poor because poor decoding skills interferes with the child's ability to appreciate the meaning of what is eventually decoded. In contrast, comprehension of spoken language is relatively good for these children.

Dyslexia may be contrasted with other forms of reading disability. For example, a child may experience difficulty learning to read because he or she has another type of developmental disorder, such as mental retardation. One of the most commonly occurring conditions associated with reading problems is specific language impairment. Many, but not all, children with specific language impairment struggle with reading as well. However, dyslexia and specific language impairment are thought to constitute separate disorders, even though they sometimes co-occur (Bishop & Snowling, 2004; Catts, Adlof, Hogan, & Ellis Weismer, 2005). Children with dyslexia, with or without specific language impairment, appear to have worse phonological skills than children with specific language impairment alone (Catts et al., 2005), whereas children with specific language impairment appear to have language deficits that are broader in nature (Bishop & Snowling, 2004). For children with specific language impairment, these broader language skills, including oral language comprehension and early phonological skills, predict reading outcome by the end of grade school (Botting et al., 2006). Like Carlos, children with specific language impairment may evidence a lack of reading comprehension when they retell the stories they read (Gillam & Carlile, 1997). Although a phonological approach to reading remediation may be effective for improving reading for children with specific language impairment (Gillon, 2002), they may also require additional support to improve reading comprehension.

For some children, oral reading seems completely divorced from reading comprehension. These children can read aloud but show no understanding of what they read. In these cases, children seem to "crack the phonological code" of written language without formal instruction. This phenomenon is known as **hyperlexia**. Hyperlexia often occurs in the context of a broader disorder such as autism or pervasive developmental disorder. Unfortunately, for the child with hyperlexia, what appears to be advanced reading ability is not actually functional for the child, because reading comprehension is very poor or absent.

## OTHER DISORDERS THAT IMPACT LANGUAGE

Children experience difficulty with language for a variety of reasons. In the 1950s, the audiologist and speech-language pathologist tended to emphasize the cause, or etiology, of the child's language disorder. With the growth of behavioral and operant psychology in the 1960s, however, emphasis switched from etiology *per se* to changing the child's behavior regardless of etiology. However, knowledge of etiology presents at least two primary advantages. The first is being able to address parents' desires to know why their child has a disorder (Aram, 1991). The second involves clinical management. The initial diagnosis can serve to orient the clinician to the likely behavioral strengths and weaknesses. Given a diagnosis of seizure disorder, for example, a clinician is alerted by the diagnostic category to examine receptive language skills. A diagnosis of dyslexia would signal a need to examine the impact of language on reading abilities. Although the diagnostic label does not predict with 100 percent accuracy an individual's profile, it can alert the clinician to what the most salient problems may be. Let us take a look at a small selection of the many conditions associated with impaired language to see how language may vary with different developmental conditions.

## Attention Deficit Disorder

Children with attention deficit disorder (ADD) are characterized by inattention and impulsivity. Hyperactivity occurs in a subset of children with ADD. Children with ADD are highly distractible, finding it difficult to focus, sustain their attention, and direct their activities toward the task at hand. These signs occur in the absence of any frank neurological deficit or acquired disorder. Parents often report that the first signs appear in the preschool years, although children may not be referred for services until their difficulties cause them problems in school. Problems with attention and impulse control are a significant handicap in the classroom, interfering with the ability to listen to directions and complete work assignments. It is not surprising, therefore, that most children with ADD have difficulty learning. The signs of ADD can persist throughout the childhood years, with an estimated one-half to two-thirds of individuals continuing to show signs in late adolescence (Claude & Firestone, 1995; McGee, Partridge, Williams, & Silva, 1991).

The distractibility and impulsivity that interfere with school work are equally disruptive in games and conversations. Other children may view the ADD child as a troublemaker who breaks both rules and toys. Children with ADD often interrupt others who are trying to talk, shift from topic to topic without warning, and appear to have general difficulties with the social aspects of language use. Other language problems may be a side effect of inattention. For example, children whose attention fluctuates may miss parts of what is said to them and appear to have a comprehension deficit. A subset of children with ADD also have coexisting speech and language disorders that are independent of attentional problems. For this reason, the American Speech-Language-Hearing Association (ASHA, 1997) recommended that speech-language pathologists and audiologists serve on multidisciplinary teams for the assessment of children with ADD.

The signs of ADD may be managed medically and behaviorally. Stimulant medications help some children by increasing attention and decreasing impulsive and hyperactive behaviors. Medication, even when beneficial, does not cure the disorder. Behavioral intervention is designed to provide the child with strategies for staying on task and minimizing the effects of ADD in his or her daily life. Some intervention techniques involve modifying the child's environment by providing routine and structure to support on-task behaviors. Rewards or recognition may also be effective in promoting appropriate behaviors. For older children, helping them develop plans for monitoring their own conduct may be effective.

## Autism

The term *autism* describes a developmental disorder that profoundly affects the child's interactions with other people and with the world. The earliest signs of the disorder include disturbed social interaction between the infant and its parents. Even as infants, these children do not seem to bond with or take comfort from others. They may seem content watching the movements of their hands or performing repetitive actions. Delayed development of language skills, as well as little use of language for play or social interactions, is typically noted. We can see the classic signs of autism in the following case:

> *Ben* was 4 years old when his pediatrician urged his parents to have him evaluated. The pediatrician noted that Ben used few words and seemed to interact with the world in an odd way. The pediatrician suspected Ben had autism. His parents took him to a university-affiliated center that specialized in the diagnosis and treatment of children with autism. The center used an integrated team approach to diagnosis, which involved a speech-language pathologist, a psychologist, and a psychiatrist. Ben and his mother were met in the waiting room by all three of these individuals, who began by talking with the mother and observing Ben. Ben had taken a train engine from the play area, which he had turned over and was slowly rolling the wheels back and forth with his finger. His mother reported that he often "plays" with toys in this repetitive manner, without using them for their actual purpose or in an imaginative way. Moreover, she reported that she often has to "tear him away" from whatever he is interested in, which was also the case today when it was time to proceed back to an exam room. Ben became quite upset but did not attempt to communicate this in words. He also did not greet any of the other adults present or interact with them when spoken to or offered toys. He did not look at the adults except fleetingly and did not look at objects with them (known as maintaining joint attention). Instead he took toys he was interested in off to the side of the room. His sole interactions with his mother involved prompting her to do things for him or grabbing her hand to make her pick up objects he could easily reach himself. His only words were repetitions of single words spoken by others (called *echolalia*). The diagnostic team agreed that the lack of social interaction, very limited language, and repetitive and restricted play all indicated that he indeed had autism. They recommended enrolling him in a therapy program that would address communication, provide behavioral management of difficult behaviors (e.g., tantrums and eating problems reported by the mother), and provide opportunities to learn group play. The mother was also given information about a local support group for families with autism so that Ben's family could meet others who were raising an autistic child.

As children with autism grow, other aspects of disturbed communication become apparent. Some of these children acquire some early language skills, only to lose them during the preschool years. For others, language development is disturbed from the start. Dunn (1997) reviewed the characteristics of autistic language, which can include deficits in language form, content, and use. Common characteristics include poor language comprehension and poor pragmatic skills. In more severe forms of the disorder, expressive language characteristics may become more apparent. A complete lack of speech, or mutism, is most likely to occur when the signs of autism are most severe (Miranda-Linne & Merlin, 1997).

The language signs most typical of this disorder involve disturbances of language *use*. Individuals with autism frequently have disturbed prosody in spoken language. They may repeat the words of others or use stereotyped speech routines rather than the context-appropriate, original utterances of normally developing children. For example, one child repeated the phrase "want juice please" over and over again as he spun in a circle. However, this was not an actual request for juice, but continued use of a phrase beyond the setting in which it was appropriate. The bizarre elements of communication in individuals with autism also extend to non-verbal pragmatics. For example, children with autism often have a flat facial affect, aberrant patterns of attention to people and objects, and abnormal gaze during conversations (Lord & Pickles, 1996; Shields, Varley, Broks, & Simpson, 1996).

A majority of children with autism fall into the mentally retarded range of intellectual functioning. However, not all cognitive domains are equally affected. Minshew, Goldstein, and Siegel (1997) tested autistic individuals whose IQ scores fell within normal limits (although many were at the low end of average) and found that these individuals' greatest deficits involved the ability to handle complex information processing in many forms (e.g., high-level language tasks, complex memory). Simple information processing and visual-spatial memory were relatively spared.

The bizarre social interactions of these children led early investigators to hypothesize that autism was the product of uncaring parents who failed to provide the emotional support children require (Kanner & Eisenberg, 1955). Later, more biological explanations of the disorder were offered (e.g., Rimland, 1964). Today, we have evidence of abnormal brain development in autistic individuals (e.g., Courchesne, Yeung-Courchesne, Press, Hesselink, & Jernigan, 1988) and preliminary evidence of a genetic role in the disorder (Petit et al., 1995).

## Mental Retardation

Language is complex and depends, in part, on other cognitive and social-adaptive skills. Children who are delayed in all aspects of development are frequently also delayed in the acquisition of language skills. The **Diagnostic and Statistical Manual of Mental Disorders** (DSM-IV; APA, 1994) defines **mental retardation** by an intelligence quotient (IQ) of less than 70 on a standardized IQ measure along with significant deficits in adaptive functioning. Even when IQ is low, an individual who shows no difficulty functioning in everyday life would not be considered to have mental retardation. The degree of mental retardation can vary considerably. DSM-IV recognizes four broad severity levels: mild, moderate, severe, and profound, which reflect a range from individuals considered "educable" to those few who require lifelong assistance.

There are many developmental conditions associated with mental retardation. Some of these are genetic (e.g., Down syndrome, Noonan syndrome, fragile X syndrome), some are due to exposure to toxins (e.g., fetal alcohol syndrome, lead poisoning), and for others the cause is unknown (idiopathic mental retardation). Given the range of conditions associated with mental retardation, it is not surprising that the language correlates can be quite variable. In general, however, children with mental retardation are typically slow to acquire communication skills. Even at the prelinguistic stage, some toddlers with retardation are less interactive and use fewer nonverbal forms of communication than normally developing children at these ages. The onset of spoken words may occur at a later chronological age.

General language ability in retarded children is sometimes reported to be like that of younger, normally developing children.

As noted, however, this general profile may not apply to all conditions associated with mental retardation. Children with different forms of mental retardation have more difficulty with certain areas of language development than others. For example, some children with Down syndrome appear to have particular problems with syntax and morphology (Stoel-Gammon, 1990). In contrast, children with Williams syndrome are unusually proficient in syntax and morphology, despite having poor semantic skills (Bellugi, Marks, Bihrle, & Sabo, 1988). Children with fragile X syndrome tend to have particular problems with verbal and nonverbal pragmatic skills (Scharfenaker, 1990). Within any group of retarded children, there is much individual variability in the acquisition of language skills. With guidance, children with mental retardation can learn to maximize their communication skills.

## Childhood Aphasia

Children who were developing normally can lose language skills because of brain damage. This acquired language disorder is known as childhood aphasia. Aphasia in children can be caused by the same disease processes that cause adult aphasia (see Chapter 9). These include relatively focal trauma to the head, stroke, infectious disease, and tumors. Also similar to the adult form of aphasia, language deficits typically occur after damage to the left hemisphere of the brain (Aram, Ekelman, Rose, & Whitaker, 1985; Cranberg, Filley, Hart, & Alexander, 1987). We see one such case with Daniel.

*Daniel* was 4½ years old when he began having daily headaches, which were soon accompanied by behavioral problems and vomiting. He was taken to the hospital and received a brain scan. This revealed a large tumor in the temporo-parietal area of his left hemisphere. He was immediately scheduled for surgery to remove the tumor. On the morning following surgery, Daniel was unable to speak and showed signs of weakness on the right side of his body. A second brain scan showed that he had had a stroke, caused by bleeding of the middle cerebral artery, which damaged the language areas of the left hemisphere (see Chapter 2 for a review).

Within days, Daniel began talking again, but his speech and language were not at the level they had been before he was hospitalized. Initially, his speech was slow and effortful, and he drooled intermittently. He had great difficulty attending to what was said and could only follow simple directions. A preschool test of general language abilities indicated low language skills compared with others his age. He had difficulty naming pictures on a vocabulary test. Many times when speaking, he would substitute nonspecific terms or pronouns for specific nouns (e.g., "push thing" for wagon; "the one" for any object). In addition, Daniel had difficulty on a test that required him to produce grammatical sentences to describe pictures. The speech-language pathologist worked with him three times a week until Daniel was released from the hospital. She also arranged to have him enrolled in a preschool program for children with language disorders after he left the hospital.

An estimated 3 in 100,000 children each year experience a stroke (NIDCD, 1991). When the stroke leads to aphasia, children show difficulty comprehending or using spoken language, despite normal intelligence. As in Daniel's case, children may initially be mute following brain damage and, as they recover, begin to show signs of fluent or nonfluent aphasia types (we will look at adult aphasia types in Chapter 9). Children with fluent aphasia may produce sentences with appropriate rate and intonation, but with nonsense words (Van Dongen, Loonen, & Van Dongen, 1985). Nonfluent aphasia is more commonly reported in children. These children use short, simple phrases and sentences. Like Daniel, they omit grammatical morphemes, creating the impression of telegraphic speech. Children may also have difficulty with reading and writing. Because reading, listening, and following directions are frequent school activities, it is not surprising that children with aphasia have academic difficulties (Cranberg et al., 1987). In contrast, appropriate language *use* is often well preserved. Language difficulties may resolve with time, so that the casual listener may be unaware that the child had experienced aphasia. However, language problems can also persist and be documented with standardized testing years after the aphasia first appeared (Vargha-Khadem, O'Gorman, & Watters, 1985; Woods & Carey, 1979).

## Seizure Disorder

Childhood **seizures** can have many different underlying causes or have no known cause at all. For many, a childhood seizure episode may cause considerable concern at the time but have no long-lasting consequences. However, when seizures are severe and persistent, behavioral deficits, including impaired language, may follow. We saw one such case with Anita, who was diagnosed as having aphasia secondary to a convulsive disorder:

> *Anita* had been having seizures since 6 months of age. Management of those seizures included drug therapy and periodic monitoring of brain electrical activity. However, this was only partially successful. Anita spoke her first words at 18 months, and speech-language development had been slow but steady since then. Following a particularly long generalized seizure at age 4, Anita lost her ability to speak, and communication was reduced to slurred sounds and gestures. Although she regained some language skills after that episode, her language remained markedly impaired.
>
> At age 5, Anita was evaluated at a university clinic. She failed to respond to sounds when her hearing was tested and seemed only somewhat aware that people were talking to her. A parent questionnaire revealed a significant delay in all areas of development, including motor, social, and self-help skills. Formal language assessment was discontinued because Anita was unable to maintain attention to the tasks and became frustrated. However, during an hourlong session with her mother, Anita used fewer than 120 words total. Most of her utterances were one or two words in length, and she often used gestures in place of words. Speech was slow and effortful; words were sometimes slurred. Anita established attention very slowly and had difficulty maintaining it. This affected her comprehension, which

was poor overall. Her mother used a number of techniques to facilitate attention and comprehension. She maintained close proximity to her daughter and touched her own lips before speaking to draw Anita's attention. The mother physically directed Anita's attention, first to her face as she spoke and then to the objects under discussion. She used short sentences and many repetitions to support the conversation. Occasionally, Anita echoed those repetitions back to her mother.

As we see in Anita's case, a prolonged period of seizure activity can lead to a deterioration of skills that were once evident. In fact, a change in language status, such as seen here, is a leading sign of an underlying neurological disturbance. For Anita, the seizure activity affected both language comprehension and expression, as well as general functioning in nonverbal domains. In other cases of seizure disorder, receptive language abilities are far more impaired than expressive skills (Rapin, Mattis, Rowan, & Golden, 1977; Worster-Drought, 1971). Receptive abilities can be so severely impaired that the child behaves as if deaf. However, the child can have normal hearing acuity, as established by an audiometric evaluation. No longer able to understand his or her own speech, the child may stop talking altogether, or speech may become garbled. However, language expression can continue if the child is introduced to sign language.

One subtype of seizure disorder is particularly associated with loss of language skills. Landau-Kleffner syndrome was first described as involving loss of language skills in children who had seizures (Landau & Kleffner, 1957). The seizure activity of these children typically involves both temporal lobes and, for some children, is managed with medication. However, the language disorder can persist even after their seizures are brought under control. Recovery of language is quite variable, ranging from a few weeks to many years (Mantovani & Landau, 1980).

## Traumatic Brain Injury

Each year, approximately 200 of every 100,000 children experience a traumatic brain injury (TBI) (NIDCD, 1991). TBI can be focal, due to a penetrating or "open-head" injury (e.g., a gunshot wound), or diffuse, as the result of force applied without penetration of the skull (i.e., a "closed-head" injury). Most commonly, it involves some combination of focal and diffuse injury. TBI can be caused by any number of events, including motor vehicle accidents, in which the injury includes both diffuse damage from the brain moving within the skull and focal contusions where the brain contacts the skull. Other events that can produce a combination of diffuse and focal injury include rough shaking (e.g., shaken baby syndrome), falls, sports injuries, assaults, and pedestrian–motor vehicle collisions.

There is considerable heterogeneity among individuals with TBI. Some of this can be accounted for by differences in the nature and severity of the injury (Chapman, 1997). Other sources of heterogeneity are related to preinjury intelligence, health, and personality, as well as family and cultural factors. Among those at highest risk for severe injury are teenaged males, primarily due to driving accidents. Because of the diffuse nature of the brain damage, the behavioral consequences range far beyond language skills. This is illustrated by the case of Gerard.

> *Gerard* was a 17-year-old high school junior when he had his car accident. He was ditching his afternoon classes with three friends when he lost control of his truck and it went off the road, flipping over several times. The two boys in the back were killed, and a third was paralyzed by the crash. Gerard was in a coma for two weeks with severe head injuries. When he emerged from his coma, cognitive and linguistic deficits were apparent. He was highly distractible and easily overwhelmed by new information or situations. Memory testing indicated that his postinjury abilities were in the fifth percentile, or below the performance of 95 percent of the normative sample for the test. He also had great difficulty understanding both written and spoken language, needing substantial amounts of time to process information and not always arriving at the correct interpretation. In contrast, his spoken language form and content appeared unaffected by his injury.
>
> Gerard's most noticeable communication deficit involved language use. His affect was flat, and he failed to use prosodic variation to convey emotion in his speech. Likewise, he did not seem to pick up on the nonverbal cues of others in conversations. His thinking had a concreteness that did not allow him to interpret jokes or sarcasm. This lack of abstract thinking had pervasive effects on his daily life as well. He was unable to conceptualize the future or plan for it effectively.

Language difficulties after TBI are different from those associated with developmental language disorders. For example, many children with TBI perform comparatively well on standardized tests of vocabulary, morphology, and syntax (Biddle, McCabe, & Bliss, 1996; Chapman et al., 1997; Ylvisaker, 1993). These tests tap knowledge gained prior to the injury. Communication breakdowns are more likely to occur in conversational or discourse contexts (Chapman et al., 1997; Chapman, Levin, Matejeka, Harward, & Kufera, 1995) or on language tasks that place particular demands on attention, information processing, and memory (Turkstra & Holland, 1988). Survivors also may have profoundly handicapping impairments in abilities referred to collectively as executive functions (Ylvisaker, Szekeres, & Feeney, 1998). These functions include the ability to plan and organize behavior, make decisions that take multiple factors into account, and regulate one's own behavior. An important difference between those with TBI and those with developmental language disorders is that individuals with TBI are likely to have had a period of normal development and must begin a new life with uncertainty about their postinjury skills and limitations (Ylvisaker, 1998). This may have a profound effect on their attitude toward therapy.

> For Gerard, therapy began in the hospital as soon as he was conscious and medically stable. Therapy was a multidisciplinary effort, with a speech-language pathologist, physical therapist, and psychologist helping Gerard address the physical, cognitive, and emotional aftermath of his injuries. By the time he was well enough to resume school, he had missed most of his junior year. The school provided a full-time classroom aide who took notes for him in class, organized his pro-

gram of study, and helped him with assignments. The school's speech-language pathologist focused on improving Gerard's basic reading and helping him learn strategies for working within the limits of his impaired memory. Other activities included role-playing practice for various social and vocational situations to improve his pragmatics in these communicative contexts. Therapy was a challenge, because Gerard did not acknowledge his language deficits and therefore did not see the point of the activities. Gerard also participated, although grudgingly, in a weekly meeting with other teens who had sustained brain injuries.

The long-term prognosis for individuals with TBI is dependent in part on which abilities were already acquired and which were still developing at the age when the injury occurred. The full effects of the injury may not be apparent until months or years later (Chapman, 1997). It has been said that after traumatic brain injury "time reveals all wounds" (DePompei, Blosser, Savage, & Lash, 1997). For example, we do not expect coherent, logical stories from 4-year-olds with or without TBI, but by 10 years of age incoherent storytelling would signal a deficit. When a brain injury is mild, the child may eventually return to normal or near-normal functioning. However, when injuries are severe, the long-term outlook may be less positive.

Two years after his injury, Gerard was finishing high school, although his graduation was uncertain. His involvement in the school's TBI program focused on vocational training to prepare him for postgraduation life. However, he had been through four jobs in as many months, quitting each time because he was bored or felt the job was beneath him in some way. He drifted away from the teens who were his friends before the injury, and his social and pragmatic problems made it difficult for him to make new social contacts.

## EVALUATION OF LANGUAGE DISORDERS

Evaluation of children with suspected language disorders takes many forms in order to accommodate the wide range of disorders that involve impaired language. The evaluation may address a number of questions of interest to the clinician and the parents. Does the child have a language disorder? Are there any factors that might account for the presence of a language disorder? How do the child's skills in various language domains compare to peers? If intervention is warranted, what aspects of language should be addressed? As we will see, components of the diagnostic process are tailored to address these types of questions.

### Language Screening

Language screenings are designed to determine whether a child's language skills warrant a full evaluation. Screenings are relatively quick to administer and often sample a range of language skills that could potentially be impaired. They may be formal measures that have been administered to large groups of children, who serve as a **normative sample**. Normative samples permit comparison of a single child's performance to a group of children who are of the same age. These children serve as a reference for the range of normal performance that can be expected. Other screenings may be informal in order to accommodate regional variations in language or dialect or to target skills of particular interest for a certain setting (e.g., conversational speech, reading readiness). Frequently, language screening is used as a cost-effective method of evaluating large numbers of children, most of whom will not have any difficulties with language skills. For example, a school district may routinely screen the language of all of their incoming kindergarten children. Only those children who fail the screening are referred for a full evaluation.

## The Case History

The case history is a way to gather background information that may be used for many purposes. It may be obtained through conversation with those who know the child best (usually the parents). In other cases, it may consist of a form that is completed prior to or during the initial evaluation. Many case histories include information concerning pregnancy, birth, and medical background. This information can be important for identifying potential causes for a language disorder. For example, if a mother reports having had rubella during her pregnancy, the clinician would be alerted to the possibility of hearing loss, which sometimes occurs under those conditions. The clinician can then plan a hearing screening during the evaluation or arrange a referral to an audiologist for a full hearing assessment, if the child's hearing has not already been tested. Information concerning developmental and family history can help determine the degree of risk for a language disorder. As we saw in earlier sections, children who have developmental language disorders are likely to have a family member who also has a language or learning disorder. In other cases, parental report of a change or cessation of language skills during the child's development would alert the clinician to explore the possibility of autism, seizure disorders, or disease processes that would impact previously normal development.

Sometimes a case history will probe for more subjective information. Parents may be asked what led them to become concerned about their child's language development. They may report what they see as their child's overall strengths and weaknesses. The parents' input may help identify those skills that, if remediated, would make the biggest improvement in their child's daily life. Parents may also be able to provide information on strategies that they have developed that seem to help their child. This type of information is invaluable for guiding subsequent therapy.

## Observation

Important diagnostic information can be gathered simply through observation. Let us consider the following case:

*Charise* was a speech-language pathologist who worked at a community clinic that handled referrals from the state's program for children with disabilities. She always made a point of meeting her clients in the lobby because, as she said, "I can always tell a lot about the way things are going to go on the walk from the front door to my office." One particular morning, she had a new referral of a child with a reported language delay. The child, a 2-year-old boy, came in hand-in-hand with his mother. He was a little overweight, and his belly peeked out beneath his T-shirt. When Charise dropped down to his eye level, he greeted her with a smile as she explained who she was. He had a round, pleasant face, with widespread, almond-shaped eyes, a broad nose, and full cheeks and lips. Overall, his face appeared soft, as if the underlying muscle tone might be low. He seemed social, and he pointed and made short one- or two-word comments about the children's paintings that hung along the hallway. There was one moment of difficulty when it came time to turn the corner and his eye caught something interesting in the opposite direction. He stamped his foot and sat down defiantly in the middle of the hallway. With a bit of cajoling, his mother got him back up and back on track. Once in the office, Charise confirmed the presence of a language delay with formal diagnostic measures. She also made a referral to a medical geneticist. The facial features, low tone, and high weight, combined with a general immaturity, made her think that a genetic syndrome might be playing a role in this child's language problems. In fact, two months later, a follow-up report was received that confirmed a diagnosis of Prader-Willi syndrome, which involves a genetic abnormality on chromosome 15.

In this case, the speech-language pathologist's initial observations contributed to this child's diagnosis. Observation is important at all stages of the diagnostic process. The speech-language pathologist may visit the child's home in order to get an idea of typical communication style within the family. A gross assessment of language functioning can be obtained by listening to a child's conversations. How the child plays can provide insight into the level of cognitive and social functioning. Classroom observations can provide insight into the specific conditions that precipitate communication problems for the school-age child. Furthermore, the speech-language pathologist may notice simple things that can greatly enhance a child's chances of success.

## Formal Measures

There are literally hundreds of commercially available, formal measures for assessing children's language. These tests vary remarkably in their focus, quality, and suitability for a specific diagnostic purpose. One method that clinicians use to select among formal measures is to consider the information that they hope to gain by administering the test. Different formal measures are developed for different purposes. For example, clinicians who wish to compare a child's performance to that of other children of the same age will select **a norm-referenced test**. If they wish to establish whether a child can use certain syntactic structures in various speaking tasks a **criterion-referenced test** would be needed.

Norm-referenced tests allow comparisons between a child's performance and that of a group of children of similar age. Beyond this common feature, however, there is great variation among norm-referenced tests. Some measure narrow domains of language functioning. For example, one norm-referenced test may examine the number of words that a child recognizes; another will evaluate broader knowledge of word meanings. Some consist of several subtests compiled into a battery that examines various components of language functioning. These may sample across the language domains of phonology, morphology, syntax, and semantics in both receptive and expressive modalities.

Criterion-referenced tests are typically more narrowly focused than norm-referenced tests. These tests are used to compare a child's performance against a standard, or criterion, for behavior. Most college course examinations, for example, are criterion-referenced tests, in that the instructor compares each student's performance against a standard for knowledge of the course content. Criterion-referenced tests may be informal, as when a clinician develops a series of "probes" to assess whether a child is able to use structures trained in therapy. Others are commercially available measures that sample language skills to determine a child's proficiency.

Once the purpose for administering a test has been determined, the clinician will examine the test's qualities. Specifically, the clinician must determine whether administering a particular test will result in valid conclusions about the child's language. Let us consider an example of why this is important.

*Brendon* was just 3½ when he was first enrolled in therapy for a language delay. At that point, his mean length of utterance (MLU) was moderately low for his age (see Chapter 7 for a review of MLU). A norm-referenced, test of expressive language placed him below the first percentile for his age, which means that 99 out of 100 children his age could be expected to score higher than Brendon on that particular test. A single-word vocabulary test was also administered, and he did not pass enough items to show that he understood even the simplest words. By contrast, his hearing, motor, and cognitive development tested well within normal limits. Based on these results, he was enrolled in a preschool program for children with specific language impairments. A little over a year later (age 4 years, 10 months), his skills were retested using a different battery of tests. At that time, all skills were well within normal limits according to the test norms. It was concluded that Brendon had overcome his earlier difficulties, and he was dismissed from the preschool program.

Two months later (age 5 years, 0 months), his mother, still concerned about Brendon's language skills, enrolled him in a university-based research project for children with specific language impairment. His language was retested with a third battery of tests. This time, Brendon received expressive language scores and receptive vocabulary scores that were once again below the first percentile for his age. How could the appearing-disappearing-reappearing language deficits be explained? The lead researcher, a speech-language pathologist, consulted the normative tables for the tests Brendon received at age 4. She discovered that the test items were so difficult that most normal 4-year-old children could not pass them. Therefore, failure to pass any items on that test battery still placed a child within normal limits of performance!

The test given to Brendon at age 4 lacked **validity**. Validity refers to the degree to which test results lead to correct conclusions concerning the skills measured (Messick, 1989). Another technical feature that clinicians will consider is a test's **reliability**. This refers to the degree to which a test provides consistent information each time it is given. An unreliable test is never valid. However, high reliability does not ensure validity. A ruler whose inch markings are too closely spaced will provide the same mismeasurement every time—highly reliable, but not at all valid! Standards for the assessment of test reliability and validity have been detailed by the combined efforts of the American Educational Research Association, American Psychological Association, and National Council on Measurement in Education (AERA, APA, & NCME, 1985). Despite such standards, many tests of child language fall short of minimal criteria for validity and reliability (e.g., McCauley & Swisher, 1984; Plante & Vance, 1994; Spaulding, Plante, & Farinella, 2006). Unfortunately, use of a psychometrically weak test can lead to erroneous conclusions. In Brendon's case, the erroneous conclusions that were based on the test results obtained when he was 4 led to the discontinuation of services that he still needed.

A final consideration in test selection is the context in which the skill domains are tested. The same items can be passed on one test and failed on another, just based on the context in which those items appear (e.g., Merrell & Plante, 1997; Wiig, Jones, & Wiig, 1996). Sabers (1996) pointed out that "the way a test measures behavior may introduce measurement aspects not intended for the test." In fact, if the simplest linguistic elements are presented in strange or difficult contexts, children will fail those items long after they are able to use and understand the elements in everyday life. For example, a child who has been using "me" since the age of 2 years will not use it in the context "You would have liked me to see the painting" until many years later. Test items designed to measure language may in fact be a stronger test of memory if the child is required to hold multiple words in memory before composing an answer using those words. Sometimes, the way test items are presented by a test is enough to influence the child's performance. Wiig and colleagues (1996) demonstrated this when they developed a computerized version of one of their tests. They found that teens' performance differed significantly on the traditional and computer-based versions of the test, even though the items were identical. For these reasons, test content and context influence how a clinician interprets the test results.

## Response to Intervention (RTI)

Response to intervention (RTI) is a method of assessing children through intervention. RTI has emerged from the field of special education in part because of concerns that standardized intelligence and academic testing do not adequately address what type of intervention is needed. Furthermore, standardized tests may not be able to differentiate between children whose poor learning is due to a learning disability and those whose poor learning may be due to inadequate instruction or lack of prerequisite knowledge on the part of the child. RTI typically utilizes a tiered system of instruction (Fuchs, Mock, Morgan, & Young, 2003). In the lowest tier, children receive the general instruction of the classroom. Children who struggle under those conditions are advanced to a second tier where more targeted instruction is provided. Children who continue to struggle under these conditions may be identified as having a learning disability, reading disability, or other educationally handicapping condition that warrants a third tier of instruction that is individualized and intensive. A speech-language pathologist may develop a response to intervention plan for a child, or serve on a team that implements such plans in school classrooms.

The current version of the Individuals with Disabilities Educational Improvement Act (IDEA 2004) allows RTI as a method of identifying children eligible for special educational services. However, some have raised concerns about this practice (e.g., Mather & Kaufman, 2006). For example, decisions about how much improvement during a treatment phase is enough to rule out a learning disability can be highly subjective. Likewise, the RTI procedures may identify children who need alternative methods of instruction to succeed, but additional and more formal testing may be needed to identify the child's strengths and weaknesses that will inform individualized instruction at the highest tier of intervention (Willis & Dumont, 2006). However, RTI can be particularly valuable in difficult-to-diagnose cases, such as differentiating between children whose language and learning difficulties are attributable to learning English as a second language and those due to a language or learning disorder in children who are bilingual (e.g., Barrera, 2006; Linan-Thompson, Vaughn, Prater, & Cirino, 2006). Furthermore, implementing RTI procedures can assist children who are struggling before being identified as having a handicapping condition.

RTI is related to procedures speech-language pathologists have also used in the assessment of children with suspected language disorders. These procedures have been referred to as *dynamic assessment*. The term "dynamic" in dynamic assessment is intended to contrast with "static" measures of assessment that measure a child's skills at one point in time. Static measures include norm-referenced and criterion-referenced measures. Dynamic assessment is designed to determine a child's potential to learn under specific conditions (like RTI) or to determine whether better performance might be obtained if the testing situation were more appropriate to a child's background experiences, cultural, or language (e.g., Gutiérrez-McClelland & Peña, 2001; Hwa-Froelich & Matsuo, 2005). For example, a young child who has never been read to at home may lack prerequisite skills for taking a vocabulary test. As in book-reading activities, a vocabulary test may require children to look at pictures on a test page, then point to a picture that is named. If a child is unfamiliar with this routine, he or she could fail the vocabulary test, not because the words are unknown, but because the task is unfamiliar. If the skills of joint attention to pictures and pointing to named pictures are trained outside of the context of the test, and the child is then retested, then a more accurate measure of vocabulary might be obtained. It is important to note that dynamic assessment should not include training with actual test materials or its exact format, because either would invalidate the test for future use with that child.

### Hearing Evaluation

As we will see in Chapter 11, hearing impairment can be an underlying cause of poor language development. Therefore, a pure-tone hearing screening is typically part of a language evaluation. If a child fails to respond during the hearing screening, a full audiological evaluation should be scheduled to rule out hearing loss as a contributing factor in the child's language difficulties.

## LANGUAGE THERAPY

Approaches to language intervention are as diverse as the children who receive services. There is no "recipe book" of procedures or one-size-fits-all method that will work with all children. In fact, therapy methods that are successful with one child may not work well with another. As we saw above, children with different types of language disorders can vary considerably in terms of their language profiles. Furthermore, children's ages, cultural backgrounds, and family situations may greatly affect the types of intervention that are best for them. Therefore, language therapy tends to be highly individualized.

When we examine different intervention methods, we first consider what the therapy approach is intended to do for the child. Wilcox (1994) reviewed major approaches to intervention: prevention, remediation, and compensation. *Preventive* services may be provided to children at risk for language disorders. These children may be at risk because they are born with conditions associated with language disorders (e.g., mental retardation, genetic disorders). Other children may receive preventive services because they are showing early signs of communication delay (e.g., late talkers). In this case, services are intended to maximize the child's potential early in development so that the impact on language can be lessened or avoided. Examples of preventive services include preschool "head start" programs and other programs designed to enrich a child's early language and educational experiences.

*Remediation* involves correction of current deficits and is perhaps the most frequent form of therapy for children. When therapy is oriented toward remediation, the clinician typically has very specific goals (e.g., increase use of target syntactic structures, morphemes, vocabulary). The clinician then devises a program to teach these linguistic targets. Let us look at an example of a therapy program designed to remediate expressive language deficits in a young boy.

> *Davin* is a 20-month-old boy who receives therapy in his home from Sue, a clinician in private practice. When therapy began recently, Davin had six "word approximations" that he used occasionally, although he understood about fifty words. Therefore, both his comprehension and expression were well below what is typical for a child his age. Sue decided that the top priority for Davin would be expressive language, specifically expanding the number of words he could use to express his needs. More words would help reduce the frustration Davin was displaying because of his poor ability to communicate. Furthermore, the fact that he had some word approximations suggested he was ready to communicate with words.

On her first visit to Davin's home, sue taught him signs for "eat," "drink," "want," "more," and "help." Sue elected to incorporate signs into Davin's therapy because children can often produce the more gross hand movements for words before they are able to produce the very precise oral-motor movements needed for intelligible speech. For many children, successful use of signs provides an immediate means for successful communication and a bridge to spoken language. Sue modeled the signs, then demonstrated them to Davin by placing her hands over his while forming the signs with him. By the second visit, it was apparent that Davin was using these first signs on his own.

A critical part of Davin's therapy program is the involvement of his parents. Sue knows that it would be unrealistic to expect Davin to catch up with his peers in the hour a week she sees him at home. It is much more effective for language therapy to be continuous throughout the week. Therefore, a large part of the therapy program involves ensuring that both parents develop techniques that they can use to continue Davin's progress after Sue leaves. Davin's mother requested that Sue come when both parents were available to participate in the therapy sessions. They learn signs along with Davin and also learn how to create opportunities for Davin to use the words he has and learn new words as well. Sue thus teaches the parents how to teach their child and gets feedback on their efforts of the previous week.

It seems obvious that parental involvement in therapy programs can be a positive thing. However, successfully bringing parents into the therapy process can be one of the biggest challenges for the clinician. Sue points out that Davin's parents were eager to be involved in the therapy process. They were also both highly educated, with college degrees, and came from middle class backgrounds. Davin is their only child, and his mother is able to stay at home with him full-time. "I don't want to overwhelm parents, and parents need to be honest with me when I suggest something that is just not possible," says Sue. For example, Sue suggested to Davin's parents that they allow him to make some choices of his own at mealtimes as a way to encourage requests. This same suggestion would not work for a working mother trying to get five young children—one with a disability—dressed and off to school on time. Sue comments, "I can tell I have gone too far when I make a suggestion and their eyes glaze over."

*Compensation* involves the introduction of strategies that assist the child to manage the effects of the disorder, rather than eliminating its signs. Compensation is often used with conditions that are not completely correctable, such as brain injury or hearing loss. For example, in our case of seizure disorder, the mother's use of visual cues provided a strategy to aid comprehension. For older children and teens, the child may be responsible for use of the strategy. A child with a learning disability, for example, may be taught how to use diagrams to summarize information from his lecture notes. For a teen, compensation may involve strategies to support academic learning. Let's look at one such example.

*Mary* works as a speech-language pathologist in a school system. Her role there is to support the children whose language deficits impact their educational progress. Jack is one of her students. In eighth grade, he still struggles with reading. It takes him a long time, and he doesn't always comprehend what he has read. Therefore, he does not learn as much from reading his textbooks as his peers do. Mary has worked with Jack on strategies that are designed to maximize his comprehension of text materials. She teaches him to recognize the cues that are used in textbooks to signal important information. These include strategies like reading the chapter and subheading titles to gain a broad idea about the content area that will be covered. Jack learns that bolded words are important, and if he doesn't fully understand them, he should look in the glossary found at the back of his book. Mary also has trained Jack on how to distinguish between a main point and the details that support it and how to spot these in text. Finally, Mary has worked with Jack's teacher to modify his homework load so that he can keep up with the content without falling behind, because of the amount of time it takes him to complete assignments.

As we saw with the cases presented in this chapter, children with language disorders often have many areas of difficulty that could benefit from therapy. However, working on everything at once would be overwhelming for both the clinician and child. Therefore, the clinician may need to prioritize the areas of need and target these sequentially. Some goals receive priority because they offer the greatest potential for positive improvement in the child's quality of life. For example, a program that provides a nonverbal child with more communicative functions (e.g., requesting, commenting) can reduce frustration for parent and child. A school-age child may benefit most from therapy that allows him or her to participate more fully in classroom activities. Occasionally, the goal that would make the greatest difference in the child's language is not necessarily the one selected. For example, one mother of a severely handicapped child was interested in her child learning social routines (e.g., greetings, "please," and "thank you"), even though other more functional aspects of communication could have been targeted. Social communication was important to the mother because she saw it as a way for her child to have positive interactions with others.

Certain therapy goals may receive priority because they help the child progress to a higher developmental stage. Wilcox (1992) developed an intervention program designed to move infants and toddlers from preverbal gestures and vocalizations to the verbal stage of communication. For a late-talking toddler, increasing the number of vocabulary words is a prerequisite for acquiring phrases and sentences. For older children, the developmental sequence for morpheme acquisition may guide selection of therapy targets. A developmental focus can combine both remediation and preventive components. For example, Dale and colleagues described a treatment method that used storybook activities to facilitate language in preschoolers (Dale, Crain-Thoreson, Notari-Syverson, & Cole, 1996). The immediate goal of this program was language facilitation. However, the treatment context of reading introduced preliteracy skills that are thought to contribute to reading success in later years.

Once the language goals are selected, the therapist must consider the structure used to train those goals. Naturalistic contexts have become very popular over the last decade. As a result, there has been an emphasis on home programs, classroom-based programs, and other intervention techniques that are incorporated into the child's daily life. For example, many programs have demonstrated that parents can be effectively trained to facilitate language development at home. Various programs have been used to teach parents to modify their speech and change how they respond to the child's attempts at communication (e.g., Eiserman, Weber, & McCoun, 1995; Gibbard, 1994; Girolametto, Pearce, & Weitzman, 1996). In fact, parent-administered programs can be as effective as clinician-administered programs, at least in the early stages of intervention (Eiserman, Weber, & McCoun, 1995; Fey, Cleave, & Long, 1997). Other programs emphasize remediation in naturalistic contexts (e.g., conversation, play) during which a clinician, parent, or teacher facilitates the learning of new linguistic forms as opportunities arise within the interaction (Figure 8.2). This technique is sometimes called "incidental teaching," because language instruction follows from natural interactions with the child. For example, a child may learn to use questions by being prompted to request toys, food, and other items encountered in his or her daily life. The effectiveness of naturalistic intervention can vary depending on the specific techniques used to facilitate language (e.g., Camarata, Nelson, & Camarata, 1994; Kaiser & Hester, 1994;

**FIGURE 8.2    A speech-language pathologist may build oral skills through activities centered around books and reading.**

Warren, Gazdag, Bambara, & Jones, 1994) and the characteristics of the child (Yoder, Kaiser, & Alpert, 1991).

Some children need more structure than is afforded by naturalistic contexts because of the nature of their disorder. For example, a child with attention deficit disorder may prove too distractible in a completely naturalistic context to benefit from incidental teaching techniques. A teenager with a traumatic brain injury may may need increased structure relative to his or her peers in order to function in school or in a work setting. Students who need assistance with language skills in the academic domain may use strategies that are explicitly taught. Finally, what is "natural" to one child may be completely unfamiliar to another. For example, in some cultures, a conversation between a child and an adult who is not a close relative is not at all natural. A clinician who uses such a "natural" context may be confronted with a child who will not talk at all under those conditions. In contrast, the use of computers as a tool for therapy may be natural for children who have been interacting with educational software programs from early ages. For these children, the high level of structure in a computer-based program may feel as natural as conversationally based therapy.

Effective therapy takes into account all of these considerations and makes adjustments to fit the needs of each child. The clinician may use a highly structured, compensatory approach with one child and a parent-administered, conversationally based approach with another. For a third child, the clinician may simply serve as a consultant to a classroom teacher who assists the language-disordered child with modifications of teaching activities and materials. This kind of flexibility allows therapy approaches to be tailored to each child's developmental stage and communicative needs.

## CLINICAL PROBLEM SOLVING

Becky is a 30-month-old girl who was brought to the clinic by her parents. They were concerned about her language development because she did not seem to use as many words as the other children at her preschool. Although Becky seemed quite interested in the toys and books in the clinic playroom, she said few words and often seemed to substitute gestures for words. All of her verbal utterances consisted of single words, with no multiword combinations. She was in good health, and other than language, the parents did not have any concerns about her development.

1. Is this child at risk for a language disorder? Why or why not?
2. What should be included in the initial evaluation of this child? What is the purpose for including each of these components?
3. Given the child's age and language level, what approach might therapy take?
4. What do we know about the long-term outlook for young children whose language lags behind their age-mates?

# REFERENCES

American Educational Research Association, American Psychological Association, & National Council on Measurement in Education. (1985). *Standards for educational and psychological testing.* Washington, DC: Author.

American Psychiatric Association. (1994). *Diagnostic and statistical manual of mental disorders* (4th ed.). Washington, DC: Author.

American Speech-Language-Hearing Association (ASHA). (1983). Social dialects. *Asha, 25,* 23–27.

American Speech-Language-Hearing Association (ASHA). (1997). Position statement: Roles of audiologists and speech-language pathologists working with persons with attention deficit hyperactivity disorder. *Asha, 39,* 14.

Aram, D. (1991). Comments on specific language impairment as a clinical category. *Language, Speech, & Hearing Services in Schools, 22,* 84–87.

Aram, D. M., Ekelman, B. L., Rose, D. F., & Whitaker, H. A. (1985). Verbal and cognitive sequelae following unilateral lesions acquired in early childhood. *Journal of Clinical and Experimental Neuropsychology, 7,* 55–78.

Barrera, M. (2006). Roles of definitional and assessment models in the identification of new or second language learners of English for special education. *Journal of Learning Disabilities, 39,* 142–156.

Bellugi, U., Marks, S., Bihrle, A., & Sabo, H. (1988). Dissociation between language and cognitive functions in Williams syndrome. In D. Bishop & M. Mogford (Eds.), *Language development in exceptional circumstances.* New York: Churchill Livingstone.

Bent, J. P., & Beck, R. A. (1994). Bacterial meningitis in the pediatric population: Paradigm shifts and ramifications for otolaryngology-head and neck surgery. *International Journal of Pediatric Otorhinolaryngology, 30,* 41–49.

Biddle, K. R., McCabe, A., & Bliss, L. S. (1996). Narrative skills following traumatic brain injury in children and adults. *Journal of Communication Disorders, 29,* 447–470.

Bishop, D. V. M., Laws, G., Adams, C., & Norbury, C. F. (2006). High heritability of speech and language impairments in 6-year-old twins demonstrated using parent and teacher report. *Behavior Genetics, 36,* 173–184.

Bishop, D. V. M., & Snowling, M. J. (2004). Developmental dyslexia and specific language impairment: Same or different? *Psychological Bulletin, 130,* 858–886.

Botting, N., Simkin, Z., & Conti-Ramsden, G. (2006). Associated reading skills in children with a history of specific language impairment (SLI). *Reading and Writing, 19,* 77–98.

Byrne, J., Ellsworth, C., Bowering, E., & Vincer, M. (1993). Language development in low birth weight infants: The first two years of life. *Journal of Developmental and Behavioral Pediatrics, 14,* 21–27.

Camarata, S. M., Nelson, K. E., & Camarata, M. N. (1994). Comparison of conversational recasting and imitative procedures for training grammatical structures in children with specific language impairment. *Journal of Speech and Hearing Research, 37,* 1414–1423.

Catts, H. W., Adlof, S. M., Hogan, T. P., & Ellis Weismer, S. (2005). Are specific language impairment and dyslexia distinct disorders? *Journal of Speech, Language, and Hearing Research, 48,* 1378–1396.

Chapman, S. B. (1997). Cognitive-communication abilities in children with closed head injury. *American Journal of Speech Language Pathology, 6,* 50–58.

Chapman, S. B., Levin, H. S., Matejka, J., Harward, H. N., & Kufera, J. (1995). Discourse ability in head injured children: Consideration of linguistic, psychosocial, and cognitive factors. *Journal of Head Trauma Rehabilitation, 10,* 36–54.

Chapman, S. B., Watkins, R., Gustafson, C., Moore, S., Levin, H. S., & Kufera, J. A. (1997). Narrative discourse in children with closed head injury, children with language impairment, and typically developing children. *American Journal of Speech Language Pathology, 6,* 66–76.

Clark, D. A. (1994). Neonates and infants at risk for hearing and language disorders. In K. G. Butler (Ed.), *Early intervention I: Working with infants and toddlers.* Gaithersburg, MD: Aspen Publishers.

Claude, D., & Firestone, P. (1995). The development of ADHD boys: A 12-year follow-up. *Canadian Journal of Behavioral Science, 27,* 226–249.

Cohen, M., Campbell, R., & Yaghmai, F. (1989). Neuropathological abnormalities in developmental dysphasia. *Annals of Neurology, 25,* 567–570.

Courchesne, E., Yeung-Courchesne, R., Press, G., Hesselink, J. R., & Jernigan, T. L. (1988). Hypoplasia of the cerebellar vermal lobes VI and VII in infantile autism. *New England Journal of Medicine, 318,* 1349–1354.

Cranberg, L. D., Filley, C. M., Hart, E. J., & Alexander, M. P. (1987). Acquired aphasia in childhood: Clinical and CT investigations. *Neurology, 37,* 1165–1172.

Dale, P. S., Crain-Thoreson, C., Notari-Syverson, A., & Cole, K.(1996) Parent-child book reading as an intervention technique for young children with language delays. *Topics in Early Childhood Special Education, 16,* 213–235.

DePompei, R., Blosser, J. L., Savage, R., & Lash, M. (1997, November). *Effective long-term management for youths with TBI.* Miniseminar presented at the annual conference of the American Speech-Language-Hearing Association, Boston, MA.

Dunn, M. (1997). Language disorders in children with autism. *Seminars in Pediatric Neurology, 4,* 86–92.

Eiserman, W. D., Weber, C., & McCoun, M. (1995). Parent and professional roles in early intervention: A longitudinal comparison of the effects of two intervention configurations. *Journal of Special Education, 29,* 20–44.

Ellis Weismer, S., Murray-Branch, J., & Miller, J. F. (1994). A prospective longitudinal study of language development in late talkers. *Journal of Speech and Hearing Research, 37,* 852–867.

Fey, M. E., Cleave, P. L., & Long, S. H. (1997). Two models of grammar facilitation in children with language impairments. *Journal of Speech and Hearing Research, 40,* 5–19.

Fischel, J. E., Whitehurst, G. J., Caulfield, M. B., & Debaryshe, B. (1989). Language growth in children with expressive language delay. *Pediatrics, 82,* 218–227.

Fuchs, D., Mock, D., Morgan, P., & Young, C. (2003). Responsiveness-to-intervention: Definitions, evidence, and implications for the learning disabilities construct. *Learning Disabilities Research & Practice, 18,* 157–171.

Gauger, L. M., Lombardino, L. J., & Leonard, C. M. (1997). Brain morphology in children with specific language impairment. *Journal of Speech, Language, and Hearing Research, 40,* 1272–1284.

Gillam, R. B., & Carlile, R. M. (1997). Oral reading and story retelling of students with specific language impairment. *Language, Speech, and Hearing Services in Schools, 28,* 30–42.

Gillon, G. T. (2002). Follow-up study investigating the benefits of phonological awareness intervention for children with spoken language impairment. International *Journal of Language & Communication Disorders, 37,* 381–400.

Gutiérrez-Clellen, V. F., & Peña, E. (2001). Dynamic assessment of diverse children: A tutorial. *Language, Speech, and Hearing Services in Schools, 32,* 212–224.

Halsey, C. L., Collin, M. F., & Anderson, C. L. (1996). Extremely low-birth-weight children and their peers. A comparison of school-age outcomes. *Archives of Pediatrics and Adolescent Medicine, 150,* 790–794.

Hwa-Froelich, D. A., & Matsuo, H. (2005). Vietnamese children and language-based processing tasks. *Language, Speech, and Hearing Services in Schools, 36*, 230–243.

Jackson, T., & Plante, E. (1997). Gyral morphology in the posterior sylvian region in families affected by developmental language disorder. *Neuropsychology Review, 6*, 81–94.

Johnson, J. M., Seikel, J. A., Madison, C. L., Foose, S. M., & Rinard, K. D. (1997). Standardized test performance of children with a history of prenatal exposure to multiple drugs/cocaine. *Journal of Communication Disorders, 30*, 45–72.

Kaiser, A. B., & Hester, P. P. (1994). Generalized effects of enhanced milieu teaching. *Journal of Speech and Hearing Research, 37*, 1320–1340.

Kanner, L., & Eisenberg, L. (1955). Notes on the followup studies of autistic children. In P. H. Hoch & J. Zubin (Eds.), *Psychotherapy of childhood*. New York: Grune & Stratton.

Landau, W. M., & Kleffner, F. R. (1957). Syndrome of acquired aphasia with convulsive disorder in children. *Neurology, 7*, 523–530.

Lewis, B. A., & Freebairn, L. (1992). Residual effects of preschool phonology disorders in grade school, adolescence, and adulthood. *Journal of Speech and Hearing Disorders, 35*, 819–831.

Linan-Thompson, S., Vaughn, S., Prater, K., & Cirino, P. T. (2006). The response to intervention of English language learners at risk for reading problems. *Journal of Learning Disabilities, 39*, 390–398.

Lord, C., & Pickles, A. (1996). Language level and nonverbal social-communicative behaviors in autistic and language-delayed children. *Journal of the American Academy of Child and Adolescent Psychiatry, 35*, 1542–1550.

Mantovani, J. F., & Landau, W. M. (1980). Acquired aphasia with convulsive disorder: Course and prognosis. *Neurology, 30*, 524–529.

Mather, N., & Kaufman, N. (2006). Introduction to the special issue, part one: It's about the what, the how well, and the why. *Psychology in the Schools, 43*, 747–752.

McCauley, R. J., & Swisher, L. (1984). Psychometric review of language and articulation tests for preschool children. *Journal of Speech and Hearing Disorders, 49*, 34–42.

McGee, R., Partridge, F., Williams, S., & Silva, P. A. (1991). A twelve-year follow-up of preschool hyperactive children. *Journal of the American Academy of Child and Adolescent Psychiatry, 30*, 224–232.

Merrell, A. W., & Plante, E. (1997). Norm-referenced test interpretation in the diagnostic process. *Language, Speech, & Hearing Services in Schools, 28*, 50–58.

Messick, S. (1989). Meaning and values in test validation: The science and ethics of assessment. *Educational Researcher, 18*, 5–11.

Minshew, N. J., Goldstein, G., & Siegel, D. J. (1997). Neuropsychologic functioning in autism: Profile of a complex information processing disorder. *Journal of the International Neuropsychological Society, 3*, 303–316.

Miranda-Linne, F. M., & Merlin, L. (1997). A comparison of speaking and mute individuals with autism and autistic-like conditions on the Autism Behavior Checklist. *Journal of Autism and Developmental Disorders, 27*, 245–264.

National Institute on Deafness and Other Communication Disorders (NIDCD). (1991). *National strategic research plan for balance and the vestibular system and language and language impairments* (NIH Publication No. 91-3217). Bethesda, MD: Author.

O'Brien, E. K., Zhang, X., Nishimura, C., Tomblin, J. B., & Murray, J. C. (2003). Association of Specific Language Impairment (SLI) to the Region of 7q31. *American Journal of Human Genetics, 72*, 1536–1543.

Paul, R. (1993). Patterns of development in late talkers: Preschool years. *Journal of Childhood Communication Disorders, 15*, 7–14.

Paul, R., & Alforde, S. (1993). Grammatical morpheme acquisition in 4-year-olds with normal, impaired, and late-developing language. *Journal of Speech and Hearing Research, 36,* 1271–1275.

Paul, R., Hernandez, R., Taylor, L., & Johnson, K. (1996). Narrative development in late talkers: Early school age. *Journal of Speech and Hearing Research, 39,* 1295–1303.

Paul, R., Murray, C., Clancy, K., & Andrews, D. (1997). *Journal of Speech and Hearing Research, 40,* 1037–1047.

Petit, E., Herlault, J., Martineau, J., Perrot, A., Barthelemy, C., Hameury, L., Sauvage, D., Lelord, G., Muh, J. P. (1995). Association study with two markers of a human homeogene in infantile autism. *Journal of Medical Genetics, 32,* 269–274.

Plante, E. (1991). MRI findings in the parents and siblings of specifically language-impaired boys. *Brain and Language, 41,* 52–66.

Plante, E., Swisher, L., Vance, R., & Rapcsak, S. (1991). MRI findings in boys with specific language impairment. *Brain and Language, 41,* 52–66.

Plante, E., & Vance, R. (1994). Selection of preschool language tests: A data based approach. *Language, Speech, & Hearing Services in Schools, 25,* 15–23.

Rapin, I., Mattis, S., Rowan, A. J., & Golden, G. G. (1977). Verbal auditory agnosia in children. *Developmental Medicine and Child Neurology, 19,* 192–207.

Records, N. L., Tomblin, J. B., & Freese, P. R. (1992). The quality of life of young adults with histories of specific language impairment. *American Journal of Speech-Language Pathology, 1,* 44–53.

Rescorla, L., Roberts, J., & Dahlsgaard, K.(1997). Late talkers at 2: Outcome at age 3. *Journal of Speech and Hearing Research, 40,* 555–566.

Rescorla, L., & Schwartz, E. (1990). Outcome of toddlers with expressive language delay. *Applied Psycholinguistics, 11,* 393–407.

Rimland, B. (1964). *Infantile autism.* New York: Appleton-Century-Crofts.

Sabers, D. L. (1996). By their tests we will know them. *Language, Speech, and Hearing Services in Schools, 27,* 102–108.

Scarborough, H. S., & Dobrich, W. (1990). Development of children with early language delay. *Journal of Speech and Hearing Research, 33,* 70–83.

Scharfenaker, S. K. (1990). The fragile X syndrome. *Asha, 32,* 45–47.

Shields, J., Varley, R., Broks, P., & Simpson, A. (1996). Social cognition in developmental language disorders and high-level autism. *Developmental Medicine and Child Neurology, 38,* 487–495.

Snowling, M. J., Bishop, D. V. M., Stothard, S. E. (2000). Is preschool language impairment a risk factor for dyslexia in adolescence? *Journal of Child Psychology and Psychiatry, 41,* 587–600.

Sparks, S. N. (1984). *Birth defects and speech-language disorders.* Boston: College Hill.

Spaulding, T. J., Plante, E., & Farinella, K. A. (2006). Do children with impaired language score at the low end of the normative distribution? *Language, Speech, and Hearing Services in Schools, 37,* 61–72.

Stoel-Gammon, C. (1990). Down syndrome: Effects on language development. *Asha, 32,* 42–44.

Tallal, P., Ross, R., & Curtiss, S. (1989). Familial aggregation in specific language impairment. *Journal of Speech and Hearing Disorders, 54,* 287–295.

Thal, D. J., Bates, E., Goodman, J., & Jahn-Samilo, J. (1997). Continuity of language abilities: An exploratory study of late- and early-talking toddlers. *Developmental Neuropsychology, 13,* 239–274.

Thal, D. J., & Tobias, S. (1992). Communicative gestures in children with delayed onset of oral expressive vocabulary. *Journal of Speech and Hearing Research, 35,* 1281–1289.

The SLI Consortium (2002). A genomewide scan identifies two novel loci involved in specific language impairment. *American Journal of Human Genetics, 70,* 384–398.

Tomblin, J. B. (1989). Familial concentration of developmental language impairment. *Journal of Speech and Hearing Disorders, 54,* 287–295.

Tomblin, J. B., Records, N., & Freese, P. (1992). Diagnosing specific language impairment in adults for the purpose of pedigree analysis. *Journal of Speech and Hearing Research, 35,* 832–843.

Tomblin, J. B., Records, N. L., & Zhang, X. (1996). A system for the diagnosis of specific language impairment in kindergarten children. *Journal of Speech and Hearing Research, 39,* 1284–1294.

Turkstra, L. S., & Holland, A. L. (1998). Working memory and syntax comprehension after adolescent traumatic brain injury. *Journal of Speech, Language, and Hearing Research, 41.*

Van Dongen, H. R., Loonen, M. C. B., & Van Dongen, K. J. (1985). Anatomical basis for acquired fluent aphasia in children. *Annals of Neurology, 17,* 306–309.

Vargha-Khadem, F., O'Gorman, A. M., & Watters, G. V., (1985). Aphasia and handedness in relation to hemisphere side, age at injury, and severity of cerebral lesion in childhood. *Brain, 108,* 677–695.

Warren, S. F., Gazdag, G. E., Bambara, L. M., & Jones, H. A. (1994). Changes in the generativity and use of semantic relations concurrent with milieu language intervention. *Journal of Speech and Hearing Research, 37,* 924–934.

Washington, J. A., & Craig, H. K. (1994). Dialectal forms during discourse of poor, urban, African American preschoolers. *Journal of Speech and Hearing Research, 37,* 816–823.

Wiig, E. H., Jones, S. S., & Wiig, E. D. (1996). Computer-based assessment of word knowledge in teens with learning disabilities. *Language, Speech, and Hearing Services in Schools, 27,* 21–28.

Wilcox, M. J. (1992). Enhancing initial communication skills in young children with developmental disabilities through partner programming. *Seminars in Speech and Hearing, 13,* 194–212.

Wilcox, M. J. (1994). Delivering communication-based services to infants, toddlers, and their families: Approaches and models. In K. G. Butler (Ed.), *Early intervention I: Working with infants and toddlers.* Gaithersburg, MD: Aspen Publications.

Willis, J. O., & Dumont, R. (2006). And never the twain shall meet: Can response to intervention and cognitive assessment be reconciled? *Psychology in the Schools, 43,* 901–908.

Woods, B. T., & Carey, S. (1979). Language deficits after apparent clinical recovery from childhood aphasia. *Annals of Neurology, 6,* 405–409.

Worster-Drought, C. (1971). An unusual form of acquired aphasia in children. *Developmental Medicine and Child Neurology, 13,* 563–571.

Ylvisaker, M. (1993). Communication outcome in children and adolescents with traumatic brain injury. *Neuropsychological Rehabilitation, 3,* 321–340.

Ylvisaker, M. (1998). Traumatic brain injury in children and adolescents: Introduction. In M. Ylvisaker (Ed.), *Traumatic brain injury rehabilitation in children* (2nd ed. pp. 1–10.). Boston: Butterworth-Heinemann.

Ylvisaker, M., Szekeres, S. F., & Feeney, T. J. (1998). Cognitive rehabilitation: Executive functions. In M. Ylvisaker (Ed.), *Traumatic brain injury rehabilitation in children* (2nd ed., pp. 221–270). Boston: Butterworth-Heinemann.

Yoder, P. J., Kaiser, A. P., & Alpert, C. L. (1991). An exploratory study of the interactions between language teaching methods and child characteristics. *Journal of Speech and Hearing Research, 34,* 155–167.

## READINGS FROM THE POPULAR LITERATURE

Dorris, M. (1996). *Broken cord.* Boston: G. K. Hall. (fetal alcohol syndrome)

Geraldi, C. (1996). *Camille's children.* Kansas City, KS: Andrews and McMeel. (foster mother of multiply handicapped children)

Gerlach, E. (1999). *Just this side of normal: Glimpses into life with autism.* Eugene, OR: Four Leaf Press. (family and autism)

Grandin, T., & Scariano, M. M. (1996). *Emergence: Labeled autistic.* New York: Warner Books. (personal account of autism)

Greenfield, J. (1980). *A place for Noah.* New York: Holt, Rinehart and Winston. (family with autistic child)

Haddon, M. (2005). *The curious incident of the dog in the night-time.* New York: Vintage Books.

Jablow, M. (1982). *Cara: Growing up with a retarded child.* Philadelphia: Temple University Press. (mental retardation)

Kaufmann, B. (1976). *Son-rise.* New York: Warner Books. (autism)

Kaufmann, S. (1995). *Retarded isn't stupid, Mom!* Baltimore: Paul H. Brookes. (mental retardation)

Lane, G., & Sagmiller, G. (1996). *Dyslexia my life.* Waverly, IA: Doubting Thomas. (dyslexia)

Maurice, C. (1994). *Let me hear your voice: A family's triumph over autism.* New York: Fawcett Columbine. (family and autism)

Papazian, S. (1997). *Growing up with Joey: A mother's story of her son's disability and her family's triumph.* Santa Barbara, CA: Fithian Press. (cerebral palsy and the family)

Rogers, D. E. (1992). *Angel unaware:* Westwood, NJ: Fleming Revell Press. (Down syndrome)

Stallings, G., & Cook, S. (1998). *Another season: A coach's story of raising an exceptional son.* New York: Broadway Books. (Down syndrome)

Williams, D. (1994). *Nobody nowhere.* New York: Perennial. (personal account of autism)

Williams, D. (1995). *Somebody somewhere: Breaking free from the world of autism.* New York: Times Books. (sequel to *Nobody Nowhere,* a personal account of life with autism).

Williams, D. (1996). *Like color to the blind: Soul searching and soul finding.* New York: Times Books. (personal account of life with autism)

# CHAPTER NINE

# DISORDERS OF LANGUAGE IN ADULTS

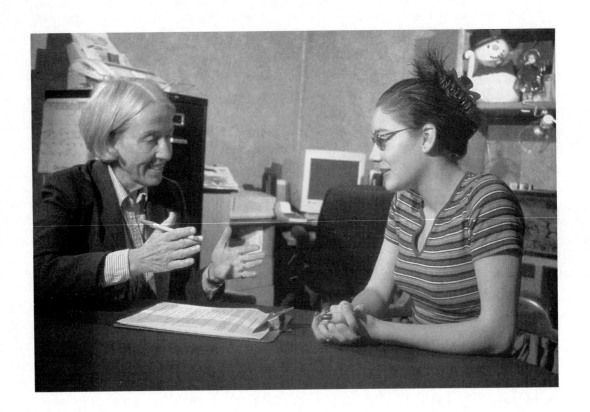

## PREVIEW

Language is well established by the adult years. Most adults have mastered the syntax and morphology of their primary language in both the spoken and written form, and language formulation and speech production occur with relatively little effort. Adult vocabularies continue to grow as life experience is gained, and adults typically become more adept at the subtleties of language use. With advanced age, language knowledge and use remain relatively stable, with the exception of some minor word-finding problems. In some adults, however, sudden or progressive damage to portions of the brain important for language and thought can significantly disturb the ability to communicate. The extent and location of brain damage influence the resulting behavior, such that various syndromes are associated with certain patterns of brain damage. Rehabilitation of adults with acquired communication disorders is challenging and rewarding work, typically accomplished in partnership with the patient, caregivers, and other professionals.

Normal language and cognition are dependent upon a healthy nervous system, and damage to the brain can disrupt those processes. When the damage specifically affects the portions of the brain that support language, the resulting impairment is referred to as **aphasia**. Because language centers are in the left hemisphere in most people, aphasia typically is associated with left hemisphere damage. Acquired language impairments may occur in children, as reviewed in Chapter 8, but aphasia is most often observed in adults. When the right hemisphere is damaged, rather than the left, the resulting syndrome of cognitive and communication impairment is quite different from aphasia. In other cases, widespread or diffuse damage to both hemispheres may occur, as is frequently observed following traumatic brain injury (TBI). As discussed in Chapter 8, teenagers and young adults are at greatest risk for TBI, but older adults may suffer the cognitive and behavioral consequences of head injury as well. With advanced age, there is increased likelihood of progressive intellectual and linguistic decline associated with various types of dementia.

## APHASIA

Aphasia is an acquired impairment of language. It results from damage to the language centers of the brain, which are typically located in the left hemisphere, as reviewed in Chapter 2. The areas of damage or injury are called **lesions**. In the case of aphasia, an individual who had normal language suddenly finds those abilities impaired or degraded. Speech-language pathologists in medical settings frequently participate in the evaluation and rehabilitation of individuals with aphasia.

*Mr. Wallace* was a right-handed man who had a bachelor's degree in engineering and retired after a distinguished career in the army. At age 67, he had a stroke in the left cerebral hemisphere. He did not suffer any physical impairment after the stroke, but his ability to communicate was markedly impaired due to aphasia. A conversational exchange with Mr. Wallace went as follows:

AUTHOR:   Tell me about the work that you did.

MR. WALLACE:   When I grew up in the army, this was my whole *fife, lar . . . light.* I was in the army, the army, and the war and everything else under the sun. Everything. And various *coun, coun, coun,* countries, and things in different places we went and in the armies. I was a colonel in the infantry. And I liked it. I was very fond of . . . I knew everybody in West Point. We all grown in our lives, grown up, and we were children. And we knew a lot of people and I think we were useful. And the people we work with. And so we did.

Mr. Wallace was having difficulty coming up with the words he needed to explain his thoughts. For example, it was obvious that he intended to say, "When I grew up in the army, this was my whole *life.*" But he did not say the word *life.* He first said the word *fife,* then he said a nonword *lar,* and finally he said an incorrect word, *light.* Mr. Wallace retained his lifelong memories and did not have an impairment of his intellect, but he had an impairment specific to language—he had aphasia.

It is important to appreciate that aphasia is an impairment of language, not simply a problem with speech production. Recall from Chapters 3 and 7 that language is a symbol system used to convey thoughts, whereas speech refers to the meaningful sounds produced by articulatory movements. Language includes the words we speak and the rules that govern how words are combined to make utterances. Mr. Wallace had trouble coming up with the appropriate words and also had difficulty combining them into meaningful sentences. Although some of Mr. Wallace's words were pronounced incorrectly, this was not due to a speech problem; it was part of his language impairment. Some individuals with aphasia *do* have difficulty articulating words because they have speech problems that coexist with their aphasia. Such acquired speech disorders include dysarthria and apraxia of speech, which were discussed in Chapter 4.

Language is distinguished not only from speech but also from thought. Patients with severe aphasia often demonstrate that they have relatively well-preserved thought processes. They retain their world knowledge, remember their life histories, and learn new things about what is going on in the world. Therefore, aphasia is not an impairment of general intellect as is observed in dementing diseases. It would be an oversimplification to suggest that individuals with aphasia possess all the cognitive abilities they had before the onset of their aphasia (see, e.g., Beeson, Bayles, Rubens, & Kaszniak, 1993; Murray, 2002), but it is the language impairment that is central to their communication problems.

## Characteristics

The difficulty coming up with words that was evident in Mr. Wallace's conversation is called **anomia**, which refers to a failure to retrieve a name. Anomia is the hallmark of aphasia in that all people with aphasia complain of difficulty coming up with the names of things. The rambling emptiness of Mr. Wallace's conversation resulted from his anomia. He overused pronouns such as *we, thing,* and *it* rather than giving specific names of people, places, or things. Individuals with aphasia may identify instances of anomia by saying something like, "oh, I can't think of the word for it," or they may describe the item that they cannot name. For example, to refer to the Veteran's Affairs hospital, a patient said, "you know, the place where I met you . . . with all the soldiers and where we did those thing with the tests." This sort of "talking around the word" is called **circumlocution**. Although circumlocution is an indicator of word retrieval problems, it is also a very useful communication strategy to compensate for anomia.

Sometimes incorrect words or nonwords are produced in place of the desired word. Such errors are called **paraphasias**. Mr. Wallace's attempts to produce the word *light* resulted in several paraphasias. They can be whole word substitutions, such as *world* for *life,* single-sound substitutions such as *fife* for *life,* or nonwords that are either closely related or totally unrelated to the target word, such as *lar* for *life.* Such nonwords are also called **neologisms**, meaning "new words," but they have no meaning to the listener. Individuals with aphasia vary as to whether they are able to detect such errors in their spoken language.

## Fluent versus Nonfluent Aphasia

Mr. Wallace's speech output was considered "fluent." It had relatively normal prosodic variations of pitch, loudness, and stress, and although there were some hesitations due to word-finding difficulties, the words flowed in a manner that sounded fairly normal. Other characteristics of **fluent aphasia** include articulation without excessive effort, utterances generally of normal length in terms of the number of words, and the presence of some syntactic structure, such as the use of articles, prepositional phrases, and appropriate word endings, such as *-ed.*

Not all individuals with aphasia speak fluently. Those with **nonfluent aphasia** produce utterances characterized by effortful, hesitant speech that may be poorly articulated. Mr. Brown provides an example of nonfluent aphasia. He was a 36-year-old man who had a congenital malformation of his vascular system that required surgery when he was 31. The surgery was complicated by a hemorrhage that occurred in the region of the left middle cerebral artery and caused extensive damage to the language areas of his left hemisphere. He had weakness on the right side of his body and a significant nonfluent aphasia. Two years after his stroke we had the following conversation.

> **AUTHOR:**   What can you tell me about the stroke?
>
> **MR. BROWN:**   Um . . . (Sighs) . . . um . . . (Sighs) . . . left . . . (Gestures to right side of body) . . . right side . . . (Shakes his head and sighs)
>
> **AUTHOR:**   And before your stroke, what did you do?
>
> **MR. BROWN:**   Um . . . resale sales (Holds up six fingers).
>
> **AUTHOR:**   Six years?

MR. BROWN:   No. Six . . . store . . . chain . . . California.

AUTHOR:   Did you do sales?

MR. BROWN:   No. No. This time . . . general . . . manager.

Mr. Brown's utterances were quite different from those of Mr. Wallace. He spoke mostly in single words and short phrases. Whereas Mr. Wallace had an excess of vague, empty words, Mr. Brown's words were almost all meaningful content words. This type of output has been called **telegraphic speech** because it lacks the little functor words, such as *is* or *the*, that are typically omitted when one sends a telegram. (In the old days people sent telegrams rather than emails, and you had to pay by the word.) The pauses and interjection of "um" give the impression that Mr. Brown was struggling to find and produce the words he wanted to say, and he had difficulty constructing complete sentences with appropriate grammatical structure. The overall speech pattern is lacking normal prosody, in that there is not the normal melodic variation of pitch, loudness, and stress. The term nonfluent is used to capture the essence of this effortful, telegraphic speech pattern. It should not be confused with the term *disfluent*, which refers to the disruption of speech fluency observed in stuttering (see Chapter 5).

The differences in fluency noted between Mr. Wallace and Mr. Brown are consistent with differences in the location of brain damage that caused their respective aphasias. To understand the relationship between fluency and lesion location, we need to briefly review brain anatomy relevant to aphasia. Aphasia typically results from damage to the left hemisphere in an area that surrounds the major horizontal fissure called the Sylvian fissure. This region, shaded in Figure 9.1, is called the perisylvian region (*peri* = around). Figure 9.2 shows a brain scan of an individual who had a stroke in this area resulting in persistent aphasia. The scan was taken several years following the stroke, and the dark regions of brain damage are clearly visible in the two images. It should be apparent from image A that the damage falls within the left perisylvian region, shown schematically in Figure 9.1.

The relatively large perisylvian region is often divided into anterior and posterior regions relative to another major fissure, the Rolandic fissure (also called the central sulcus) that runs roughly perpendicular to the Sylvian fissure, as seen in Figure 9.1. The primary motor area and the areas important for motor planning are located in the frontal lobe, which is anterior to the Rolandic fissure. Broca's area is a frontal lobe region important for the motor planning of speech movements. It makes sense that brain damage to those anterior regions of the left hemisphere are likely to affect motor control and planning and thus contribute to a disruption of speech production like that observed in nonfluent aphasias. As observed with Mr. Brown, anterior lesions often damage the motor areas for the right arm and leg as well, such that individuals with nonfluent aphasia often have right-sided weakness or paralysis, which is called right **hemiparesis**. Conversely, lesions that spare the anterior motor regions (i.e., lesions that are posterior to the Rolandic fissure) are typically associated with fluent aphasia and no hemiparesis, as observed in Mr.

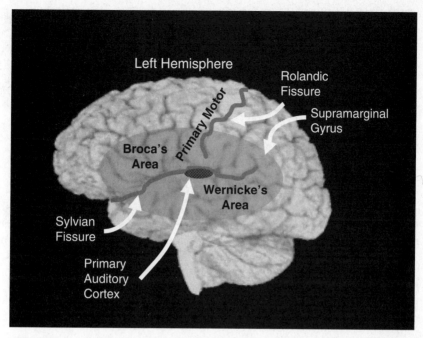

**FIGURE 9.1    A schematic drawing of the left hemisphere indicates the language centers in the perisylvian region. Note that the primary auditory area is actually hidden from view inside the Sylvian fissure; the arcuate fasciculus is a white matter pathway that is deep within the hemisphere.**

Wallace. In general, anterior lesions are associated with nonfluent aphasia, and posterior lesions are associated with fluent aphasia. Large lesions that encompass both anterior and posterior regions would result in nonfluent aphasia because damage includes the critical anterior motor regions.

Beyond the distinction between fluent and nonfluent aphasias, classification systems have been used over the past century to distinguish identifiable aphasia subtypes. The Boston classification system is commonly used in North America (Goodglass, 1993; Helm-Estabooks & Albert, 2004; Kertesz, 2006). In general, the aphasia types reflect performance profiles that indicate (1) whether the aphasia is fluent or nonfluent, (2) whether auditory comprehension is relatively good or impaired, and (3) whether the ability to repeat sentences is preserved or impaired. Just as fluency characteristics offer some insight regarding lesion location, some inferences can be drawn from the status of auditory comprehension and verbal repetition abilities. An understanding of those processes is helpful before examining some aphasia types in more detail.

**FIGURE 9.2** An MRI (magnetic resonance imaging) scan of the head showing a large perisylvian lesion in the left hemisphere that resulted in significant aphasia. Image A shows the dark region of damage from a lateral perspective (in a vertical plane), with the patient looking to the left. Image B shows an image in a horizontal plane near the Sylvian fissure. Note that the lesion is on the right side in image B because radiologic films are often flipped so that right and left are reversed.

## Auditory Comprehension

Auditory comprehension requires the extraction of meaning from spoken words and the processing of grammatical structures in connected utterances. Auditory comprehension problems are common in aphasia, but the degree of impairment can vary considerably. Some individuals have trouble understanding the meaning of single words and simple commands, such as when they are instructed, "Show me the table." Others can respond to simple requests but have trouble when understanding depends on careful processing of each word in relation to other words in an utterance. For example, the following verbal request would challenge most individuals with aphasia: "Do you want chicken or steak for dinner? Because if you want chicken, you need to get it out of the freezer."

Auditory comprehension is dependent upon information processing in the posterior, superior temporal lobe in the region called Wernicke's area, which is adjacent to the primary auditory region (Figure 9.1). Damage to Wernicke's area does not impair the ability to hear but interferes with the understanding of spoken language. Lesions to Wernicke's area are considered "posterior" because they are posterior to the Rolandic fissure and do not include the frontal motor regions. Mr. Wallace's stroke damaged Wernicke's area, and he had trouble understanding what was said in conversation. He also made errors on yes/no questions such as "Do you eat a banana before you peel it?" Mr. Wallace's comprehension was assessed using a variety of tasks that included pointing to items in response to their name, simple and complex commands, yes/no questions, and more difficult tasks such as comprehending a paragraph read aloud.

## Repetition

Although the ability to repeat what other people say is not a particularly important or meaningful use of language, it is a useful diagnostic task when examining for aphasia. The ability to repeat words, phrases, and sentences requires auditory processing by posterior regions of the left hemisphere as well as verbal formulation by the anterior regions of the left hemisphere. So, the ability to repeat sentences is a good test of the integrity of the entire left persylvian region. Difficulty with verbal repetition can arise for several reasons. The attempts by Mr. Wallace (with fluent aphasia) to repeat sentences resulted in errors because of his auditory comprehension problems and his many paraphasic errors. Mr. Brown (with nonfluent aphasia) had trouble repeating sentences because he omitted the little grammatical words, just like he did in his conversational speech. Repetition can also be disrupted by damage to the **arcuate fasciculus**, a collection of fibers that connect the posterior and anterior perisylvian regions (see Figure 9.1). Damage to these fibers, as well as to other posterior regions in the left hemisphere, disrupts repetition abilites even when Broca's and Wernicke's areas are spared (Damasio & Damasio, 1980). Such lesions appear to disconnect the posterior and anterior language regions, such that auditory input processed in Wernicke's area is not conveyed to Broca's area for speech production.

Relatively good verbal repetition is observed in some aphasias that result from lesions on the periphery of the left perisylvian region, or from isolated lesions within the perisylvian region that do not disturb the input and output processes necessary for repetition. In such cases, it is somewhat surprising to observe a patient who can repeat full sentences but cannot formulate a sentence on his or her own.

## Summary of Neuroanatomical Principles
## Related to Aphasia

Several neuroanatomical principles have been introduced that highlight the relation between brain regions and language behaviors. Before summarizing those principles, it is important to remember that successful communication requires participation of many parts of the brain and that damage to a particular area does not mean that *only* the damaged area is responsible for the impaired function. Also, it is known that people vary in terms of their precise brain organization, such that identical lesions in two people may result in slightly different language profiles. With those caveats in mind, the following generalizations can be made:

1. Large anterior lesions interfere with fluent speech production, so nonfluent aphasias are associated with anterior lesions and fluent aphasias are associated with posterior lesions.
2. Lesions in and around Wernicke's area interfere with auditory comprehension, so posterior lesions tend to be associated with poor auditory comprehension and anterior lesions may leave auditory comprehension relatively well preserved.

3. Lesions within the perisylvian region disrupt the ability to repeat sentences, but lesions on the periphery of the perisylvian region result in relatively preserved ability to repeat.
4. Lesions throughout the left hemisphere can disrupt naming abilities, resulting in anomia, so the presence of anomia is not predictive of lesion location.

## Aphasia Types

We have noted the general predictability of language performance based on lesion location and have suggested that patients with similar lesions tend to have similar language characteristics. Aphasia classification systems are useful for identifying such clusters of language behaviors. We will review some of the more common aphasia types. The syndromes are labeled according to the Boston classification system, which characterizes aphasia type on the basis of fluency, auditory comprehension, and repetition abilities. Such classification systems are clinically useful, but not all individuals with aphasia will fit a specific type. In a large aphasia recovery study, Wertz and colleagues (1981) found that about 75 percent of the individuals with aphasia were classifiable by aphasia type, leaving 25 percent who were considered unclassifiable. In those cases, it is still useful to characterize the aphasia in terms of fluency, auditory comprehension, and repetition.

Figure 9.3 shows the decision process for classifying four of the more common aphasia types: Broca's, global, conduction, and Wernicke's. This simplified classification is based on the observed fluency of spontaneous speech (fluent versus nonfluent) and the status of auditory comprehension (good or poor). The figure also includes schematic drawings intended to depict a typical lesion location for each aphasia type. As indicated in Figure 9.3, the aphasia types differ with regard to observable language characteristics and likely lesion location. The nonfluent aphasias include damage to anterior portions of the brain, and the fluent aphasias are restricted to posterior lesions. As mentioned, however, there is considerable variation from person to person, so the predicted relations between lesion location and language behavior are not without many exceptions.

**Broca's Aphasia.**    Broca's aphasia is a nonfluent aphasia characterized by slow, hesitant, telegraphic speech. We saw an example of **Broca's aphasia** in Mr. Brown, the 36-year-old with nonfluent aphasia. As apparent in his conversational sample, utterances are of reduced length, typically fewer than four words, and have little syntactic complexity. The utterances are mostly isolated productions of nouns with some adjectives and verbs, and they are notably lacking in articles, prepositions, and other grammatical function words (called *functors*). Broca's aphasia is sometimes referred to as "motor aphasia" or "expressive aphasia," terms that highlight the observed production problems. Auditory comprehension is dependent upon understanding of complex grammar or the little functor words. Repetition ability is limited to a few words. When asked to repeat full sentences, individuals with Broca's aphasia may simply repeat the content words, such as the nouns. Reading

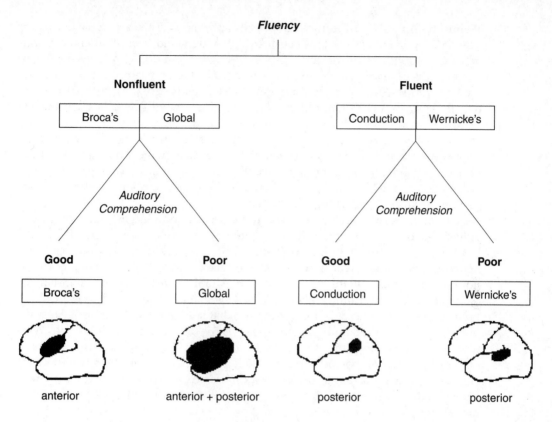

**FIGURE 9.3   A decision tree used to guide the classification of four common aphasia types based upon fluency of spontaneous speech (fluent vs. nonfluent) and auditory comprehension (good vs. poor). Schematic drawings depict typical brain lesions associated with each aphasia type and indicate whether the lesion extends anteriorly or posteriorly relative to the Rolandic fissure.**

and writing are also impaired in individuals with Broca's aphasia, because the aphasia affects all language modalities.

Broca's aphasia results from lesions affecting the posterior portion of the left inferior frontal lobe. These are considered anterior lesions because they extend anteriorly relative to the Rolandic fissure (see Figure 9.3). When a lesion is small and restricted to Broca's area, the individual may have Broca's aphasia for only a short time following the brain damage and then recover to a more fluent aphasia. Persistent Broca's aphasia typically results from larger lesions that not only affect Broca's area but also extend posteriorly to the anterior parietal lobe. An extensive anterior lesion often results in right hemiparesis due to damage to the primary motor cortex in the frontal lobe, as noted with Mr. Brown.

**Wernicke's Aphasia.**  In contrast to Broca's aphasia, **Wernicke's aphasia** is characterized by fluent speech that is difficult to understand because it contains numerous paraphasias (incorrect words or nonwords) and is relatively devoid of content. Mr. Wallace, the man who was introduced as an example of fluent aphasia, has Wernicke's aphasia. Immediately following his stroke, his utterances were heavily sprinkled with paraphasias in place of meaningful words, such that he made comments like "Oh, and there is a *kusbit* and a *wuzman*." Other individuals with more severe Wernicke's aphasia produce strings of neologisms (nonwords), so they may sound like they are speaking a foreign language. They have a normal flow of speech with variations in prosody but few real words. This type of output is sometimes called **jargon aphasia**, and it sounds similar in some ways to the jargon of a young child learning a language.

In addition to their fluent, paraphasic speech, individuals with Wernicke's aphasia have significant impairment of auditory comprehension (Figure 9.3). They have difficulty understanding spoken sentences and even have trouble comprehending many single words. This was the case for Mr. Wallace. When asked to point to the table, he blankly repeated, "table, table, I should know what that is." Another patient with more severe Wernicke's aphasia responded to the task by pointing to the door and saying something that sounded like "*illotime*." An additional sign of impaired auditory processing is the failure of individuals with Wernicke's aphasia to recognize their production errors. When asked to repeat words or sentences spoken by the clinician, their performance is no better. Repetition abilites are impaired due to the poor auditory processing and production problems. Reading and writing are also typically impaired in individuals with Wernicke's aphasia.

As might be expected, Wernicke's aphasia is associated with lesions in what is known as Wernicke's area (Figure 9.1). This region in the posterior, superior portion of the left temporal lobe is adjacent to the primary auditory cortex and is thought to be critical for auditory comprehension of language. Such posterior lesions typically spare the cortical areas important for motor control of the body, so individuals with Wernicke's aphasia rarely have hemiparesis.

**Conduction Aphasia.**  **Conduction aphasia** is somewhat similar to Wernicke's aphasia in that the verbal output is fluent, paraphasias are common, and repetition is impaired. However, individuals with conduction aphasia have better auditory comprehension than those with Wernicke's aphasia, presumably because much of Wernicke's area is spared (Figure 9.3). It is not uncommon for these individuals to attempt to self-correct their own errors, and frequently they are successful after several attempts. The self-corrections and hesitations associated with word-finding problems cause some disruption of the flow of speech, but the verbal output retains a sense of fluency in that articulation is accomplished with relative ease. Because the lesion spares the anterior motor regions, conduction aphasia typically is not associated with hemiparesis.

Conduction aphasia is associated with lesions in the left temporo-parietal region, particularly in an area immediately posterior to the Sylvian fissure called the supramarginal gyrus. As mentioned earlier, such a lesion disrupts the communication between the anterior and posterior language regions, resulting in the poor repetition of spoken utterances that is a hallmark of this aphasia type.

**Global Aphasia.** **Global aphasia** refers to severe language impairment affecting all domains. It is associated with large left-hemisphere lesions that essentially damage the entire perisylvian region (Figure 9.3). In global aphasia, meaningful verbal output is typically extremely limited. In some cases, it is limited to repetitive utterances, such as "one, two, three" or "I can see." In other cases, the utterances are repetitive jargon such as "nanna nanna nanna." Utterances that are repeated are called **perseverations**. It is worth noting that even individuals with global aphasia are capable of communicating wants, needs, and opinions if the listener provides a supportive communication environment.

**Anomic Aphasia.** A common aphasia type not shown in Figure 9.3 is **anomic aphasia**. This syndrome is characterized by word retrieval difficulty in conversation and in the context of naming tasks, with relative preservation of fluency, auditory comprehension, and repetition abilities. Athough all aphasia types exhibit word-finding difficulty, in the case of anomic aphasia, it is the primary deficit. Anomic aphasia can result from relatively isolated lesions in the posterior temporoparietal region, but it has also been associated with lesions throughout the left hemisphere. Some of the other aphasia types may evolve to anomic aphasia after a period of recovery if the brain damage is not extensive. Therefore, the presence of anomic aphasia does not provide information about the location of the aphasia-producing lesion.

## Causes of Aphasia

There are about one million Americans with aphasia and about 80,000 new cases of aphasia every year (National Aphasia Association, 1988). It is a disorder most often associated with older age, with the average age of people with aphasia being about 67 years (Hier et al., 1994). Stroke is the most common cause of brain damage resulting in aphasia. A **stroke**, also called a cerebrovascular accident, is an interruption of blood flow to the brain caused by blockage of an artery or the bursting of an artery (hemorrhage). When blood flow to brain cells is interrupted, they are deprived of oxygen, which ultimately results in cell death. Those brain cells do not regenerate, so the functions subserved by the damaged cells are impaired. Other causes of brain damage, such as traumatic accident, brain tumor, or infection, can also result in aphasia.

It has long been known that in right-handed people language problems tend to occur after damage to the left hemisphere. It is damage to the left perisylvian region that typically results in aphasia. The major blood vessel that serves the perisylvian region is the middle cerebral artery; therefore, stroke affecting the left middle cerebral artery is the most common cause of aphasia (Benson & Ardila, 1996).

The onset of aphasia is typically abrupt, but some etiologies may be associated with a slowly progressive onset. Brain tumors can cause slow onset of aphasia as they either infiltrate or compress critical language areas. **Primary progressive aphasia** is a relatively rare syndrome in which aphasia develops in the absence of a documented neurological event (McNeil & Duffy, 2001; Mesulam, 1982). In other words, the aphasia is not caused by a stroke or head injury, but rather by a progressive loss of brain cells in the cortical areas important for language.

## Assessment

The initial evaluation of a person with aphasia may take place at the bedside in an acute care hospital. Informal interaction with the patient allows observation of some aspects of verbal fluency, auditory comprehension, and word retrieval. A few structured tasks can further inform the speech-language pathologist of the patient's ability to understand spoken and written language, to repeat sentences, and to communicate by writing. The initial assessment goals are typically to characterize the nature of the impairment and to appraise the functional abilities of the patient. A more comprehensive language assessment is usually deferred until a few days or weeks later, when the patient is able to sit at a table and tolerate the demands of sustained, structured interaction. However, the speech-language pathologist can be of considerable assistance to the patient and family during the first few days after the onset of aphasia as they seek to understand this strange disorder. Most important, the speech-language pathologist can facilitate successful communication with the patient and begin the process of training compensatory strategies to be used on a temporary or long-term basis.

*Mrs. Victor* awoke one morning and fell as she tried to get out of bed. She realized that her right side was weak and that she felt odd. After dragging herself to the nightstand, she telephoned her daughter using her left hand. As she tried to respond to her daughter's "hello," Mrs. Victor realized that she could not speak. Her daughter recognized her mother's phone number on her caller ID and was alarmed by her unintelligible speech. She assured her that she would call for help and come right over. Later that day, after a trip to the emergency room and admission to the medical center, Mrs. Victor lay in a hospital bed with her daughter at her side. It had been a hectic five hours of medical examinations, a brain scan, and admission paperwork. When the hospital speech-language pathologist arrived for her first bedside visit, she found Mrs. Victor's daughter upset and confused about her mother's condition.

After ten minutes of informal interaction with Mrs. Victor, it was apparent to the speech-language pathologist that Mrs. Victor had global aphasia: She produced very little meaningful speech and appeared to have difficulty understanding what was said to her. In order to support Mrs. Victor in her attempts to communicate, the speech-language pathologist provided a pad of paper and began to write single words as possible responses to questions she was asking. For example, to help Mrs. Victor respond to the question, "Where are you from?" the speech-language pathologist wrote (and said) *Tucson?* When Mrs. Victor shook her head no, the speech-language pathologist offered *Green Valley?* To which Mrs. Victor smiled and said, "yes." After several successful exchanges of information using the written support, Mrs. Victor and her daughter were obviously showing some relief. This initial visit ended with the speech-pathologist explaining to the daughter about aphasia and providing some written information about the nature of the communication impairment. Over the next several days, the daughter and nursing staff became adept at supporting Mrs. Victor's communication by offering written words, pictures, and objects as needed to clarify her intentions. Mrs. Victor was then transferred to a rehabilitation facility where she would receive aphasia treatment for several months. During her initial session with the speech-language pathologist at the rehab facility, she received a more extensive evaluation of her language abilities.

Comprehensive language assessment is frequently accomplished by the use of standardized tests of aphasia. Most of the tests take an hour or less to administer. They sample language behaviors of varying complexity and allow the examiner to create a summary profile of aphasia type and severity. There are many supplemental tests that may also be used to characterize patient performance, as well as informal measures constructed by the speech-language pathologist. Some protocols are specifically designed to examine the impact of the language impairment on everyday communication situations and are considered functional communication measures. The overall goal of assessment is to document the current status of the patient and provide direction for the treatment plan.

## Treatment

**Individual Therapy.**   The goals of aphasia treatment are to maximize the recovery of impaired language functions, to assist in the development of alternative and compensatory communication strategies, and to help the patient adjust to the residual deficits. There are countless approaches to achieving such goals. It is the responsibility of the speech-language pathologist to either select an existing treatment approach or design a unique approach that is appropriate for the specific patient. The treatment plan should take into consideration the nature and extent of the language impairment as well as the residual language and cognitive abilities. Treatment plans are influenced by additional factors such as the time since the onset of aphasia and the patient's functional needs, motivation, and desires. Although the classification by aphasia type is useful to characterize the overall aphasia profile, it does not offer specific direction for treatment, because individuals with the same aphasia type may differ in many ways.

There is a large body of literature to guide speech-language pathologists toward appropriate treatment approaches for a particular set of symptoms (see, e.g., Chapey, 2001; Helm-Estabrooks & Albert, 2004; Holland & Forbes, 1993; Robey, 1998). Clinicians update their knowledge of the evidence-based treatment approaches by reading professional journals and attending continuing education presentations.

The experienced clinician knows that a given treatment can be effective for patients with different impairments and that not all patients with similar impairments will respond to the same treatment approach (Hillis & Caramazza, 1994). Therefore, each patient's response to treatment should be carefully monitored and documented in order to evaluate its therapeutic effect and to make adjustments as needed.

When selecting or designing a treatment plan, the speech-language pathologist may approach treatment from several different perspectives. One approach is to stimulate the return of language abilities that are impaired but appear to have potential to improve or be restored. Many treatment protocols are designed to stimulate language by following a task hierarchy that requires progressively more difficult responses (some protocols are reviewed in Helm-Estabrooks & Alberts, 2004). The speech-language pathologist may determine what support or cues are necessarily to help the patient respond correctly and then systematically withdraw the support as the patient progresses. This approach incrementally shifts the burden from the clinician to the patient in order to achieve the desired response.

When implementing a treatment plan, the speech-language pathologist is challenged to find appropriate tasks that help the patient improve to a higher level of functioning. Although patients or family members may initially set a goal for completely normal language without any intermediate steps, the speech-language pathologist charts a realistic path that moves toward normal language but has intermediate goals along the way.

Some treatment approaches take advantage of residual abilities that can be used to substitute or compensate for impaired abilities. For example, a patient may be able to write a word or part of a word that he or she is unable to say. The use of writing to supplement spoken output may be an effective strategy. However, another possibility is that the written word may facilitate the spoken production of the word.

> After several months of language therapy, Mrs. Victor showed significant improvement of her comprehension of spoken and written language. Her spoken language remained severely impaired, however. She had several words and phrases that she typically uttered, such as "yes, but I don't know" and "oh my, oh my." The speech-language pathologist implemented treatment to improve Mrs. Victor's ability to write meaningful single words to communicate her thoughts. Mrs. Victor was able to relearn the spelling of many words, such that after several months of treatment she was able to write more than fifty words. It was noteworthy that on occasion Mrs. Victor was able to say the word that she was writing, despite the fact that she rarely spoke meaningful words in other contexts.

Individual treatment plans may include several goals that variously address auditory comprehension, speech production, reading, writing, and gestural communication. The treatment for Mrs. Victor focused on written rather than spoken language, due to the severity of her aphasia. Figure 9.4 shows another patient who responded well to a writing treatment (Beeson, 1999; Beeson, Rising, & Volk, 2003).

Obviously, the return of spoken language is the treatment goal whenever possible. A variety of treatment approaches to improve spoken language have

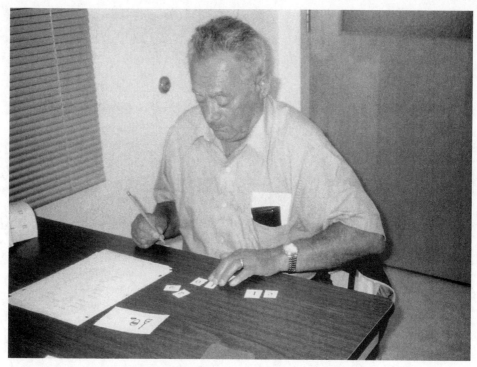

FIGURE 9.4   Individual therapy to improve writing for single words that includes arranging of letters to spell the word and copying the word.

been shown to be effective (e.g., see Chapey, 2001; Helm-Estabrooks & Albert, 2004). Many individuals with aphasia are able to say a word if they hear the first sound or syllable of the word. This responsiveness to phonemic cueing (as it is called) can be particularly useful if the patient can learn to provide his or her own phonemic cue for the word (Nickels, 1992). Therapy goals are selected so that they are appropriate for the particular patient and have immediate or eventual impact on their functional communication abilities.

**Group Therapy.**   Aphasia may result in social isolation and reduced opportunity to engage in conversation. Group therapy for individuals with aphasia provides a setting where conversation is facilitated and supported by the clinician, and patients can learn to maximize their communication skills (see Figure 9.5). In a small group of three to five individuals with aphasia, the speech-language pathologist can work with the patients to (1) facilitate successful communication despite their residual language impairment, (2) encourage communication using all modalities, and (3) teach and elaborate specific communication strategies (Beeson & Holland, 2007). In the small group setting, patients can learn from the clinician and from each other how to compensate for language difficulties. When appropriate, group

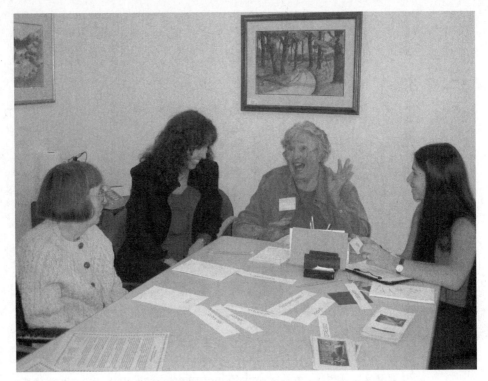

**FIGURE 9.5    Group therapy for aphasia focuses on conversational language supplemented by writing and gestures.**

members are encouraged to use alternative communication strategies, including gestures, drawing, and writing to supplement the spoken utterances. Groups also can offer considerable psychological and social support for members as they adjust to their impairment. Many examples of structured and informal conversational activities have been reported in recent literature regarding group therapy (Elman, 2007), and there is evidence that many individuals with aphasia can continue to improve language abilities long after the time of their strokes (Beeson & Holland, 2007).

## ACQUIRED READING AND WRITING IMPAIRMENTS

As previously noted, most individuals with aphasia have difficulty reading and writing as well as listening and speaking, so aphasia treatment frequently includes intervention for all language modalities. On relatively rare occasions, damage to the left posterior temporo-parietal region results in isolated impairments of reading and writing in the absence of significant aphasia. The speech-language pathologist is involved in the assessment and treatment of written language disorders.

*Alexia* refers to an acquired impairment of reading, and *agraphia* refers to an acquired impairment of writing. **Pure alexia**, also known as *alexia without agraphia*, is an unusual syndrome wherein the patient is able to write but cannot read. It is thought to result from a disruption of the transfer of visual information to the part of the brain that recognizes the word as a meaningful unit. The individual with pure alexia can see the words and may even be able to identify the letters of the word, but fails to recognize the word as a whole. Many individuals with pure alexia compensate for their lack of word recognition by reading the individual letters aloud; when they hear the word spelled aloud, they can recognize it. This letter-by-letter reading approach is useful, but painfully slow.

> One day *Mr. Lincoln* answered the telephone and wrote down a message from the caller for his wife. Later, when his wife called home, Mr. Lincoln picked up the note to read her the message. To his surprise, the letters made no sense to him; he could not read his own handwriting! He told his wife that there was something wrong with his eyes and that he thought he should go see his eye doctor. The eye doctor found nothing wrong with Mr. Lincoln's eyes but recognized that a stroke had affected his ability to recognize written words.
>
> Within a week, Mr. Lincoln was in treatment with a speech-language pathologist to improve his reading. He could recognize single letters and figure out most words by spelling them letter-by-letter, but he had great difficulty recognizing written words as whole units. The speech-language pathologist implemented a treatment that involved reading written passages multiple times in order to increase his rate for the practiced text (Beeson & Hillis, 2001). Over the course of treatment, Mr. Lincoln showed improved reading rate for the practiced text, and, more important, his reading rate and accuracy improved for new reading material. In other words, the treatment appeared to improve his ability to recognize written words. Ultimately, Mr. Lincoln was able to read with adequate accuracy and speed to meet his daily needs.

Some individuals with acquired alexia also have difficulty spelling. They experience a syndrome called *alexia with agraphia*. The term **agraphia** refers to an acquired impairment of spelling. Individuals with acquired agraphia vary with regard to their residual writing abilities (Rapcsak & Beeson, 2002). Some may be able to sound out words they cannot recall how to spell, relying on their preserved knowledge of the relations between sounds and letters. In such cases, it is not uncommon to make errors on irregularly spelled words. For example, "school" might be spelled *skool*. Given that individuals vary with regard to the nature of their reading or writing difficulties, treatment approaches for acquired alexia and acquired agraphia are tailored to the specific nature of the impairment (Beeson & Hillis, 2001).

## RIGHT-HEMISPHERE COMMUNICATION DISORDERS

Damage to the right hemisphere may result in some word retrieval difficulties similar to that observed in left-hemisphere damage. However, the prominent features of right-hemisphere damage (RHD) tend to be quite different from those associated with left-hemisphere damage. Individuals with RHD may have a host of subtle impairments in their thought organization, mental flexibility, and use of language that affect their ability to understand and communicate effectively (Lehman Blake, Duffy, Myers, & Tompkins, 2002). Although individuals with RHD typically understand the content of individual sentences, they often fail to understand the gist of the conversation or appreciate humor or figures of speech. For example, when a patient with right-hemisphere damage was asked to explain what it means when someone says, "You can't have your cake and eat it too," he responded, "It means you have share it, I guess. You can't eat the whole thing." These difficulties with the abstract use of language are accompanied by reduced use of facial expression and prosody to convey emotion while speaking, so that individuals with RHD appear to be disinterested during conversational exchange. They are also less perceptive of the nonverbal communication cues provided by other speakers and often fail to keep up with the natural give-and-take and shift of topic in conversation. These functions are referred to as extralinguistic aspects of communication, meaning that they are features other than the actual words used to speak. These problems sound rather vague, and, in fact, individuals with RHD simply may be perceived as odd, rude, or inattentive, rather than brain-damaged. However, their change in cognitive and communication abilities is clearly evident to friends and family who know them well. One of the patients at our clinic, Mr. Rice, explained his perception of one of the effects of his right-hemisphere stroke as follows:

> Taking turns in talking conversation was very difficult . . . because I would interrupt and have something to say in the middle of the conversation and interrupt everything. Train of thought and everything else. I thought I had to jump in otherwise I'd lose what I was trying to say.

Mr. Rice was 66 years old when he experienced a right-hemisphere stroke. One year after his stroke he still had weakness of his left arm and leg, but he could walk without assistance and communicate effectively. His speech was easy to understand, but the prosody sounded somewhat flat, as if lacking emotion; even when he joked, his voice and facial expression were difficult to interpret. It was notable that Mr. Rice was able to provide some insight into the nature of his problem, because many individuals with RHD do not recognize their deficits.

Mr. Rice also experienced **left neglect**, in that he tended to orient his gaze away from the left and was relatively unaware of sensory input on the left side of his body and the left side of his visual field. Left neglect is relatively common following right-hemisphere damage, and it occurs even when there is no loss of sensory or motor function on the left side and no loss of vision on the left (Heilman, Watson, & Valenstein, 2003). In other words, the visual images are getting to the brain, but they are essentially ignored.

These effects of brain damage have shown that the right hemisphere plays a special role in maintaining attention to the space around us and our intrapersonal space as well. Left neglect may interfere with communication, in that people to the patient's left are ignored and the left half of the page may be ignored when reading and writing. It is likely that the attentional problems associated with left neglect also relate to the impaired ability to attend to the extralinguistic information provided during conversation (Myers, 1999). Future research may help to clarify the relation between neglect and the cognitive-communication impairment associated with right-hemisphere damage.

## Incidence of Right-Hemisphere Damage

Given the relatively subtle nature of the cognitive-communication problems associated with RHD, it is not surprising that the incidence and prevalence are not well documented. The American Heart Association (2006) reported that there were about 500,000 new strokes each year in the United States, with about half affecting the right hemisphere. About half of those adults with right-hemisphere damage will have communication impairments, so we would estimate 125,000 new cases of right-hemisphere-related communication impairments caused by stroke per year (Benton & Bryan, 1996; Tompkins, 1995). Stroke is the most common cause of damage isolated to the right hemisphere, but other causes include traumatic injury or tumor.

## Assessment and Treatment

Assessment of the patient with RHD typically includes sampling language in conversation and picture description tasks, assessing the extralinguistic aspects of communication, and examining for evidence of neglect or attentional problems (Myers, 1999; Tompkins, 1995). Examination of extralinguistic deficits includes tasks such as interpretation of a story or a pictured scene that requires integration of the component parts into one main idea. Patients may be asked to explain the meaning of figures of speech or to produce the certain expressions with appropriate prosodic variation to convey different emotions. They may also be asked to produce or understand narrative stories. All of these tasks share the common goal of probing comprehension and use of language in a flexible, abstract manner that comes naturally to most adults but may be problematic for those with RHD. Numerous tasks can be used to examine for neglect, including a very simple request for patients to put a mark on a line to divide it in half. Individuals with left neglect often bisect the line to the right of the midline because they do not perceive the leftmost part of the line. The ability to sustain attention is also assessed using tasks that increase from focused attention on one stimulus to divided attention on two stimuli. Some standardized tests are available to examine the RHD patient.

Treatment for cognitive and communication deficits associated with RHD is challenging, particularly because individuals with RHD often do not recognize their deficits. In contrast to individuals with aphasia due to left-hemisphere damage, who are often highly motivated to improve their language skills, it is common for individuals with RHD to deny that they have had a change in their communication abilities. Treatment for RHD may be directed toward facilitating recovery of the underlying impairment or toward the development of compensatory strategies to overcome the problems. Greater understanding of the underlying causes of the communication deficits observed in RHD is needed, but it is currently assumed that the extralinguistic deficits are related to the features of neglect and inattention (Myers, 1999). For that reason, some treatment tasks are directed toward improving performance on attention tasks. For example, patients may be asked to listen or look for specific stimuli such as a particular number or word in the midst of other numbers or words (Sohlberg & Mateer, 2001). These types of attention tasks are also used with individuals with traumatic head injury because they often have problems with attention too. Tasks that are directed toward improving extralinguistic abilities may be similar to those used for assessment. After observing the patient's deficits, the speech-language pathologist may structure the language tasks in such a way that a hierarchy of cues provides support for the patients. As discussed in aphasia therapy, the clinician's goal is to assist the patient to make small sequential gains in the direction of normal performance. This may require providing feedback when the patient fails to produce or comprehend the extralinguistic features, such as prosodic variation to mark emotion, followed by a model of the appropriate response. The treatment goals are directed toward improved performance in a variety of settings and communication environments, not simply in the therapy room. This is true for all treatments for speech, language, and hearing disorders, but is especially relevant for the problems associated with RHD, because these problems often affect the social aspects of communication.

## DEMENTIA

**Dementia** refers to an acquired, progressive impairment of intellectual function that is chronic and affects several aspects of mental activity, including memory, cognition, language, and the processing of visual-spatial information (Cummings & Benson, 1992; Kaszniak, 2002). Dementia may also result in changes in emotion or personality. It is distinguishable from temporary conditions that impair mental function such as confusional states that may last for a few hours or a few days. The progressive intellectual decline in dementia is distinct from isolated, specific impairments such as aphasia due to focal brain damage. Numerous diseases can cause the diffuse brain damage that results in dementia, and the characteristics of the dementia vary to some extent depending on the disease process.

### Types of Dementia

The most common type of dementia is **Alzheimer's disease** (AD) (Cummings & Benson, 1992; Dugué, Neugroscl, Sewell, & Marin, 2003). AD affects about 4.5 million Americans, and it accounts for more than half of all dementias (Alzheimer's Association, 2006). It is characterized by language, memory, and cognitive impairments that include poor judgment and difficulty with calculation, reasoning, and higher level thinking. Caregivers note that the early signs of dementia include memory and concentration problems, such as forgetting the location of things, poor recall for recent events, and trouble handling finances and performing complex tasks. Speech is typically well articulated and fluent and may have good grammatical structure, but the content is increasingly empty as the disease progresses. In the early stages, the language impairment may appear similar to anomic aphasia in that there are many instances of word-finding difficulties. In later stages, it may resemble the empty ramblings observed in some individuals with Wernicke's aphasia. At the end stages, there may be little verbal output at all.

Alzheimer's disease can only be confirmed after death, by the presence of specific brain changes observable if an autopsy is performed. For that reason, the diagnosis of AD prior to death is tentative, referred to as "probable" AD, based on the presenting symptoms and the exclusion of other causes of dementia. The criteria for the behavioral diagnosis of Alzheimer's disease and other types of dementia are described in detail in a manual published by the American Psychiatric Association (2000).

In addition to Alzheimer's disease, there are some forty or fifty other causes of dementia. One of the more common causes is vascular disease resulting in multiple strokes that produce diffuse brain damage. Whereas Alzheimer's disease tends to have a steadily progressive course, the cognitive decline associated with vascular, or **multi-infarct**, dementia may cause a stair-step decline as subsequent strokes occur. Other types of dementia are associated with Pick's disease, Parkinson disease, and Huntington's disease. **Pick's disease** is characterized by brain abnormalities in the frontal and temporal lobes and typically results in marked changes in personality. Parkinson disease is a relatively well-known progressive disorder of movement that is accompanied by dementia in about 35 to 40 percent of cases (Kaszniak, 2002). Huntington's disease is a genetic disorder that results in progressive onset of a movement disorder and eventual dementia.

Memory impairment is often the initial symptom of dementia; however, in some cases the language decline may be the first sign. At our clinic, Mr. Dean brought his 67-year-old wife for an evaluation because, as he explained, her language "was becoming more and more confused." Her speech was well articulated and easy to understand, but it was devoid of meaningful content and contained many perseverative thoughts. A report of a head scan indicated there was a generalized loss of brain substance but no evidence of a stroke.

When shown a toy gun and asked to name it, Mrs. Dean said:

MRS. DEAN:   This is to put. Um, you can put a thing inside the . . .

AUTHOR:   Can you tell me the name of it?

MRS. DEAN:   Well, it's supposed to be, to do. But that, that's musty. It's hard, when you're on the table and the table is dirty, I take the longer thing, like this, and get the end. I don't, don't go by this thing. No, this I, see it always in my house. Oh here I can do this, I can do this. It goes if you go.

Mrs. Dean's verbal output sounded in many ways like an individual with aphasia. However, there were some features of her behavior that were unlike those observed in aphasia. She showed anxiety and perseverative thoughts as she repeatedly asked where her husband had gone and how she was going to get home. Mrs. Dean indicated during a private interview that his wife had become paranoid about her money. She no longer used the bank but had begun stuffing money under the mattress at home. Six months following the interview, Mrs. Dean's neurologist observed that her behavior had become increasingly bizarre, showing signs associated with frontal lobe damage, such as lack of inhibition and modesty. The neurologist rejected a diagnosis of Alzheimer's disease in favor of a working diagnosis of Pick's disease. Like AD, Pick's disease is a cortical dementia, meaning that there is a progressive loss of neurons in the cortex. In Pick's disease, brain changes occur primarily in the frontal and temporal lobes, resulting in changes in personality that accompany the changes in intellect, memory, and language. As with Alzheimer's disease, the diagnosis of Pick's disease is not actually confirmed unless the brain is studied after death.

## Prevalence

Although the exact prevalence of dementia is not known, there is a clear increase with age. It has been estimated that the syndrome affects approximately 5 to 8 percent of individuals over 65 years, 15 to 20 percent of individuals over 75 years, and 25 to 50 percent of those over 80 years (American Psychiatric Association, 2000). The prevalence of dementia is expected to increase as the older segment of our population continues to grow in number.

## Assessment and Intervention

A comprehensive examination of cognitive function is critical to the diagnosis of dementia and may be performed by a neuropsychologist. Several standardized rating scales are used to screen for dementia. These scales include tasks that look at general knowledge, memory, communication, and visual-spatial skills (such as drawing). Other scales rate the severity of dementia using observational criteria, rather than direct testing. Comprehensive tests of cognitive function evaluate attention, initiation, visual-spatial construction, conceptualization, language, and memory. In many settings, a speech-language pathologist is involved in the assessment of language and communication abilities and contributes to the understanding of language function relative to other cognitive abilities. Individuals with dementia may also have concomitant hearing impairment that interferes with daily function and performance on cognitive assessments, so an audiological evaluation is an important component of the diagnostic process.

Speech-language pathologists are taking an increasingly active role in the care of individuals with dementia. Although dementia is an irreversible process, therapeutic approaches may be employed that maximize communication and cognitive performance (Bayles & Kim, 2003). There are numerous sources of information regarding environmental and linguistic manipulations that positively influence the behavior of individuals with dementia (Bayles & Tomoeda, 1995;

Davis, 2005; Hopper, 2001; Small & Perry, 2005). For example, communication performance can be improved by minimizing distractions and using familiar objects or pictures to stimulate recollections. Auditory comprehension may be improved with the use of simplified syntax and vocabulary. Memory demands can be minimized by making use of a memory book that contains biographical information, pictures of family and friends, and schedule information (Bourgeois, 1992).

The patient's performance profile on a test battery can be examined to determine his or her relative strengths and weaknesses. This information, combined with observation and experimentation, may help clinicians discover the cognitive, language, and environmental manipulations that minimize the effects of the dementia (Tomoeda, 2001). It is often the role of the speech-language pathologist to develop a program that outlines strategies for communicating with specific dementia patients. The speech-language pathologist works with caregivers, including family members and nursing home staff, to implement the plan and thus provide consistent support to maximize the performance of the dementia patient. In the case of Mrs. Dean, it was apparent that her husband was exhausted by his failure to communicate successfully with his wife. He stated, "She can't even tell me what she wants to eat for dinner." One easy solution to that problem was discovered: If Mr. Dean wrote down three choices for dinner and asked his wife which one she would like, she was able to respond by pointing to one of the options. Other suggestions were made to Mr. Dean to adapt his communication style in such a way as to maximize his wife's ability to communicate.

In closing this chapter, we want to emphasize that acquired impairments of language and cognition may have profound implications for the lives of the affected individuals and their families. Patients may experience significant limitations in their daily activities and restrictions on their participation in society. Thus, speech-language pathologists who work with adults with acquired language disorders are concerned not only with the acquired impairment but also with the consequences of that impairment. Evaluation and treatment approaches are sensitive to the specific needs of a given individual in his or her unique life situation.

## CLINICAL PROBLEM SOLVING

Mrs. Anderson was a 55-year-old woman who suffered a left-hemisphere stroke that resulted in aphasia. She was administrated the *Western Aphasia Battery* (Kertesz, 1982) to sample her language abilities. As part of the test, she was asked to describe what was happening in a pictured scene of a man and a woman having a picnic near a lake. Her spoken response follows:

> Is family, um, picnic. And fish, and man is, um, oh, um reading, and, and, um lady, is pouring and set, um, son is, is, ha . . . is, um, is, um flying kite. And neighbor is dishing and neighbor is um, sailing, and boy, um, playing in water, and man, and lady in, listen to radio. And daughter, I mean, dog, oh . . . oh . . . stave, is lady, is man, is stave, oh, stay. I don't know.

1. Would you classify Mrs. Anderson's aphasia as fluent or nonfluent?
2. In what lobe of the brain is the lesion most likely to be located? Why?
3. Mrs. Anderson had trouble repeating sentences longer than four words. Would you expect her lesion to be in the perisylvian region or outside the perisylvian region? Why?
4. Would you guess that Mrs. Anderson had right hemiparesis? Why or why not?

## REFERENCES

Alzheimer's Association. (2006). Alzheimer's disease statistics. Retrieved December 4, 2006, from http://www.alz.org/resources/fact sheets/FSAlzheimerstats.pdf

American Heart Association. (2006). Heart disease and stroke statistics—2006 update: A report from the American Heart Association Statistics Committee and Stroke Statistics Subcommittee. *Circulation, 113,* e85–e151.

American Psychiatric Association. (2000). *Diagnostic and statistical manual of mental disorders.* (DSM-IV-TR). Washington, DC: Author.

Bayles, K. A., & Kim, E. S. (2003). Improving the functioning of individuals with Alzheimer's disease: Emergence of behavioral interventions. *Journal of Communication Disorders, 36*(5), 327–344.

Bayles, K., & Tomoeda, C. (1995). *The ABCs of dementia.* Tucson, AZ: Canyonlands Publishing.

Beeson, P. M. (1999). Treating acquired writing impairment: Strengthening graphemic representations. *Aphasiology, 13,* 367–386.

Beeson, P. M., & Hillis, A. E. (2001). Comprehension and production of written words. In R. Chapey (Ed.), *Language intervention strategies in adult aphasia* (4th ed., pp. 572–595). Baltimore: Lippincott, Williams & Wilkins.

Beeson, P. M., & Holland, A. L. (2007). Aphasia groups in a university setting. In R. Elman (Ed.), *Group treatment of neurogenic communication disorders: The expert clinician's approach* (2nd ed.) San Diego: Plural Publishing.

Beeson, P. M., & Rapcsak, S. Z. (2006). The aphasias. In P. J. Snyder & P. D. Nussbaum (Eds.), *Clinical neuropsychology: A pocket handbook for assessment* (2nd ed., pp. 436–459). Washington, DC: American Psychological Association.

Beeson, P. M., Bayles, K. A., Rubens, A. B., & Kaszniak, A. W. (1993). Memory impairment and executive control in individuals with stroke-induced aphasia. *Brain and Language, 45,* 253–275.

Beeson, P. M., Rising, K., & Volk, J. (2003). Writing treatment for severe aphasia. *Journal of Speech, Language, and Hearing Research, 46,* 1038–1060.

Benson, D. F., & Ardila, A. (1996). *Aphasia: A clinical perspective.* New York: Oxford University Press.

Benton, E., & Bryan, K. (1996). Right cerebral hemisphere damage: incidence of language problems. *International Journal of Rehabilitation Research, 19*(1), 47–54.

Bourgeois, M. S. (1992). *Conversing with memory impaired individuals using memory aids: A memory aid workbook.* Gaylord, MI: Northern Speech Services.

Chapey, R. (Ed.). (2001). *Language intervention strategies in adult aphasia* (4th ed.). Baltimore: Lippincott, William & Wilkins.

Cummings, J. L., & Benson, D. F. (1992). *Dementia: A clinical approach.* Boston: Butterworth.

Damasio, H., & Damasio, A. (1980). The anatomical basis of conduction aphasia. *Brain, 103,* 337–350.

Davis, L. A. (2005). Educating individuals with dementia: Perspectives for rehabilitation professionals. *Topics in Geriatric Rehabilitation, 21*(4), 304–314.

Dugué, M., Neugroscl, J., Sewell, M., & Marin, D. (2003). Review of dementia. *The Mount Sinai Journal of Medicine, 70,* 45–53.

Elman, R.J. (2007). *Group treatment for neurogenic communication disorders: The expert clinician's approach* (2nd ed.). San Diego, CA: Plural Publishing.

Goodglass, H. (1993). *Understanding aphasia.* San Diego: Academic Press.

Heilman, K. M., Watson, R. T., & Valenstein, E. (2003). Neglect and related disorders. In K. Heilman & E. Valenstein (Eds.), *Clinical neuropsychology* (4th ed., pp. 296–346). New York: Oxford University Press.

Helm-Estabrooks, N., & Albert, M. L. (2004). *Manual of aphasia and aphasia therapy* (2nd ed.). Austin, TX: Pro-Ed.

Hier, D. B., Yoon, W. B., Mohr, J. P., Price, T. R., & Wolf, P. A. (1994). Gender and aphasia in the stroke data bank. *Brain and Language, 47,* 155–167.

Hillis, A. E., & Caramazza, A. (1994). Theories of lexical processing and rehabilitation of lexical deficits. In M. J. Riddoch & G. W. Humphries (Eds.), *Cognitive neuropsychology and cognitive rehabilitation* (pp. 449–484). Hillsdale, NJ: Lawrence Erlbaum Associates.

Holland, A. L., & Forbes, M. (Eds.). (1993). *Aphasia treatment: World perspectives.* San Diego: Singular Publishing.

Hopper, T. (2001). Indirect interventions to facilitate communication in Alzheimer's disease. *Seminars in Speech and Language, 22,* 290–304.

Kaszniak, A. W. (2002). Dementia. In V. S. Ramachandran (Ed.), *Encyclopedia of the human brain* (pp. 89–100). San Diego: Elsevier Science.

Kertesz, K. (2006). *Western Aphasia Battery–Revised.* San Antonio, TX: Harcourt Assessment.

Lehman Blake, M., Duffy, J. R., Myers, P. S., & Tompkins, C. A. (2002). Prevalence and patterns of right hemisphere cognitive/communicative deficits: Retrospective data from an inpatient rehabilitation unit. *Aphasiology, 16,* 537–547.

McNeil, M.R. & Duffy, J.R. (2001). Primary progressive aphasia. In R. Chapey, *Language Intervention Strategies for Aphasia.* 4th ed., pp. 472–486. Baltimore: Williams and Wilkins.

Mesulam, M-M. (1982). Slowly progressive aphasia without generalized dementia. *Annals of Neurology, 11,* 592–598.

Murray, L. L. (2002). Attention deficits in aphasia: Presence, nature, assessment, and treatment. *Seminars in Speech and Language, 23,* 107–116.

Myers, P. (1999). Right hemisphere damage: Disorders of communication and cognition. San Diego: Singular.

National Aphasia Association. (1988; reviewed 2005). *Impact of aphasia on patients and families: Results of a needs survey.* New York: Author.

Nickels, L. (1992). The autocue? Self-generated phonemic cues in the treatment of a disorder of reading and naming. *Cognitive Neuropsychology, 9,* 155–182.

Rapcsak, S. Z., & Beeson, P. M. (2002). Neuroanatomical correlates of spelling and writing. In A. E. Hillis (Ed.). *Handbook on adult language disorders: Integrating cognitive neuropsychology, neurology, and rehabilitation.* (pp. 71–99). Philadelphia: Psychology Press.

Robey, R. R. (1998). A meta-analysis of clinical outcomes in the treatment of aphasia. *Journal of Speech, Language, and Hearing Research, 41,* 172–187.

Small, J. A., & Perry, J. (2005). Do you remember? How caregivers question their spouses who have Alzheimer's disease and the impact on communication. *Journal of Speech, Language, and Hearing Research, 48*(1), 125–136.

Sohlberg, M. M., & Mateer, C. A. (2001). *Cognitive rehabilitation: An integrative approach.* New York: Guilford.

Tomoeda, C. K. (2001). Comprehensive assessment for dementia: A necessity for differential diagnosis and management. *Seminars in Speech and Language, 22*(4), 275–290.

Tompkins, C. A. (1995). *Right hemisphere communication disorders: Theory and management.* San Diego: Singular Publishing Group.

Tröster, A., & Woods, S. P. (2003). Neuropsychological aspects of Parkinson's disease and parkinsonism syndromes. In R. Pahwa, K. E. Lyons, & W. C. Koller (Eds.), *Handbook of Parkinson's disease* (3rd ed., pp. 127–157). New York: Marcel Dekker.

Wertz, R. T., Collins, M. J., Weiss, D., Kurtzke, J. F., Friden, T., Brookshire, R. H., Pierce, J., Holzapple, P., Hubbard, D. J., Proch, B. E., West, H. A., Davis, L., Matlvitch, V., Morley, G. K., & Resurreccion, E. (1981). Veteran's Administration cooperative study on aphasia: A comparison of individual and group treatment. *Journal of Speech and Hearing Research, 24,* 580–594.

## READINGS FROM THE POPULAR LITERATURE

Bauby, J-D. (1997). *The diving bell and the butterfly.* New York: Random House. (locked-in syndrome)

Bayley, J. (2000). *Elegy for Iris.* New York: St. Martin's Press. (Alzheimer disease)

Bryant, B. (1992). *In search of wings: A journey back from traumatic brain injury.* South Paris, ME: Wings Press. (traumatic brain injury)

Crimmins, C. (2000). *Where is the mango princess?* New York: Random House. (traumatic brain injury)

Davidson, A. (1997). *Alzheimers, a love story. One year in my husband's journey.* Secaucus, NJ: Carol Pub. Group. (Alzheimer disease)

DeMille, A. (1981). *Reprieve.* New York: Doubleday. (famous dancer's account of her stroke)

Douglas, K. (2001). *My stroke of luck.* New York: W. Morrow. (actor's experience with stroke, aphasia, and dysarthria)

Edsall, S. (2004). *Into the blue: A father's flight and a daughter's return.* New York: St. Martin's Press. (a daughter's story about her father who had a stroke)

Ellison, B., & Ellison, J. (2001). *Miracles happen: One mother, one daughter, one journey.* New York: Hyperion. (spinal cord injury)

Fishman, Steve. (1988). *A bomb in the brain: A heroic tale of science, surgery and survival.* New York: Scribner. (brain hemorrhage, subsequent epilepsy)

Harper, M. S. (2001). *The worst day of my life, so far.* Athens, GA: Hill Street Press. (Alzheimer disease)

Klein, B. S. (1998). *Slow dance: A story of stroke, love and disability.* Berkeley, CA: Page Mill Press. (stroke and aphasia)

McGowin, D. F. (1994). *Living in the labyrinth: A personal journey through the maze of Alzheimer's disease.* New York: Dell Publishing. (early Alzheimer's disease from patient's perspective)

Newborn, B. (1997). *Return to Ithaca.* Rockport, MA: Element. (young woman with aphasia)

Osborne, C. (1998). *Over my head: A doctor's own story of head injury from the inside looking out.* Kansas City, MO: Andrews McMeel Pub. (traumatic brain injury)

Shiplett, Jane Lund. (1996). *A glass full of tears.* Aurora, OH: Writer's World Press. (dementia)

Swanson, K., & Chrunkra, M. (1999). *I'll carry the fork.* Los Altos, CA: Rising Star Press. (traumatic brain injury)

# CHAPTER TEN

# THE BIOLOGICAL
# FOUNDATIONS OF HEARING

## THEODORE J. GLATTKE

## PREVIEW

Sound is a form of energy that is present everywhere in our environment. In Chapter 3, we learned that sound can be described in terms of frequency and intensity and the characteristics of the sounds associated with speech. In this chapter, we consider how the sounds around us are received and processed by the auditory system. We will see how the structures of the outer and middle ear transmit sound to the inner ear. We will learn how the structure of the inner ear contributes to our ability to hear sounds of different pitches and how the nervous system further shapes sound perception.

## STRUCTURE AND FUNCTION OF THE EAR

### The Outer Ear

The ear usually is described as having three distinct divisions: outer, middle, and inner. As illustrated in Figure 10.1, the outer ear consists of a visible portion, the **auricle**, or **pinna**, and a canal that leads from the pinna to the eardrum, or tympanic membrane. The canal between the pinna and tympanic membrane is the **external ear canal**.

The shape of the pinna is created by pieces of cartilage that form ridges and depressions that are peculiar to each person. In fact, pinna configurations are so unique that we could identify people using "pinna prints" instead of fingerprints. In adults, the pinna is about 3.5 inches in height and about 1.5 inches wide. It is a sound collector and also serves to enhance the sound pressure of certain frequencies. You can exaggerate this effect by cupping your hand behind your pinna and thus increasing the dimension of the sound collector. For most people, the pinna acts to increase high-frequency sounds by about 5 dB SPL. It also helps us to locate the sources of high-frequency sounds that are overhead, such as those produced by flying insects.

The external ear canal is about 1 inch long and about 0.4 inch in diameter. Cartilage forms the foundation of the canal near the pinna. The inner portion of the canal is framed by hard bone. If you place your finger slightly into the canal and move your jaw, you can feel your jawbone moving against the flexible portion of the external ear canal. The canal protects the tympanic membrane from physical trauma due to nearly everything except for cotton swabs pushed into the canal by the owner! Specialized cells in the floor of the ear canal produce a waxy substance called **cerumen** that helps to keep the skin of the canal moist and traps debris that might normally fall against the tympanic membrane. Like the pinna, the length and shape of the ear canal also serve to enhance sound pressure. The canal produces a boost in SPL of about 15 dB for sounds in the frequency region of 2500 to 3500 Hz and for multiples of those frequencies. Taken together, the effects of the pinna and external ear canal provide a helpful boost in the mid- and high-frequency region of the sound spectrum. Without those structures, we would have a slight loss of hearing.

**FIGURE 10.1    A schematic drawing of the divisions of the hearing mechanism.**

## The Middle Ear

The **middle ear** consists of a cavity, a ventilating tube that connects the cavity to the pharynx, and several moving parts that work together to boost the pressure created by the sound energy that arrives at the eardrum, or tympanic membrane. The middle ear apparatus is called a **transformer** because of the change in pressure that it creates. You probably use transformers every day: The small adapters that are found on the electrical cords of CD players, computer accessories, and video cameras are transformers that change the voltage supplied by the power company to a value that is required by the device. By analogy, the middle ear provides a boost in pressure to drive the inner ear system.

The principal parts of the middle ear are illustrated in Figure 10.2. The middle ear cavity is formed of bone that is covered by thin mucosa similar to the lining of the nasal cavities. The volume of the cavity is small, less than about 2 cc. The eardrum, or **tympanic membrane**, is stretched across the opening of the external canal so that nearly all of the sound energy entering the canal pushes on the eardrum. It is thin, flexible, and yet strong enough not to burst when humans dive

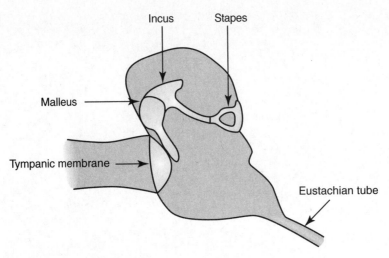

**FIGURE 10.2    The middle ear.**

100 or more feet below the surface of the ocean. The eardrum is roughly circular in shape and has a diameter of about 1 cm, a little less than ½ inch.

It is connected to three bones, or **ossicles**, that span the middle ear cavity between the eardrum and the inner ear. The names of the ossicles were inspired by their shapes. The hammer, or **malleus**, is the first of the ossicles. It is about 9 mm long, and its long arm is attached firmly to the eardrum. The anvil, or **incus**, is the second ossicle and is about 7 mm in size. The head of the incus and head of the malleus are covered by tissue that holds them together so that they move together. In this way, they form two arms of a lever. The difference in the length of the two bones helps to create the transformer effect of the middle ear. The third ossicle is the stirrup, or **stapes**. The footplate of the stapes looks like the bottom of a stirrup. The footplate is oval, and it is about 3 mm in length and about 1 mm in width. It fits into an opening called the oval window of the inner ear system.

The principles by which the middle ear transformer works are illustrated in Figure 10.3. The transformer boosts the pressure by a significant amount. The largest boost is due to the differences in the areas of the eardrum and stapes footplate. The part of the eardrum that moves in response to the incident sound has an area that is about twenty times the area of the stapes footplate. The force that collects on the eardrum is transmitted directly to the footplate, and so the force per square mm of area at the stapes is boosted by a factor of about 20 to 1. This boost in pressure, or *force per unit of area*, is the same effect that occurs when a thumbtack is used. The force applied to the large head is sufficient to enable the tack to penetrate a piece of wood because the area of the point of the tack is much smaller than the area of the head.

The second mechanism that helps to boost the pressure is found in the lever action resulting from the difference between the lengths of the malleus and incus. The ratio of 9 mm (malleus) to 7 mm (incus) is equivalent to about 1.3 to 1. Force applied to the long arm of the lever is increased by an amount equal to the ratio of

Area ratio of TM/stapes is approx 20:1

Length ratio of malleus/incus is approx 1.3:1

TM

Stapes

Malleus

Incus

Pressure at stapes is about 20 X pressure at TM

Pressure is increased by about 1.3:1

Combination of area ratio and lever system = pressure boost of 26:1

**FIGURE 10.3    Mechanisms that create the transformer effect of the middle ear.**

the lengths of the long and short arms, or about 1.3 to 1. The combination of the ratio of the areas of the eardrum and stapes (20:1) and the lever action of the ossicles (1.3:1) provides a boost of about 26 to 1, or about 28 dB. The combined effects of the outer and middle ear systems allow us to hear sounds that are about 30 to 60 dB below the intensities that would be needed if our outer and middle ear apparatus did not exist or was destroyed. Individuals born without an external ear canal or middle ear apparatus, or persons who have an ear infection that leaves the middle ear full of thick fluid, will experience a loss of hearing of about 60 dB for airborne sounds.

This middle ear transformer will work properly only *when the eardrum is intact* and when the *cavity is filled with air*. The **Eustachian tube** connects the middle ear cavity with the pharynx, and it opens each time a swallow occurs. When the tube opens, air passes from the back of the throat into the middle ear, and fluid that is secreted by the lining of the middle ear is allowed to drain into the throat. If the tube is blocked, the exchange of air and drainage of fluid will be affected. The tube may become blocked due to upper respiratory allergies, a cold, or another condition that causes an increase in secretion or swelling of the tissue that lines the middle ear, Eustachian tube, or pharynx. If the air is not refreshed, the air in the middle ear cavity will be absorbed by the tissue, and the eardrum will be pushed inward by the difference in air pressure between the atmosphere and the middle ear cavity. A clinician looking at the eardrum will say that it is "retracted." Many people experience a temporary retraction of the eardrum when they are passengers in an airplane that descends rapidly for a landing. The increase in air pressure associated with the loss of altitude must be matched by the middle ear—this usually is accomplished by swallowing. If an air passenger has a cold, it may be difficult to balance the pressure. The result may be a painful experience and a temporary loss of hearing. The pain is a signal that the eardrum is pushed inward, or retracted, and the loss of hearing is due to the fact that the stiffness of the eardrum is increased when the pressure in the middle ear does not match the pressure in the ear canal. The increased stiffness resulting from a pressure imbalance will cause the eardrum to respond poorly to low-frequency sounds and the result may be a loss of hearing in the low-frequency region.

If the Eustachian tube remains blocked for a long period of time, the clear fluid that is secreted by the lining of the middle ear cavity will collect in the cavity. The fluid replaces the air, and the fluid level can rise to a point where it can be seen by a clinician using an otoscope to examine the eardrum. The addition of the fluid increases the stiffness of the eardrum considerably because of the reduction of the volume of air in the middle ear cavity and the incompressibility of the fluid. This produces a greater hearing loss that may eventually include both low- and high-frequency sounds if the cavity fills completely. The disorder caused by fluid in the ear is called *otitis media* (see also Chapter 11). It not only creates a hearing problem but it also is a serious medical problem that requires attention. If the fluid remains for a long period of time, it serves as a fertile medium for infection that can lead to serious consequences, including spontaneous rupture or perforation of the eardrum. A middle ear that is filled with fluid combined with a perforated tympanic membrane loses its ability to work as a transformer.

The middle ear ossicles are attached to two small muscles. The tensor tympani muscle pulls the malleus inward, toward the center of the head. The muscle is named because it tenses or stiffens the eardrum or tympanum. The tensor tympani muscle is innervated by the Vth cranial nerve (trigeminal), which is the principal sensory nerve of the face and controls the muscles that are involved in chewing. The tensor tympani contracts when we swallow, yawn, and chew, and it also responds to tactile stimulation of the skin of the face. The second muscle is the stapedius. When it contracts, it pulls the stapes outward. The stapedius muscle is innervated by the VIIth cranial nerve (facial), which controls the muscles of facial expression. The stapedius muscle contracts in response to sounds that are about 60 to 80 dB SPL in persons with normal hearing thresholds.

When the stapedius muscle contracts in response to sound, it adds stiffness to the middle ear transformer system. The change in stiffness can be measured by a clinical instrument known as a tympanometer. The change in stiffness resulting from contraction of the stapedius is known as the *acoustic reflex*. The reflex is bilateral, which is to say that it appears on both sides during stimulation of either ear. In this way it is like the change in pupil diameter that occurs when a bright light is presented to either eye. Traditionally, the acoustic reflex was thought to serve to protect the ear from intense sound. However, few sounds found in nature (such as thunder, the roar of waterfalls, rockslides, an imminent predator) are of sufficient intensity to activate the acoustic reflex. It is noteworthy that our world became very noisy long after middle ear muscles were created. Therefore, it is unlikely that these muscles were designed to protect against the industrial noises of gunpowder, steam, internal combustion, and jet engines.

A modern view of the action of the acoustic reflex is that, although it may help to protect the ear from intense sounds, its principal role is to alter the transmission characteristics of the middle ear to enable us to hear important sounds, such as speech, in noisy situations. The tensor tympani muscle may serve the same role when we are generating noise by eating, swallowing, or talking. Neither muscle can react with sufficient speed to protect us from the most dangerous sounds in our world: the explosive reports of firearms.

In Chapter 2, we considered how the biological systems that support speech and language were affected in a child with Down syndrome. This genetic disorder also affects the hearing mechanism as well. We can see how the outer and middle ear mechanisms are affected in the case of Alicia.

> Alicia underwent a full audiologic evaluation to determine hearing function. Like most children with Down syndrome, she has small and irregular pinnas. The audiologist used an otoscope in order to examine the appearance of the ear canal and tympanic membrane. For some children with Down syndrome, the ear canal is narrower than usual. In the case of Alicia, the ear canals have a normal appearance and are open and clear. However, she appears to have some fluid in the middle ear. This is common in children with Down syndrome, who have a high rate of middle ear infections. Alicia's mother reports that her child has been plagued by these infections. On this day, the presence of middle ear fluid was accompanied by a mild degree of hearing loss because the fluid changed the mechanical workings of the tympanic membrane and ossicles. The fluid caused an increase in the stiffness of the moving parts of the middle ear apparatus.

## The Inner Ear

The inner ear converts energy to a code that can be interpreted by the brain. In this way, it serves the same role as the retina of the eye, touch receptors in the skin, and olfactory receptors in the nose and taste buds. The process of conversion is called *transduction*. The inner ear has three separate transduction systems: (a) the vestibule, (b) the semicircular canals, and (c) the cochlea. Transducers in the vestibule help us to maintain our orientation with respect to gravity, or the center of the earth. The semicircular canal systems provide us with information about head position and help us to maintain a fix on visual targets when we are moving. The cochlea contains the transducers for hearing. The three parts of the inner ear share important features. The first is that the inner ear is filled with fluid. Forces acting on the inner ear due to gravity, acceleration of the head or body, or sound ultimately create motion of the fluid in the inner ear system. The fluid couples the energy of the stimulus to the transducers that convert the stimulus to responses of neurons. The second shared feature is that the transducer mechanisms are similar in all three parts of the inner ear. They consist of a mechanical receptor, called a *hair cell*, and a *covering membrane* that causes or otherwise enhances the motion of the hairlike cilia found on the top of the hair cells. The remainder of the chapter will focus on how these principles apply in the cochlea—the end organ for hearing.

## Cochlear Structure and Function

The fundamental arrangement of several important parts of the cochlea is illustrated in the series of drawings in Figure 10.4 (after Kiang, 1975). The cochlea is a hard-walled chamber that is filled with fluid (Figure 10.4A). There are two flexible "windows." The **oval window** is the location at which the stapes connects to the inner ear. The **round window** is a second opening on the body of the cochlea, and it is also covered with a flexible membrane. When the stapes forces the oval window inward, the round window is forced outward by the pressure of the fluid in the chamber. In Figure 10.4B the stapes has been added, and a "basilar" (basement), or supporting, membrane is stretched across the cavity. The inward motion of the stapes causes the **basilar membrane** to move in response to fluid displacement because it lies in the pathway of the fluid.

Sensory cells are added in Figure 10.4C. These are hair cells that sit on the basilar membrane. An opening called the helicotrema allows the fluid in the top

**FIGURE 10.4    Schematic drawing to illustrate the components of the cochlea (after Kiang, 1975). As shown in drawings A and B, the cochlea is likened to a hard-walled container with flexible membranes on the top and bottom and another membrane stretched across the middle (C). Drawings D and E elongate the container to better represent the structure of the true cochlea.**

channel to flow directly into the bottom channel. (Note that the helicotrema is located at the top, or apex, of the cochlea in its true, coiled shape.) Fluid will flow through this channel only when the stapes moves very slowly, such as in the case in which a change in air pressure within the middle ear causes the oval window to be pushed inward or pulled laterally. When stapes vibrations occur rapidly, such as at the lower limit of our range of hearing, then it is the basilar membrane that responds to the forces applied by the stapes.

There are about 12,000 hair cells in the cochlea of humans with healthy ears. The structure is designed to accommodate the hair cells along a length of about 36 mm (from the base close to the stapes to the opposite end, called the apex). To illustrate this point, Figure 10.4D extends the length of the fluid chamber. Figure 10.4E shows the fluid chamber coiled into a shell shape, approximating the true configuration of the cochlea.

Sitting on the basilar membrane is the **organ of Corti,** named for the anatomist who provided an early description of its structure. In Figure 10.5, we see its components, which include supporting structures, hair cells, and an overlying membrane called the *tectorial membrane* (tectum = roof). This is the view you would have if you unrolled the cochlea as in Figure 10.4D and then sliced it as if you were slicing salami. There are two sets of hair cells—a single row of inner hair cells and three rows of outer hair cells. These cells are so named because they contain hairlike projections called **cilia**. Hair cells are delicate and can be easily damaged through aging, disease, or exposure to certain drugs, or by prolonged exposure to loud noise. Once damaged, the hair cells can regenerate in some species, such as birds, but they do not repair themselves in mammals. Movement of the basilar membrane sets off a shearing motion of the hair cell cilia. This motion is translated by the receptor cells into a chemical-electrical signal that is carried to the brain via auditory nerve fibers.

The shape of the basilar membrane influences how sound energy is analyzed by the cochlea. The membrane is relatively narrow at the base, the end near the stapes. It is about ten times wider at the apex. A change in stiffness accompanies the change in width of the basilar membrane so that the base end is about 100 times stiffer than the apex end. The gradation in stiffness is important because it helps to determine how sounds are represented in the cochlea. The stiffness of the basilar membrane near the base of the cochlea creates an efficient response for high-frequency sounds. The more flaccid region near the apex cannot respond to high-frequency energy, so its responses are limited to low frequencies.

The stiffness change from the base to the apex of the cochlea allows the cochlea to analyze the sounds transmitted by the stapes, much like the spectrum analyzer discussed in Chapter 3. The basis of this analysis was described by Georg von Békésy in 1928. He examined the behavior of the cochleas of several species of animals. The bone containing the cochlea was removed from the animal's skull and drilled to expose the membranes in the fluid spaces of the ear. The preparation was placed under a conventional light microscope and then driven mechanically by a sound source. von Békésy described the motion patterns of the basilar membrane and noted that a *traveling wave* developed along the membrane in response to

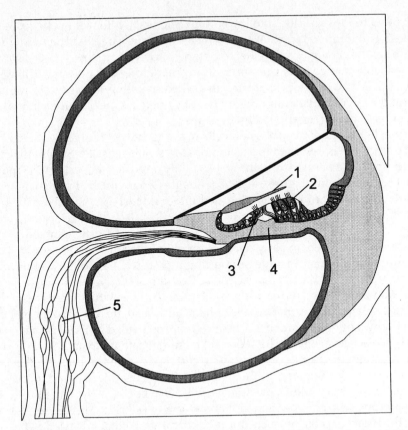

**FIGURE 10.5   Cross-section the cochlea and organ of Corti: (1) tectorial membrane, (2) outer hair cells, (3) inner hair cells, (4) basilar membrane, (5) cell body of the auditory nerve.**

sound. When high-frequency sounds were employed, the disturbance traveled only a few millimeters from the base of the cochlea. When low frequencies were used, the traveling wave spread from the base to the apex. The place of maximum vibration of the traveling wave was determined by the frequency of the sound. Because each frequency was associated with a specific place of stimulation, the cochlea was said to be *tonotopically organized*.

The illustrations in Figure 10.6 are based on von Békésy's observations (von Békésy, 1960). Three sketches of the basilar membrane are shown. The membrane is "unrolled" as in Figure 10.4D, with the base of the cochlea on the right and the apex on the left. The dashed lines represent the gross patterns of the traveling wave disturbances for 5000, 1000, and 200 Hz, respectively. The numerical scales below the three schematics provide an indication of the distance along the basilar membrane in millimeters and the places where individual frequencies would create the maximum disturbances. The traveling waves described by von Békésy appeared to move from base to apex. Frequencies between about 1000 and 20,000 Hz are represented along the 18 mm of the membrane closest to the base of the cochlea. Frequencies between about 100 and 1000 Hz are represented in the "upper" half of the cochlea, between about 18 and 36 mm from the base. Frequencies below about 100 Hz probably result in a wave that sweeps the basilar membrane from end to end without developing a peak in the disturbance pattern.

von Békésy's work ushered in a new understanding of how the inner ear analyzed sound. His continuing efforts over the next thirty years led to the Nobel Prize in Medicine and Physiology, awarded to him in 1961. Two physicists, Gold and Pumphrey, examined the von Békésy studies and studies of human threshold sensitivity and frequency discrimination and concluded that there had to be some active amplifier process that actually added energy to the signal delivered to the inner ear by the stapes footplate (Gold, 1948, 1989). They reasoned that this amplifier might occasionally become unstable and develop a shrill whistle, like one hears when a public address system produces feedback. They also reasoned that the amplifier elements must be highly tuned. Gold and Pumphrey presented their ideas to scientific experts around 1948, twenty years after von Békésy's report, but they were unable to convince anyone of the merit of their theory and so they pursued other scientific ventures.

**FIGURE 10.6  Traveling waves corresponding to different sound frequencies as described by von Békésy.**

About twenty years after Gold and Pumphrey's brief visit to auditory science, evidence for the leakage of energy from the ear back into the air was discovered by David Kemp, who also had a background in physics. Kemp was listening to low-intensity sounds and realized that some unknown source of sound was interacting with the external sound. When he placed a miniature microphone in the ear of a listener, he was he was able to record the "whistle" that reflects the feedback predicted by Gold and Pumphrey (Kemp, 1978). The tones recorded by Dr. Kemp, and from thousands of other subjects since 1978, must reflect an energy source within the inner ear and some disturbance that is transmitted backward through the fluid of the inner ear and middle ear cavity to the eardrum. In this case, the eardrum works like a loudspeaker diaphragm, producing vibrations in the air rather than responding to them! These sounds are called **otoacoustic emissions**. Emissions occur both spontaneously and in response to stimulation and are present in virtually every healthy ear. Kemp found the evidence needed to support the notion that an active amplifier exists inside of the cochlea.

For a power source, we must look at the details of the organ of Corti. Recall that there are three rows of outer hair cells and only a single row of inner hair cells. Therefore, the outer hair cells outnumber the inner hair cells by about 3:1 (9,000 to 3,000 in humans). There are also a number of other differences between these two types of cells (see Table 10.1). The hair cells differ in shape: The outer hair cells are relatively cylindrical in shape, whereas the inner hair cells are jug-shaped. The position and structural support of the two types of cells also differs. The outer hair cells are in contact with the tectorial membrane, but the cilia of the inner hair cells are free of attachments above their cell bodies. Outer hair cells are situated over the flexible basilar membrane, whereas the inner hair cells sit on a rigid bony shelf. The inner hair cells are firmly encased in supporting structures that surround each inner hair cell, but the outer hair cells are situated on supporting cells at their base. Finally, the inner hair cells receive nearly all of the afferent, or sensory, nerves leading from the ear to the brain. In contrast, the outer hair cells receive nearly all of the efferent or control nerves leading from the brain back to the ear.

These differences point to important functional differences between the outer and inner hair cells. Today, most theories of inner ear function argue that the inner hair cells are the actual sensory transducers. The nerve supply attached to the inner hair cells and measures of their electrical properties during stimulation of the

**TABLE 10.1   Differences Between Inner and Outer Hair Cells**

| OUTER HAIR CELLS | INNER HAIR CELLS |
| --- | --- |
| Three rows of cells | One row of cells |
| Cylindrical in shape | Jug-shaped |
| Contact with tectorial membrane | No contact with tectorial membrane |
| Sit on flexible basilar membrane | Sit on bony shelf |
| Support cells at hair cell base | Support cells surround hair cells |
| Receive efferent nerve fibers from the brain | Send afferent nerve fibers to the brain |

ear are compatible with this notion. The outer hair cells are thought to contribute to the amplification of motion in the inner ear in response to low intensity sounds. No one has actually "seen" the outer hair cells in operation inside of the ear, but we do know several things about how they work. If outer hair cells are missing, hearing loss occurs in that region. When outer hair cells are compromised or destroyed, the inner hair cells do not function normally. However, if the outer hair cells return to normal function, the inner hair cells do so as well. Likewise, otoacoustic emissions disappear when outer hair cells are compromised, only to reappear if the outer hair cells are restored to normal function.

Outer hair cells have been studied *in vitro*, that is to say, in artificial environments after being removed from an ear. Studied this way, Brownell and his coworkers (1983) discovered a startling fact in the early 1980s: They demonstrated that the outer hair cells changed their lengths in response to chemical stimulation. Other investigations demonstrated that changes in cell length of 5 to 10 percent of the original length can occur in response to electrical, chemical, or mechanical (acoustic) stimulation. When the cell is activated, or depolarized, by a stimulus, *it becomes shorter*! If the cell is returned to its resting electrical (chemical) state, then *its length is restored*! Finally, if the cell is hyperpolarized, the opposite of depolarization, then *its length increases*! As illustrated in Figure 10.7, depolarization of the outer hair cells occurs when the cilia are tilted toward the tallest row. Hyperpolarization would occur if the cilia are forced to move in the opposite direction beyond their normal resting positions. In a sense, the outer hair cells act like small biological motors or muscles, changing length with each cycle of the stimulus that is effective in driving them. If the *in vitro* observations predict what is occurring in the living ear, then it is possible that the outer hair cells enhance the motion of the organ of Corti structures by alternately compressing and then expanding. During upward motion of the basilar membrane, as illustrated in Figure 10.7, the outer hair cells become shorter, effectively pulling the tectorial membrane and other structures closer together and forcing endolymph to stream across the inner hair cell cilia. Basilar membrane motion in the opposite direction is associated with a lengthening of the cells, exaggerating the motion and amplifying the motion of the fluid across the inner hair cell cilia.

It is clear that the analysis of incoming sounds performed by the cochlea is very precise and sensitive to exquisitely low levels of stimulus intensity. A leading scientist and physician of the nineteenth century, Helmholtz (1885) predicted today's theory by suggesting the cochlea contained highly tuned resonators that could vibrate to enhance the response of the basilar membrane. The earlier observations of von Békésy (1960), based on dead ears, took auditory theory in the right direction, toward recognition of the importance of a traveling wave in the analysis of sounds by the inner ear. When the highly tuned devices (the outer hair cells) become unstable, spontaneous otoacoustic emissions are created in a way that is probably similar to the creation of feedback in a conventional hearing aid. The inner hair cells are probably the actual sensory transducers that provide information about sound. The outer hair cells appear to enhance the performance of the cochlea so that minute amounts of energy can create a sensation of sound. The

**FIGURE 10.7** Action of the outer hair cells (OHC) relative to movement of the basilar membrane. Note the change in length of the outer hair cells and the change in position of the hairs, or cilia, of these cells as the basilar membrane rises or falls. IHC-inner hair cell.

outer hair cells work very hard to help us to hear, and they are very vulnerable to noise, certain medications, and systemic problems that compromise their energy supply. When outer hair cells are damaged temporarily by loud noise, we experience a loss of otoacoustic emissions and a temporary loss of hearing. When outer hair cells are destroyed, the loss of emissions and hearing become permanent. No other sensory system comes with its own built-in amplifier. If it did, you would find energy leaking from the system back to the environment (like emissions): Eyes would emit light, noses would emit odorants, temperature receptors might emit heat!

## AUDITORY CONNECTIONS IN THE BRAIN

We hear with our brains, not our ears. Each ear communicates with the central nervous system (CNS) through afferent (ascending) and efferent (descending) connections. The outer hair cells receive nearly all of the efferent connections from the brain to the ear. The inner hair cells are connected to nearly all of the afferent neurons. The afferent neurons travel from the ear to the CNS in the VIIIth cranial nerve, referred to as the auditory nerve. The auditory nerve also contains the neurons from the vestibular system. The neurons from the auditory portion of the VIIIth cranial nerve end when they reach the brainstem. They make connections with neurons in the cochlear nucleus.

As illustrated in Figure 10.8, the neurons that leave the cochlea travel to other places in the CNS, where they make connections. In the figure, ascending pathways from the right and left ears are shown as solid and dashed lines, respectively. The ascending nerve fibers connect with several groups of neurons (called nuclei) within the brainstem, where auditory information is processed. These nuclei are shown in light gray. There are two sets of nuclei in the brainstem, and some of the ascending auditory information crosses from one side of the brainstem to the other. Neurons in the brainstem send information to the cerebrum, first through subcortical nuclei (dark gray), and from there nerve pathways radiate diffusely to the primary auditory cortex, which is found in the temporal lobe of the brain (see Chapter 2).

It is important to note that the right and left ear inputs are mixed together in the brainstem and that each of the nuclei and fiber tracts above the cochlear nucleus contains neurons that can be traced to both ears. This *binaural* representation helps us to locate sounds in space by comparing the information received from one ear with the information received from the other. The function of each of the major CNS structures that contain auditory neurons is not understood completely. However, we know that all of the structures maintain the tonotopic organization that was established in the cochlea. In other words, individual frequencies in simple and complex sounds are represented at specific places within the nervous system from the ear to the cortex.

**FIGURE 10.8   The central auditory pathways (components not to scale). The nerve fibers (solid and dashed lines) from the cochlea of each ear travel to nuclei in the brainstem (light gray). Nerve fibers from nuclei on each side cross, and information from each ear reaches nuclei on both sides of the cerebrum (areas in dark grey).**

Much of what we know about the function of individual parts of the auditory nervous system comes from studying humans who have experienced damage to structures due to physical trauma or disease. Mr. Viner provides one such example.

*Mr. Viner* suffered a small stroke (blockage of blood flow within the brain). This damaged the tissue of the primary auditory cortex on the left side of his brain. However, the surrounding language areas within the left hemisphere were left intact. Because the auditory cortex in his right hemisphere was intact, he could still process sounds and his hearing was normal. Two years later, he suffered a second stroke, this time in the right hemisphere. It was much more extensive, damaging the primary auditory cortex and surrounding cortical regions. Suddenly, Mr.

Viner's hearing changed drastically. He could detect when sounds occurred, but he could not "make sense" of them. His wife now had to write notes to communicate, because when she spoke he heard jibberish. In fact, his own speech sounded so abnormal to him, he soon stopped talking as well, resorting to the use of a writing pad to communicate with others.

In Mr. Viner's case, the blood supply to the auditory cortex was interrupted on both sides of the brain. When damage affects only one side, the patient may not experience a hearing loss and may reveal only subtle problems associated with understanding speech in noisy situations. If the auditory cortex is destroyed on both sides, then the patient may have a loss of hearing but will not be deaf. Rather, he or she may have difficulty finding the sources of sounds in space, understanding speech, and making sense of musical sequences.

At the lower end of the system, damage to the auditory nerve will affect hearing in the ear served by that nerve. The amount of hearing loss due to damage to the nerve is not easy to predict. Persons with auditory nerve damage often have difficulty understanding speech, even without a significant hearing loss for pure tones. In addition, they may not hear intense sounds with appropriate loudness. In contrast, persons who lose outer hair cells reveal a hearing loss and an abnormal growth of loudness when sounds become intense. Reports of subtle symptoms by patients will help a clinician arrive at a clearer picture of the causes of the individual's problems.

In summary, the auditory system is exquisitely designed to help us become aware of and to use the sounds that occur in our environment. The design enhances our ability to hear by virtue of three important features: (1) resonance properties of the outer ear, (2) transformer action of the middle ear, and (3) active amplification of the energy that arrives at the inner ear. The cochlea analyzes sounds into the individual frequencies that are present in a way that is similar to a spectrum analyzer. Individual inner hair cells are responsive to very narrow ranges of frequencies in the spectrum through a process that creates *tonotopic organization* in the cochlea. Neurons carrying information from the inner hair cells to the CNS maintain the tonotopic organization. The CNS is also organized so that information about individual tones projects to specific places in the brain. All of the elements of the auditory system operate constantly, because we are never free of auditory stimulation. At a primitive level, the auditory system helps us to ward off danger and to find sources of survival. At a more advanced level, the auditory system connects us with the people in our world through speech, music, and other sounds that we associate with them.

Our most important link with people is language, and our most important link in language that develops normally is hearing. The auditory system is uniquely designed to allow us to be aware of sounds, locate them, and recognize them. Its acoustical, physical, and psychological features are unique, sensitive, and structured to enhance our listening abilities. The most vital parts can be permanently injured by intense stimulation. Once gone, they cannot be repaired. The best hearing aids that we have today cannot restore normal quality to sound, though they provide remarkable assistance to persons with hearing impairments. The best action to take is to avoid situations that are dangerous to your hearing so that you can preserve the unique human link that is associated with the auditory system.

## CLINICAL PROBLEM SOLVING

Mr. Johnson is 65 years old and has worked for a road construction company for forty years. Although he has been using ear plugs to protect his hearing for ten years, he did not think about protecting his hearing when he was much younger. Today, he has a permanent hearing loss, mainly in the high-frequency region.

1. What region of the basilar membrane (base, middle, apex) is likely to be damaged in Mr. Johnson's ears?
2. Which cells in the organ of Corti are likely to be affected by a forty-year history of noise exposure?
3. Give some examples of speech sounds that Mr. Johnson might not be able to recognize because of his hearing loss.

## REFERENCES

Brownell, W. E. (1983). Observations on a motile response in isolated hair cells. In W. Webster & L. Aitkin (Eds.), *Mechanisms of hearing* (pp. 5–10). Clayton, Australia: Monash University Press.

Gold, T. (1948). Hearing: II. The physical axis of the action of the cochlea. *Proceedings of the Royal Society, 135,* 492–498.

Gold, T. (1989). Historical background to the proposal 40 years ago of an active model for cochlear frequency analysis. In J. P. Wilson & D. T. Kemp (Eds.), *Cochlear mechanisms: Structure, function and models* (pp. 299–306). London: Plenum Press.

Helmholtz, H. L. von (1954). *On the sensations of tone as a physiological basis for the theory of music.* A. Ellis, Trans. (Original published in 1885 by Longmans, Green)

Kemp, D. T. (1978). Stimulated acoustic emissions from within the human auditory system. *Journal of the Acoustical Society of America, 64,* 1386–1391.

Kiang, N. Y-S. (1975). Stimulus representation in the discharge patterns of auditory neurons. In D. B. Tower (Ed.), *The nervous system: Volume 3: Human communication and its disorders* (pp. 81–96). New York: Raven Press.

von Békésy, G. (1960). *Experiments in hearing.* New York: McGraw Hill.

# CHAPTER ELEVEN

# DISORDERS OF HEARING
# IN CHILDREN

ANNE MARIE THARPE

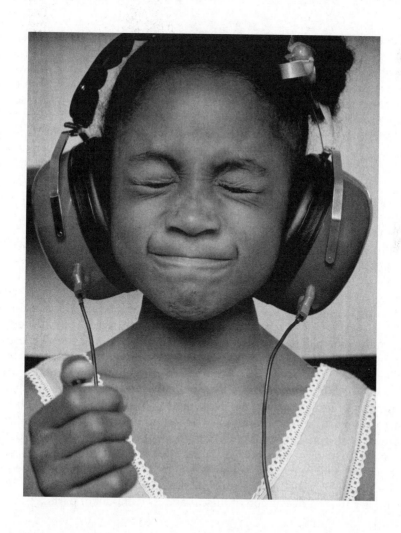

■ ■ ■ ■ ■ ▬▬▬▬▬▬▬▬▬▬▬▬▬▬▬▬▬▬▬▬▬▬▬▬▬▬▬▬▬▬▬▬▬

**PREVIEW**

For the vast majority of children, listening and learning through the auditory modality is a passive and natural process. However, some children experience a hearing loss that impairs their ability to communicate and may require some level of habilitation. Audiologists are uniquely trained professionals with the skills to evaluate the hearing of children of any age, even newborns. Audiologists are also prepared to initiate intervention, provide support and counseling to families, and work with educators and other professionals to design habilitation and educational programs for children with hearing loss. This chapter will begin with a discussion of the various causes, types, and degrees of hearing loss in children. We will investigate the identification and impact of hearing loss on the receptive and expressive communication of children.

Between 1 and 6 per 1,000 children experience a hearing loss that impairs their ability to communicate and may require some level of habilitation (Parving, 1993; Watkin, Baldwin, & McEnery, 1991). The presence of a hearing loss can create challenges related to communication, education, and socialization. To understand the potential impact for a child, the following questions must be addressed: Which frequencies are affected by the hearing loss? How severe is the hearing loss? Is it permanent or temporary? A hearing test will begin to answer these, and other, questions. To test hearing, we use an electronic instrument called an **audiometer**. The audiometer generates pure-tone frequencies at different levels of sound intensity. The goal of hearing testing is to determine the lowest intensity level at which various pure tones and speech are detected (called thresholds). The person's thresholds are plotted on an **audiogram**. A sample audiogram of a person with normal hearing can be seen in Figure 11.1. It shows the test frequencies labeled along the horizontal axis at the top of the audiogram, with the lowest frequency representing 125 cycles per second, or 125 hertz (Hz) and the highest representing 8000 Hz. The intensity is represented in decibels (dB) and is labeled on the vertical axis on the left side of the audiogram. A normal threshold is between −10 and 25 dB, and the most intense signal that can be produced by most audiometers is 120 dB. The right-ear response is plotted with a circle (red, if color is used). We can remember this with the mnemonic "red, right, round." The left-ear response is plotted with an X (blue, if in color). In Figure 11.1, the audiogram shows thresholds for the right and left ear are between 0 and −5 dB, indicating normal hearing.

　　**Air conduction audiometry** refers to the presentation of speech or pure-tone stimuli via earphones to the patient. The test signal travels through the ear canal, across the eardrum and middle ear space, to the inner ear and is ultimately transmitted to the auditory centers in the brain. You can follow the path of an air-conducted signal by viewing Figure 11.2A. As you can see, if someone has difficulty hearing a signal by air conduction, the problem could be in any of the areas through which the signal travels, from the ear canal to the inner ear (see Chapter 10 for a discussion of the ear and its component parts).

**FIGURE 11.1   An audiogram displays results of hearing testing. An individual's responses to pure tones of varying frequencies (labeled across the top of the audiogram) are plotted according to the lowest intensity level at which they heard those tones (labeled along the vertical axis). Round symbols correspond to responses to tones in the right ear; the Xs correspond to responses to tones in the left ear. The gray region represents the range frequencies and intensities over which most speech sounds occur.**

 **Bone conduction audiometry** refers to the transmission of sounds presented to the individual by a bone vibrator that is typically placed behind the ear on the mastoid bone. The vibrator causes the bones of the skull to vibrate, which in turn stimulate the inner ear, or **cochlea**. The cochlea is a labyrinth carved into the skull that is lined with a membranous surface and filled with fluid. When a signal causes the skull to vibrate, the cochlea is stimulated by the vibrations, and hearing does not depend on the outer and middle ears. You can follow the path of a bone-conducted signal by viewing Figure 11.2B. If someone has difficulty hearing by bone conduction, the damage must be in the inner ear or auditory nerve. Such hearing losses result in fairly equal air and bone conduction thresholds, and the condition is known as a **sensorineural hearing loss** (see Figure 11.3A).
 When someone demonstrates normal hearing by bone conduction, but has difficulty hearing signals presented by air conduction, the problem must be in the outer or middle ear. This condition is known as a conductive hearing loss (see Figure 11.3B). The difference between the air and bone conduction responses is referred to as an air-bone gap. When an individual has both a sensorineural and a conductive hearing loss it is referred to as a **mixed hearing loss** (see Figure 11.3C).

**(A)**                                                            **(B)**

**FIGURE 11.2    The two pathways of sound in the ear. Broken arrows demonstrate the route of (A) air conduction hearing and (B) bone conduction hearing.**

In addition to classifying the type of hearing loss, the audiogram is also used to classify the degree of hearing loss. Figure 11.4 illustrates a widely accepted classification of the degree of hearing loss.

As valuable as the audiogram is for describing the type and degree of hearing loss, it is important to note that we cannot predict academic, social, or communicative success or limitations from the audiogram alone. It simply defines the line between hearing and not hearing at various frequencies. It does not describe the quality of what is heard or the difficulties that the hearing loss may impose on an individual. Those issues will be addressed later in this chapter.

## AUDITORY PATHOLOGIES

Disorders associated with hearing loss in children can be **congenital** (present at birth), or acquired at any time after birth. In addition, hearing loss can be genetic or caused by other factors that damage the auditory system, such as diseases or toxins. It is important to note that not all genetic disorders are congenital and not all congenital disorders are genetic. For example, mucopolysaccharidoses syndrome (MPS) is a genetically inherited metabolic disorder, but children with MPS are healthy at birth. The genetic effect of this disorder results in a progressive hearing loss with age. On the other hand, children whose mothers abuse alcohol during

**FIGURE 11.3** Pure-tone air and bone conduction audiograms. (A) Severe high-frequency sensorineural hearing loss. (B) Mild conductive hearing loss. (C) Moderate to severe mixed hearing loss.

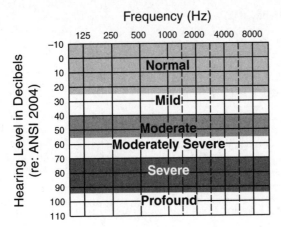

**FIGURE 11.4    Classification of pure tone hearing loss by degree.**

pregnancy may incur damage to the auditory mechanism in utero as one of several symptoms of fetal alcohol spectrum disorder. The resulting hearing loss is congenital, acquired during prenatal development, but not genetic. We will review a variety of disorders using the following categories: *genetic without associated abnormalities, genetic with associated abnormalities, acquired prenatally, acquired perinatally,* and *acquired postnatally.*

## Genetically Inherited Hearing Loss

Over the last decade, our knowledge of genetic hearing impairment has increased dramatically. Approximately forty auditory genes have been identified, and hereditary hearing loss occurs as a result of mutations in these genes. It is estimated that 50 percent of all congenital hearing loss is genetically transmitted (or **endogenous**). Approximately two-thirds of genetic hearing losses occur as the only abnormality, and one-third occur in association with additional abnormalities or as part of a *syndrome.* Some of the most common types of genetic conditions associated with hearing loss can be found in Table 11.1. Pediatric audiologists frequently must draw on knowledge of genetics to counsel families. We see this in the following case:

> *Caesar's* parents were taken totally by surprise when they were told that he had a moderate sensorineural hearing loss in both ears. After several weeks of thinking and talking with each other about the hearing loss, they returned to Caesar's audiologist and asked him whether their future children were at risk for hearing loss. Although not a geneticist, their audiologist knew that because Caesar had no other risk factors for hearing loss, there was a high likelihood that the hearing loss was the result of a recessive mode of genetic inheritance. After explaining the possible causes of hearing loss to Caesar's parents, they were referred for further genetic counseling.

**TABLE 11.1  Genetic Disorders Associated With Hearing Loss**

| DISORDER | CLINICAL SIGNS |
|---|---|
| **AUTOSOMAL DOMINANT DISORDERS** | |
| Waardenburg's syndrome | Pigment abnormalities including a white forelock and different-colored irises; unilateral or bilateral sensorineural hearing loss. |
| Alport's syndrome | Nephritis; ocular lesions; progressive hearing loss. |
| Stickler syndrome | Ocular anomalies; cleft palate; progressive hearing loss. |
| Treacher Collins syndrome | Facial malformations including depressed cheek bones, deformed pinna, receding chin; conductive or mixed hearing loss. |
| Branchio-oto-renal syndrome | Ear malformation; renal anomalies, mixed hearing loss. |
| Neurofibromatosis | Tumor disorder; variable audiological findings. |
| **AUTOSOMAL RECESSIVE DISORDERS** | |
| Usher syndromes | Retinitis pigmentosa; congenital sensorineural hearing loss. |
| Friedrich's ataxia | Nervous system disorder; ocular abnormalities; abnormal movement; progressive sensorineural hearing loss. |
| Hurler's syndrome | Growth failure; mental retardation; progressive hearing loss. |
| **X-LINKED DISORDERS** | |
| Hunter's syndrome | Growth failure; mental retardation; mixed or conductive hearing loss. |
| Norrie's syndrome | Progressive visual impairment; mental retardation; progressive sensorineural hearing loss. |
| Alport's syndrome | Renal disorder; ocular abnormalities; progressive sensorineural hearing loss. |

Genes occur in pairs and are located on twenty-three pairs of **chromosomes**. One member of each gene pair is inherited from each parent. Each egg and sperm carries one-half of the chromosomes from each parent, so that, when the egg is fertilized by the sperm, a child inherits half of the genes from the father and half from the mother. There are three primary patterns of inheritance: *autosomal dominant, autosomal recessive,* and *X-linked.*

Hearing loss that is genetically based may result from any of these three modes of inheritance. The pattern of inheritance associated with each mode will determine the probability that a child will develop a hearing loss. For example, when genes for hearing loss are inherited in an autosomal dominant manner, only one copy of the affected gene (inherited from either parent) is required for hearing loss to occur in the child who inherits the gene. As illustrated in Figure 11.5, one parent typically exhibits a hearing loss, and each offspring has a 50 percent chance of inheriting the gene for hearing loss. This does not mean that half of the children of a parent with an autosomal dominant gene will be affected. It does mean, rather, that each child has a 50 percent chance of being affected. Approximately 20 percent of genetic hearing loss is the result of dominant inheritance (Morton, 1991).

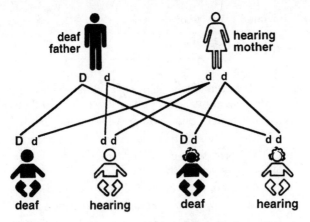

FIGURE 11.5   Persons with dominant deafness have one dominant gene that leads to deafness (D) and a corresponding normal gene (d). Each child has a 50/50 chance of inheriting the deafness gene (D) from the parent who has this trait.

From Shaver (1988). Reprinted with permission.

Most inherited hearing loss is autosomal **recessive**, which accounts for approximately 80 percent of genetic hearing loss (Shaver, 1988). A child must receive two copies of the gene for **hearing loss** in order for the trait to be expressed. This means the parents of a child with recessive hearing loss each carry one affected and one nonaffected gene in the pair, so both have normal hearing. However, if their child receives both copies of the affected gene, a hearing loss will occur. As shown in Figure 11.6, when both parents are carriers of the recessive gene for hearing loss,

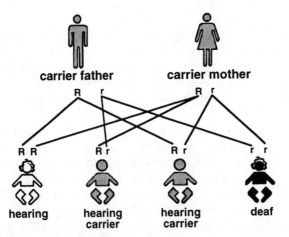

FIGURE 11.6   Persons with recessive forms of deafness have a double dose of the deafness gene (r), one inherited from each of the parents. The parents are hearing carriers and have a 25 percent chance of producing a deaf child with each pregnancy.

From Shaver (1988). Reprinted with permission.

each child of that union has a 25 percent chance of having hearing loss. Because each parent carries only one of the recessive genes, and therefore has normal hearing, the parents may be unaware that their offspring are at risk of inheriting a hearing loss. To date, twenty-two autosomal-recessive genes for nonsyndromic hearing loss have been discovered. Nearly all genes for autosomal recessive genetic hearing loss identified thus far cause **prelingual** (before the development of speech) severe-to-profound loss (Sundstrom, Van Laer, Van Camp, & Smith, 1999).

In the case of X-linked inheritance, the genes responsible for hearing loss are located on the X chromosome. Females inherit an X chromosome from each parent, whereas males inherit an X chromosome from their mother and a Y chromosome from their father. As shown in Figure 11.7, a female with a recessive gene for hearing loss on one of her X chromosomes will not exhibit hearing loss herself. However, each son has a 50 percent chance of having the trait, and each daughter has a 50 percent chance of being a carrier. If a father has an X-linked gene for hearing loss (with a mate who is *not* a carrier), he must pass his X chromosome to his daughters, and therefore all of his daughters will be carriers, and all of his sons will have normal hearing because they only inherit the Y chromosome from their father. Approximately 2 to 3 percent of hearing loss is the result of X-linked transmission making it the least common method of inheriting a genetic hearing loss.

It is important to understand that genetically inherited hearing losses are not invariant in terms of the clinical picture they present. In fact, the same genetic cause can give rise to different degrees of hearing loss in different children. In some cases, hearing loss may be so mild that the child functions well without any intervention at all. In other cases, hearing loss may be severe to profound and may co-occur with other features of a genetic syndrome.

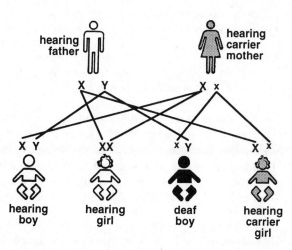

**FIGURE 11.7** **X-linked recessive deafness is caused by a gene on the X chromosome and occurs only in males. The sons of a woman who is a carrier of x-linked deafness have a 50 percent chance of being deaf and the daughters have a 50 percent chance of being carriers.**

From Shaver (1988). Reprinted with permission.

## Acquired Hearing Loss

Acquired hearing losses are those that are caused by **exogenous** (outside the genes) factors, such as disease, toxicity, or trauma. These factors can occur during pregnancy (**prenatally**), shortly before, during, or shortly after delivery (**perinatally**), or after birth (**postnatally**).

It is important for pediatric audiologists to be familiar with the consequences of these insults to the auditory system in order to appropriately counsel families regarding expectations for their children. For example, some infections result in hearing losses that are progressive, and audiologists should prepare families for that eventuality. Some prenatal infections result in hearing losses that are not present at birth but appear later in childhood. The maternal infections that can impact the developing fetus in the pre- and perinatal periods are known as the STORCH complex of infections. **STORCH** is an acronym for *s*yphilis, *t*oxoplasmosis, *o*ther, *r*ubella, *c*ytomegalovirus, and *h*erpes simplex. All of these diseases put infants at high risk for hearing loss. The pediatric audiologist is alert to these possibilities and can arrange for periodic audiological monitoring of these children.

**Prematurity.**    Approximately 11 percent of all births are at fewer than 37 weeks' gestation and are considered preterm. Low birthweight resulting from preterm delivery is a strong predictor of developmental problems including hearing loss (Wilson-Costello, Friedman, Minich, Fanaroff, & Hack, 2005). For a premature infant, there may be multiple factors that raise the risk for hearing loss. Therefore, all premature infants requiring a stay in the neonatal intensive care unit should have their hearing screened prior to discharge. In order to understand the many concerns that can co-occur with a premature birth, let us look at the case of Maya.

> *Maya* weighed only 1,450 grams (approximately 3.2 pounds) at birth and could be held in the palm of one hand. Maya's mother knew from her prenatal classes that premature babies are about thirty times less likely to survive than are full-term infants, and those who survive are at high risk for health and developmental problems. Immediately after birth, Maya had her first test—the APGAR. Fortunately, her scores were within normal limits on this measure.

A low APGAR score can signal that an infant is severely stressed and in need of resuscitation (Apgar, 1953). The score is based on five signs, which form the mnemonic APGAR: *a*ppearance, *p*ulse, *g*rimace, *a*ctivity, and *r*espiration. A low APGAR score may indicate that the infant received insufficient oxygen prior to or during delivery, which results in asphyxia. Simmons (1980) identified asphyxia as the most common high-risk factor in the medical histories of babies with hearing loss.

> Maya's mother noticed her daughter's skin was a yellowish color. She was told by her nurse that this was caused by hyperbilirubinemia, the result of excessive *bilirubin* (a bile pigment in the blood). Maya seemed to enjoy lying naked under warm lights for her phototherapy (treatment by exposure to light), and in a few days the yellow tinge to her skin was gone.

If Maya had had a more serious case of hyperbilirubinemia, she would have required a blood transfusion and may have been at risk for hearing loss. Although some researchers have reported that up to 80 percent of infants surviving hyperbilirubinemia demonstrate some degree of sensorineural hearing loss, others have reported no such relationship (Bergman et al., 1985; deVries, Lary, & Dubowitz, 1985; Sabo, Brown, & Watchko, 1992; Salamy, Eldredge, & Tooley, 1989).

In addition to these medical concerns, preterm infants are susceptible to bleeding within the skull, or *intracranial hemorrhage*. Mental retardation and hearing loss are common sequelae of intracranial hemorrhage (Krishnamoorthy, Shannon, DeLong, Todres, & Davis, 1979).

> In Maya's case, a brain scan showed no evidence of intracranial hemorrhage. Other than being very small, Maya was in good health overall. Once it was clear that Maya's health was not in any danger, her physician recommended that she receive a hearing evaluation by the audiologist. The results of her evaluation were normal. (Later in this chapter, information on hearing testing techniques for infants will be described.) Maya was required to stay in the hospital until her weight was increased, and then she went home with her mother to begin her new life.

As we see from Maya, not all children who are born prematurely will develop a hearing loss or other significant problems. Other premature infants are not as lucky as Maya. Some infants, because they are born before their immune systems are fully developed, are susceptible to a variety of infections. Because of this, they are given medications to help them fight off the bacteria. Some antibiotics (e.g., streptomycin, kanamycin) are known to cause sensorineural hearing loss by damaging structures of the inner ear. In addition, diuretics, commonly used with neonates who have chronic lung disease, have been shown to have a negative effect on hearing (Sabo et al., 1992), and when used with other ototoxic drugs the effects may be multiplied (Salamy et al., 1989). The typical hearing loss associated with ototoxicity is bilateral, sensorineural, and high frequency.

**Postnatal Infections.**   In contrast to Maya, Cole had an uneventful pre- and postnatal course.

> *Cole* was the product of a full-term gestation and normal delivery. After 24 hours in the hospital, he and his mother went home. Cole continued to develop normally, babbling and sitting up around 6 months of age, walking and producing his first words around 1 year of age. By the time Cole was in kindergarten, he was quite a precocious child. He seemed to be into everything and was always full of stories about his latest adventures to tell his mother. One day during his first year of kindergarten, Cole had flulike symptoms. He ran a fever and slept a great deal. After several days with no break in his fever, Cole's mother took him to the doctor. Following a brief examination, his pediatrician instructed Cole's mother to take him to the emergency room at the hospital. A test at the hospital confirmed that Cole had *bacterial meningitis*.

The age at which children are most likely to contract meningitis is 6 to 12 months. However, it is possible for older children to contract the disease as well. Approximately 15 percent of meningitis survivors have neurologic sequelae that may include seizures, paresis, learning or developmental disabilities, and hearing loss (Kallio, Kilpi, Anttila, & Peltola, 1994). The hearing loss is usually bilateral, sensorineural, mild to profound in degree, and permanent.

> With this knowledge in mind, when Cole was feeling better, his physician ordered a hearing test. A pediatric audiologist found that Cole demonstrated a profound hearing loss in both ears.

Audiologists should be seeing fewer cases like Cole in the future. The availability preventive vaccines should result in a marked decline in hearing loss secondary to meningitis (Klein, 1994; Stein & Boyer, 1994).

Viral infections can also lead to hearing loss. A common viral cause of unilateral sensorineural hearing loss in children is *mumps.* The associated hearing loss occurs suddenly and can range in severity from mild to profound. Approximately 5 percent of mumps patients acquire hearing loss (Vuori, Lahikainen, & Peltonen, 1962). *Measles* is another viral cause of sensorineural hearing loss in children. Approximately 10 percent of those with measles have resulting hearing loss. The pattern is typically a bilateral severe-to-profound, high-frequency hearing loss (Bergstrom, 1984).

## Other High-Risk Factors for Hearing Loss

A number of other medical conditions can lead to hearing loss. Each can give rise to hearing losses of various types and severity. To illustrate, we will consider three conditions that can produce conductive, sensorineural, or mixed hearing loss.

**Otitis Media.**   Inflammation of the middle ear space, or **otitis media**, is the most frequent cause of hearing loss in young children. Approximately one-third of children in the United States have recurrent and severe middle ear disease by age 3; the peak age for acute otitis media is 7 to 12 months (Klein, 1992). Hearing loss associated with otitis media when fluid is present in the middle ear (called otitis media with **effusion** [OME]) is conductive, unilateral, or bilateral. This loss typically fluctuates. The average hearing loss caused by otitis media is between approximately 25 and 30 dB (Brookhouser, Worthington, & Kelly, 1993; Fria, Cantekin, & Eichler, 1985). Several factors contribute to the likelihood of the occurrence of otitis media (Table 11.2). These include placement in day care centers (Alho, Koivu, Sorri, & Rantakallio, 1990; Pukander, 1982; Sipila, Karma, Pukander, Timonen, & Kataja, 1988), parental smoking (Sipila et al., 1988; Stahlberg, Ruuskanen, & Virolainen, 1986), and the autumn season (Alho, Oja, Koivu, & Sorri, 1995). Antibiotic therapy is the most common form of treatment for OME. The insertion of tubes into the eardrums for treatment of OME usually eliminates the conductive

**TABLE 11.2  High Risk Factors for Otitis Media in Children**

1. First episode of acute otitis media prior to 6 months of age
2. Infants who are bottle-fed
3. Children with craniofacial anomalies, stigmata, or other findings associated with syndromes known to affect the outer and middle ear
4. Ethnic populations with documented increased incidence of outer and middle ear disease (e.g., Native American and Eskimo populations)
5. Family history of chronic or recurrent otitis media with effusion
6. Children in group day care settings or crowded living conditions
7. Children exposed to excessive cigarette smoke
8. Children diagnosed with sensorineural hearing loss, learning disabilities, behavior disorders, or developmental delays and disorders

From Bluestone & Klein (1996).

hearing loss by allowing drainage of middle ear fluid and is the most common operation for children in the United States (Kleinman, Kosecoff, DuBois, & Brook, 1994).

**Persistent Pulmonary Hypertension of the Newborn (PPHN).**  Also known as persistent fetal circulation, PPHN is a physical abonormality of the blood vessels connected to the heart that results in deficient oxygenation of the blood, or severe hypoxemia. Twenty to forty percent of infants diagnosed with PPHN have sensorineural hearing loss (Leavitt, Watchko, Bennett, & Folsom, 1987; Sell, Gaines, Gluckman, & Williams, 1985; Walton & Hendricks-Munoz, 1991). The onset of hearing loss is thought to be related to the combined effects of the very medical procedures (e.g., drug therapy, ventilation) used to keep babies with this condition alive (Hendricks-Munoz & Walton, 1988; Walton & Hendricks-Munoz, 1991). Hearing loss associated with PPHN has been described as bilateral, progressive, and sensorineueral, with variability in degree and the possibility of delayed onset (Hendricks-Munoz & Walton, 1988; Naulty, Weiss, & Herer, 1986).

**Fetal Alcohol Syndrome (FAS).**  FAS is the most common preventable cause of birth defects today and is estimated to occur in 1 of every 750 live births (Streissguth, Landesman-Dwyer, Martin, & Smith, 1980). FAS results from drinking alcohol during pregnancy. The timing and amount of consumption will influence the severity of the consequent disorders. FAS is characterized by a constellation of physical, behavioral, and cognitive abnormalities. Only a few investigations of hearing status in this population have been conducted; however, they suggest a high incidence of recurrent otitis media and a possibly higher than average incidence of bilateral sensorineural hearing loss (Church & Gerkin, 1988; Streissguth, Clarren, & Jones, 1985).

## DEGREE OF HEARING LOSS AND ITS EFFECT ON COMMUNICATION

The classification of hearing loss is usually a bit different for children than for adults. Hearing loss in adults has been defined as an average of greater than 25 dB thresholds at the frequencies 500, 1000, 2000, and 3000 Hz (American Academy of Otolaryngology & American Council of Otolaryngology, 1979). In children, however, hearing loss is frequently regarded as an average threshold of greater than 20 or even 15 dB over the same range of frequencies (Northern & Downs, 1991). After all, young children are in the process of learning speech and language and cannot always "fill in the gaps" of conversation the way that adults can. If some words or sounds are missed in conversation, an adult can often determine what was said by the context. For example, if an adult hears "The *ole* of my shoe needs repairing," he or she will figure out that the misunderstood word must be "sole" based on the other key words in the sentence. Children, on the other hand, do not have the extensive vocabularies, linguistic experiences, or strategies to assist them in interpreting misunderstood words. This means that even a slight hearing loss can result in speech perception that is missing critical consonant or vowel sounds. Some of the unvoiced consonants (e.g., th, f, k, t) are produced with intensities that are barely audible or not audible at all in soft conversational speech (see Figure 11.8).

**FIGURE 11.8** **Effects of a mild hearing loss on ability to hear conversational levels of speech. The connected circles reflect the air conduction thresholds. For simplicity, only the right ear is shown.**

An audiogram will provide a good starting place for understanding the impact of a hearing loss, because greater degrees of loss are typically associated with more severe consequences to the individual. We can see this relationship in Table 11.3. However, it is impossible to characterize the type or severity of communication problems an individual child with hearing impairment will have from the audiogram alone. Many factors contribute to communication ability, such as severity, configuration, and age of onset of hearing loss. Additional factors, such as intelligence, extent and quality of intervention, and family support, also influence a child's communication development. With those factors in mind, we will attempt

**TABLE 11.3  Impact of Hearing Loss**

| | |
|---|---|
| **BILATERAL HEARING LOSS** | |
| Minimal Hearing Loss (16 to 25 dB HL) | At 15 dB a student can miss up to 10 percent of the speech signal when a teacher is at a distance greater than 3 feet and when the classroom is noisy. |
| Mild Hearing Loss (26 to 40 dB HL) | With a 30 dB loss, a student can miss 25 to 40 percent of a speech signal. Without amplification, the child with 35 to 40 dB loss will miss at least 50percent of class discussion. |
| Moderate Hearing Loss (41 to 55 dB HL) | Child understands conversational speech at a distance of 3 to 5 feet (face-to-face) only if structure and vocabulary are controlled. Without amplification, the amount of speech signal missed can be 50 to 75 percent with a 40 dB loss, and 80 to 100 percent with a 50 dB loss. |
| Moderate-to-Severe Hearing Loss (56 to 70 dB HL) | Without amplification, conversation must be very loud to be understood. A 55 dB loss can cause a child to miss up to 100 percent of speech information. |
| Severe Hearing Loss (71 to 90 dB HL) | Without amplification, may hear loud voices about 1 foot from ear. When amplified optimally, children with hearing ability of 90 dB or better should be able to identify environmental sounds and detect all the sounds of speech. |
| Profound Hearing Loss (≥ 91 dB HL) | Aware of vibrations more than tonal patterns. May rely on vision rather than hearing as primary avenue for communication and learning. |
| **UNILATERAL HEARING LOSS** (Normal hearing in one ear with the other ear exhibiting at least a mild permanent loss.) | May have difficulty hearing faint or distant speech. Usually has difficulty localizing sounds and has greater difficulty understanding speech in background noise. |

to describe general effects of different degrees of hearing loss on communication in the following scenarios.

> *Julia*, age 7, has a mild conductive hearing loss (15–30 dB) bilaterally. Julia's hearing loss is the result of otitis media with effusion. This temporary loss should disappear as the middle ear fluid resolves. As can be seen in Figure 11.8, Julia has a mild hearing loss that is "flat" in that all frequencies are affected to a similar degree. She can hear vowels clearly but has difficulty hearing some voiced consonants. For example, Julia cannot hear the fricatives f, th, v, z because they are below her threshold. This type of hearing loss would be similar to trying to listen with cotton balls in your ears. Her teachers noticed that Julia seemed to have difficulty paying attention in class and frequently appeared to daydream.

Numerous studies suggest that some children with recurrent bouts of otitis media are at risk for language delays or disorders. However, the research has not been clear regarding the long-term effects of otitis media on speech and language, that is, after the otitis media has cleared up.

> *Suzanne*, age 10, has a mild to moderate hearing loss (30–50 dB) bilaterally. As illustrated in Figure 11.9, without her hearing aids, Suzanne misses almost all of the speech sounds at normal conversational loudness levels. She can hear vowels better than consonants and has difficulty discriminating between consonants. Therefore, she misunderstands similar-sounding words such as *sue, shoe, two, coo*. In addition,

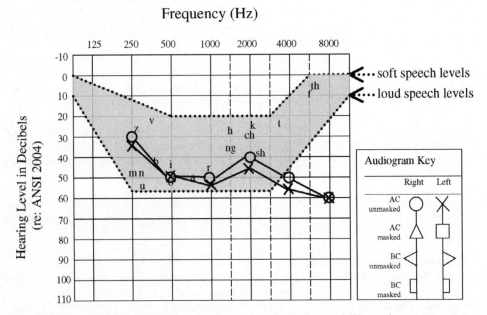

**FIGURE 11.9    Effects of a mild-to-moderate hearing loss on ability to hear conversational levels of speech. The thresholds fall above the intensity of many speech sounds.**

her speech is sometimes difficult to understand because she frequently distorts or omits consonants when speaking. Suzanne is considered at risk for academic problems even though her hearing loss is relatively mild (Tharpe & Bess, 1991).

*Catherine*, age 2, has a severe-to-profound sensorineural hearing loss (80 sloping to 100 dB) bilaterally. Catherine's parents initially requested a hearing test because they were concerned about her lack of speech and language development. As illustrated in Figure 11.10, she cannot hear conversational-level speech or many environmental sounds. Catherine can hear loud environmental sounds and loud speech if the speaker is close by. Without the use of hearing aids, Catherine will not develop speech. Even though she now uses hearing aids, she still exhibits severe speech and language deficits. Her speech is characterized by excessive nasality, substitutions, omissions, restricted range of voice pitch, and extended duration of phonation.

*Roy*, age 9, has a profound hearing loss (greater than 90 dB) in his right ear with normal hearing in his left ear. His parents never noticed that he had difficulty hearing until age 4, when they observed that he would always switch the telephone to his left ear when his grandparents called. When Roy started school at age 5, his teacher reported problems of inattention and daydreaming. Figure 11.11 illustrates Roy's unilateral hearing loss. It was once believed that such losses would result in few if any problems as long as a child was seated preferentially in the classroom, with the normal-hearing ear toward the teacher. Unilateral hearing losses, however, have been found to put children at risk for communication and academic problems

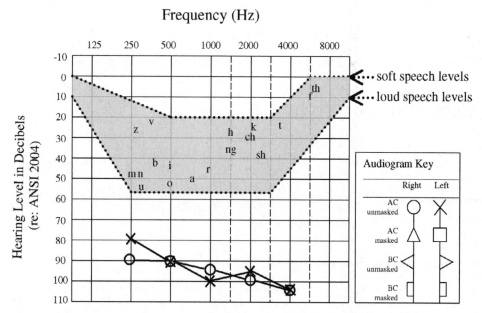

**FIGURE 11.10   Effects of a severe-to-profound hearing loss on ability to hear conversational levels of speech. Note that the thresholds fall well below the level of even loud speech. For simplicity, only right ear thresholds are shown.**

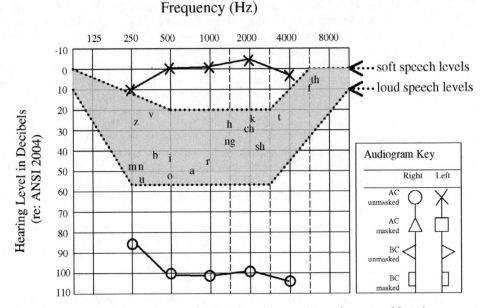

**FIGURE 11.11** Unilateral hearing loss of the right ear. Note the normal hearing thresholds for the left ear as indicated by the *x*s.

(Bess & Tharpe, 1986). In fact, approximately 30 percent of children with unilateral hearing loss have been found to need grade repetition or resource assistance in school (Bess & Tharpe, 1986; Oyler, Oyler, & Matkin, 1988).

## AUDIOLOGICAL TESTING

In the last decade, several organizations and lawmakers have called for earlier identification and intervention of infants with hearing impairment (Healthy People 2000, 1990; Joint Committee on Infant Hearing, 2000; NIH, 1993). As a result, audiologists are identifying and evaluating children at younger ages than ever before. This evaluation of infants and children requires both behavioral and electrophysiological test procedures.

### Behavioral Testing

Even with the widespread use of advanced technological evaluation tools, behavioral testing remains a valuable part of hearing assessment for children. The behavioral technique employed depends largely on the age and developmental level of the child. Some general principles hold across all behavioral tests. Testing is conducted in sound-treated rooms that meet the requirements for accurate measurements set forth by the American National Standards Institute (1991). Test signals are increased and decreased systematically until the softest level at which the infant or child responds (usually 50% of the time) is reached. This level is called the *threshold* or, in the case of young infants, *minimum response level* (*MRL*), because they may actually hear a sound at a lower level than that to which they are able or willing to respond. Thresholds or MRLs can be determined via earphones for air conduction testing, via a bone vibrator for bone conduction testing, or via loudspeakers for soundfield testing.

When testing is conducted via earphones or a bone vibrator, one problem that must be addressed is *cross-over* of sound presented to the opposite ear. This refers to the fact that the two ears are not totally isolated, and sometimes a sound going to one ear can cause the skull to vibrate and actually stimulate the other, or nontest, ear. The audiologist must eliminate participation of the nontest ear during testing. To do so, noise is delivered to the nontest ear with a frequency spectrum similar to the test signal, but at a higher intensity, so that any sound crossing over from the test ear will not be heard. This is called masking noise, and responses obtained in this manner are referred to as *masked thresholds*.

For children, behavioral testing usually begins with the use of speech stimuli. A *speech reception threshold* is determined by asking the child to repeat two-syllable words that have equal stress on each syllable, called **spondaic words**. These are words such as *baseball, hotdog,* or *airplane*. Children who are shy or whose speech is difficult to understand may point to the picture of the word that they heard rather than say the word. If a child is unable to repeat words or identify pictures, a *speech awareness threshold* is obtained that simply identifies the softest intensity level at which a child responds. Pure-tone air conduction testing is typically conducted next. Several techniques for obtaining pure-tone thresholds from children of different ages are discussed below.

**Behavioral Observation Audiometry (BOA).**   For infants from birth to approximately 5 months of age, *behavioral observation audiometry* is typically employed. Rather than measuring the softest sound that infants can hear, audiologists measure the lowest level at which they respond to sound (the *minimum response level*). With this technique, the audiologist looks for gross body movements such as eye-widening, startles, breathing changes, facial grimaces, or cessation of movements that are time-locked with sound presented through speakers. Although BOA is a useful clinical procedure for infants, responses are highly variable and often difficult to interpret (Moore & Wilson, 1978). Also, only a limited number of responses can be obtained before the infant gradually adapts, or **habituates**, to the sound. With maturation, the child responds to lower and lower signal intensity levels, until approximately 2 years of age (Thompson & Weber, 1974). These factors contribute to a wide range of results in typically developing infants, so it is impossible to define hearing loss as a change or deviation from this "norm" (Thompson & Weber, 1974). Therefore, BOA is probably best viewed as a hearing screening assessment procedure that allows one to conclude that an infant's hearing is grossly within or outside the range of normal hearing.

**Visual Reinforcement Audiometry (VRA).**    *Visual reinforcement audiometry* is a procedure that addresses many of the problems inherent in BOA. Used for infants and young children from approximately 6 months to 2 years of age, VRA depends on the child's natural inclination to turn toward a sound source. The schematic in Figure 11.12 illustrates the VRA test arrangement. An infant (I) is seated in a high chair or parent's lap facing an observation window. Examiner 1 ($E_1$) is in a darkened room and cannot be seen by the infant. When $E_1$ determines that the infant is in a quiet state, an auditory signal is delivered through earphones or speakers. When the infant turns in response to the signal, the visual reinforcer (VR) (a toy in a Plexiglass box) is animated and lights up on the side where the sound emanated. Examiner 2 ($E_2$) (perhaps the infant's parent) serves as an assistant who is needed to keep the infant content and sitting quietly during the test. Figure 11.13 illustrates several aspects of the VRA procedure.

**Conditioned Play Audiometry (CPA).**    At approximately 2 to $2\frac{1}{2}$ years of age, play audiometry becomes the behavioral technique of choice. *Tangible reinforcement operant conditioning audiometry (TROCA)* is one form of play audiometry developed by Lloyd and colleagues (Lloyd, Spradlin, & Reid, 1968). For this technique, the child is conditioned to push a button when a sound is heard. The button push is followed by the delivery of an edible reinforcement controlled by the examiner. The reinforcement is small, preferably sugarless, and quick to eat. The treat may be varied to keep a restless child's interest. More traditional conditioned play audiometry techniques include placement of a peg in a pegboard or a block in a box when the child hears the sound. The audiologist chooses tasks that are fun and interesting to the child.

**Speech Discrimination Testing.**    As discussed earlier in this chapter, the pure-tone audiogram does not tell precisely how well a person understands the most important sound stimulus, speech. For that reason, *speech discrimination* testing is usually

**FIGURE 11.12    Typical two-room test suite arrangement for conducting visual reinforcement audiometry. $E_1$ = Examiner 1, $E_2$ = Examiner 2, I = Infant, VR = Visual Reinforcer.**

FIGURE 11.13   Illustration of various aspects of visual reinforcement audiometry (VRA). Panel A illustrates the assistant wearing masking earphones while the child is being tested through speakers. Panel B illustrates the infant head-turn in response to sound and the subsequent animation of the mechanical toy as reinforcement. Panel C illustrates the VRA procedure with the infant wearing earphones.

conducted after pure-tone testing for children who are approximately 3 years of age or older. Unlike threshold tests, speech discrimination testing is conducted at a comfortable loudness level in an attempt to determine the child's ability to understand conversational speech. Typical materials for discrimination testing consist of monosyllabic words that can be repeated or pointed to on picture cards.

### Auditory Brainstem Response Testing

Sometimes valid behavioral tests cannot be obtained from children. This may be because the child is too young (under 4 or 5 months of age) or uncooperative due to behavioral or developmental disabilities. For those children, alternative testing procedures that do not require voluntary responses are quite useful. You will recall from Chapter 10 that information about sounds must be transmitted from the inner ear to the brain via the brainstem pathways. The **auditory brainstem response** (ABR) reflects the electrical activity along the auditory pathway. Electrodes are placed on the scalp and on the earlobes or mastoids of the patient in order to record this electrical activity. The electrical activity is recorded as a waveform that occurs in response to acoustic stimuli. The normal waveform consists of five waves that occur at specific time intervals or latencies. At high intensity levels (approximately 80 dB), all five waves should be observable. The peak of the fifth wave can be observed at intensity levels that are within approximately 10 dB of true auditory threshold. It is this feature of the ABR that is useful for estimating hearing threshold. Since a child does not provide a voluntary response and can even be asleep for this test, the ABR makes a valuable contribution to the pediatric test battery, particularly for children who are unable or unwilling to cooperate for behavioral testing (see Figure 11.14).

### Immittance Audiometry

A standard component of the pediatric test battery is **immittance audiometry**, which includes *tympanometry* and *acoustic reflex thresholds*. Tympanometry is a measurement of the mobility of the middle ear system as air pressure is varied in the external auditory canal. It is a valuable tool for identifying the presence of middle ear fluid associated with otitis media and other middle ear pathologies commonly seen in children. The procedure is quick and painless, making it ideal for children. A rubber-tipped probe is inserted gently into the child's ear canal, and air pressure is pumped into the cavity formed between the end of the probe and the eardrum (tympanic membrane). As the air pressure in the cavity is varied above and below ambient air pressure, the mobility of the tympanic membrane is measured and plotted on a graph called a *tympanogram*. In a normally functioning ear, maximum mobility should occur at or near ambient air pressure. This is an important measurement because pathology, such as otitis media, will influence the movement of the eardrum.

The acoustic reflex threshold is the lowest intensity required to elicit a contraction of the stapedius muscle (see Chapter 10). This contraction can be evoked

**FIGURE 11.14   An audiologist prepares an infant for auditory brainstem response testing by placing an electrode on her scalp.**

by introducing a loud sound (usually a pure tone) to the ear canal either through the probe or through an earphone placed on the opposite ear from the probe. This test provides information about the functioning of the middle and inner ear as well as the auditory nerve. In a normal functioning ear, a reflex is elicited when the sound is between about 65 and 95 dB. A hearing loss may result in an elevation of the sound level needed to evoke the acoustic reflex or an absence of the reflex altogether. The presence of middle ear fluid or damage to the acoustic nerve may also affect the acoustic reflex. The acoustic reflex thresholds, viewed in conjunction with the tympanogram and audiogram, can assist the pediatric audiologist in determining the type and degree of hearing loss.

## Otoacoustic Emissions

Evoked otoacoustic emissions (OAEs) were discovered in 1978 (see Chapter 10) and were quickly incorporated into the audiologist's clinical armamentarium. Although there are several types of evoked OAEs, they are all produced by presenting sound to the ear and then examining the ear's response recorded by a miniature microphone in the ear canal. The presence of OAEs suggests a normally functioning cochlea; absent or reduced OAEs are the result of conductive or cochlear hearing loss. Like immittance audiometry, this tool is particularly useful for children because it is quick and painless, and requires no voluntary response.

It is important to note that no one test should be depended upon when testing infants or young children. Rather, a battery of tests is used by pediatric audiologists. Let us look at a typical evaluation.

*Juan's* mother brought him in for a hearing evaluation at age 2 because of concern about his lack of speech and language development. Juan had several aunts and uncles on his mother's side of the family with hearing loss, so she was particularly concerned that his hearing might be a factor in his communication problems. His medical history included a normal gestation and delivery, a few colds and upper respiratory infections, and several episodes of otitis media that had been treated with antibiotics. When testing began, Juan refused to wear earphones, repeatedly yanking them off and crying. As an alternative to the earphones, Juan was tested in soundfield through speakers utilizing visual reinforcement audiometry. Responses were consistent with a mild (35–45 dB) hearing loss for all of the test frequencies and speech. In an effort to determine if the hearing loss was conductive or sensorineural, the audiologist attempted to put a bone vibrator on Juan. Again, he resisted the placement of anything on his head, so the audiologist had to abandon that tactic. By having an assistant blow bubbles to distract him while he sat on his mother's lap, the audiologist was able to place the probe for tympanometry in his ear canal and obtain a tympanogram. The results were consistent with the presence of middle ear fluid in both ears. Even though the audiologist was not able to obtain all of the test results that she wanted, the overall pattern of the test results (i.e., the mild hearing loss and abnormal tympanograms) suggested that the hearing loss was conductive. She then recommended that Juan be seen by his pediatrician for treatment of the middle ear fluid and then return for another hearing test to determine if his hearing loss had resolved following medical treatment.

## Hearing Screening

One of the many responsibilities of the pediatric audiologist is to organize and oversee the screening of neonates, infants, preschoolers, and school-age children for hearing loss and middle ear disease (otitis media). The process of screening involves identifying those at risk for hearing loss or ear disease so they can be referred for further evaluation. Screening tests provide a quick, simple, safe, valid, reliable, and cost-effective means of identifying children in need of further evaluation; they are not intended to diagnose hearing loss.

Guidelines are available for screening children at various ages. For infants, both brainstem response testing and evoked otoacoustic emissions are used for screening purposes. The Joint Committee on Infant Hearing (2000) and the American Speech-Hearing-Language Association (ASHA, 1997) recommend screening infants who have known indicators associated with sensorineural or conductive hearing loss, if screening for all newborns is not available. As recently as 2002, thirty-seven states had mandated newborn hearing screening statutes or regulations (ASHA, 2002).

ASHA (1997) recommends screening preschoolers who have any indicators associated with late-onset or progressive hearing loss or parental or health care provider concerns regarding hearing, speech, language, or developmental delay. Play audiometric techniques are recommended, although visual reinforcement audiometry may be used if necessary. ASHA (1997) recommends screening school-age children upon initial entry to school, annually in kindergarten through third grade, and in seventh and eleventh grades. Furthermore, all children entering special education, repeating a grade, or entering the school system without evidence of having passed a previous hearing screening are typically screened. In addition, school-age children reporting exposure to high levels of noise should receive a hearing screening. The recommended screening procedure is play or conventional audiometry with earphones.

There has been considerable debate on the issue of *who* should be screened for middle ear disease. Some professionals feel that *all* children should be screened, while others believe only those considered at greatest risk for middle ear disease should be screened. ASHA has left that decision to each individual screening program (1997). ASHA recommends a middle ear screening protocol that includes a case history from the parent or guardian; visual inspection of the ears to identify risk factors for outer and middle ear disease, and any contraindications for performing tympanometry; examination of the external ear canal and tympanic membrane; and tympanometry with a screening or diagnostic tympanometer (ASHA, 1997).

## MANAGEMENT OF CHILDREN WITH HEARING IMPAIRMENT

Once hearing loss has been identified and described in terms of type and degree, a decision must be made regarding the most appropriate intervention: medical or audiological, or both. Consideration is given to medications, surgical interventions, or the use of amplification devices including hearing aids. As a general rule, conductive types of hearing loss are most likely to benefit from surgical approaches or amplification, whereas the options for sensorineural hearing losses are usually limited to amplification.

### Amplification

The early identification of hearing loss in children has little value if intervention is not initiated in a timely manner. The first, and perhaps the most important, step in intervention is the fitting of appropriate sound amplification. It is the role of the pediatric audiologist to ensure that children receive a consistent and audible speech signal at intensity levels that are safe and comfortable. The Pediatric Working Group (1996) developed recommendations for fitting amplification on infants and children. Although no hard and fast rules exist regarding the specific degree of hearing loss for which amplification should be used, the group concurred that any child with thresholds exceeding 25 dB HL should be considered a candidate for hearing aids. This includes children with unilateral or bilateral hearing loss.

There are several different types of hearing aids available today. These include the (1) *body aid,* (2) *behind-the-ear aid,* (3) *in-the-ear aid,* and (4) *in-the-canal aid.* These are worn by both adults and children (see Chapter 12 for a photograph of these types of aids). By far the most common hearing aid type for children is the behind-the-ear aid (see Figure 11.15). All of these hearing aid types contain similar internal components and function similarly. A microphone picks up the acoustic signal and converts it to an electrical signal that is amplified (made louder), filtered, and converted back to an acoustic signal by a receiver. In behind-the-ear hearing aids, the amplified sound is routed to the child's ear by tubing that leads to an earmold. The earmold, made specifically for an individual child's ear, allows the sound to be directed to the ear canal and keeps the hearing aid in place.

It is particularly important when fitting children to know exactly how much the sound is being amplified, since it is difficult or impossible for an infant or young child to tell you when the amplified sound is too loud or not loud enough. Although initial hearing aid settings can be made with computerized prescriptive formulae, amplified sound levels are typically verified by an audiologist using *probe microphone measures.* A probe microphone is one that is small enough to be inserted into the ear canal of a child while the hearing aid is worn (see Figure 11.16). A sound signal is presented from a small speaker, and the probe microphone system records the intensity level of the test signal amplified through the hearing aid from within the child's ear canal. Several techniques are available for making needed measurements quickly from a child.

Sometimes, traditional hearing aids are not sufficient to overcome the hearing deficits of those with profound hearing losses. An alternative to traditional

**FIGURE 11.15    Schematic of a behind-the-ear hearing aid. Dashed lines indicate the path of sound as it is received by the microphone and processed through the hearing aid components before delivery to the ear.**

**FIGURE 11.16   Probe microphone measurements with a cooperative child.**

hearing aids for those children is the **cochlear implant**. The cochlear implant is a surgically implanted device that uses electrodes inserted into the cochlea to stimulate the auditory nerve with electrical current (see Figure 11.17). A microphone, worn on the child's ear in a casing that looks like a hearing aid, converts the acoustic signal to an electrical signal. The electrical signal is modified by a processor, which may be in a body-worn or behind-the-ear case, and then sent to a receiver worn behind the child's ear. The signal is then transmitted through the skin to an internal receiver implanted in the mastoid bone, from which it is transmitted to electrodes implanted in the cochlea. Although cochlear implants do not restore normal hearing, children vary markedly in terms of the benefits received from the implant. Most children experience a minimum of sound awareness, and some develop excellent speech recognition ability. The pediatric audiologist assists in

**FIGURE 11.17    Schematic of a cochlear implant.**

determining whether a child is an appropriate candidate for the cochlear implant, counsels families on the benefits and limitations of the implant, and sets the stimulus levels of the speech processor after implantation. An audiologist or speech-language pathologist works with the child to develop or improve listening skills.

## Communication and Education Approaches

One of the most difficult decisions facing parents of a child newly identified with hearing loss is how to communicate effectively with their child. The most common communication options are *auditory-oral, total communication,* and *manual* modes. Auditory-oral communication emphasizes listening and oral communication. A total communication approach includes listening, speech reading, signing, finger spelling, and oral expression. A manual mode of communication uses one of the signed languages, typically without oral speech. The decision regarding which communication mode to adopt usually is highly influenced by the degree of the child's hearing loss. Children with mild or moderate hearing losses generally use an auditory-oral approach because they have a considerable amount of residual hearing. Children with severe-to-profound hearing loss, however, may have a more difficult time acquiring spoken language and may require the additional visual input afforded by a total or manual communication approach. It is not uncommon, however, for children or their parents to adopt communication modes for cultural reasons. For example, when a child with moderate hearing loss is born to parents who are deaf and who use a manual communication approach, the child is most likely to use a manual approach also. Many factors—audiological, educational, and cultural—are considered when choosing the communication mode that is best for an individual family.

Federal law has strongly influenced the education of children with hearing loss. Public Law 108–446, or Individuals with Disabilities Education Improvement Act (IDEA), was intended to fulfill four primary purposes: (1) to ensure that all children with handicaps have available to them a *free, appropriate public education* that emphasizes special education and related services designed to meet their unique needs; (2) to ensure that the rights of handicapped children and their parents or guardians are protected; (3) to help states pay for education of all children with handicaps; and (4) to ensure and assess the effectiveness of educational programs. Children who are deaf or hard-of-hearing are covered by this legislation. Under IDEA, *deaf* means "a hearing impairment that is so severe that the child is impaired in processing linguistic information through hearing, with or without amplification, which adversely affects educational performance." *Hard-of-hearing* means a hearing loss, permanent or fluctuating, that adversely affects a child's educational performance. Children with handicaps from birth to age 3 and their families are provided with early intervention programs, and appropriate public education and related services to children with disabilities 3 to 5 years of age are provided under the law.

In the past, children with hearing loss received their education in segregated schools and classrooms. Now most are enrolled in general education programs in local schools with normal hearing peers. This trend is referred to as *inclusion* and may occur on a full-time or part-time basis. If additional services are needed for these children, they may attend resource classrooms by leaving their general education classroom for short periods during the day. Another alternative is to receive additional support from an itinerant teacher who travels from class to class. Special services are designed to meet the unique needs of children with hearing loss and maximize the benefit they receive from their educational program. These special services may include speech-language pathology, audiology, psychology, counseling, or physical therapy, among others.

The role of the audiologist in the schools is an important one. Duties include developing and supervising the school's hearing screening program, monitoring the hearing of children identified with hearing loss, participating in the educational planning for children with hearing loss, monitoring individual hearing aids or other assistive devices to ensure their proper function, and educating teachers and other school personnel regarding hearing loss, hearing aids, and communication with children having hearing loss.

## Counseling

Counseling is an important component of the overall services that audiologists provide to children and their families and, more specifically, a critical part of the management process. Counseling can include explaining test results, making recommendations for habilitation services, and assisting families as they work through feelings of confusion and disappointment about their child's hearing loss.

Although not trained as professional counselors, audiologists can provide educational and supportive counseling to help families make practical life changes to ease the unexpected disruptions that hearing loss can cause.

Most counseling takes place informally while discussing test results or responding to a parent's phone call. Support groups can provide a more structured setting where families share their feelings of fear, confusion, and perhaps guilt, with other parents of children with hearing impairment. It is through communication with other families that parents learn that they are not alone. Support groups may include parents, siblings, and even extended family members such as grandparents, aunts, and uncles.

## CLINICAL PROBLEM SOLVING

The parents of 4-year-old Josh were shocked to learn that his articulation problems were the result of a moderate sensorineural hearing loss in both ears. After all, neither of them had a hearing loss, nor did any of their parents or siblings. The pregnancy with Josh was normal, as was his entire postnatal course.

1. What are some possible causes of Josh's hearing loss?
2. Is it more likely that Josh's hearing loss will be treated medically or with hearing aids?
3. What receptive communication difficulties might you expect with this degree of hearing loss?
4. Might expressive communication difficulties also occur with this degree of hearing loss? If so, why?

## REFERENCES

Alho, O. P., Koivu, M., Sorri, M., & Rantakallio, P. (1990). Risk factors for recurrent acute otitis media and respiratory infection in infancy. *International Journal of Pediatric Otorhinolaryngology, 19,* 151–161.

Alho, O. P., Oja, J., Koivu, M., & Sorri, M. (1995). Risk factors for chronic otitis media with effusion in infancy. *Archives of Otolaryngology Head and Neck Surgery, 121,* 839–843.

American Academy of Otolaryngology & American Council of Otolaryngology. (1979). Guide for the evaluation of hearing handicap. *Journal of the American Medical Association, 241,* 2055–2059.

American National Standards Institute. (2004). *Specifications for audiometers* (ANSI S3.6-R2004). New York: Author.

American Speech-Language-Hearing Association Panel on Audiologic Assessment. (1997). *Guidelines for audiologic screening.* Rockville, MD: ASHA.

American Speech-Language-Hearing Association (ASHA). (2002, June 27). *Early hearing detection and intervention action center.* Retrieved June 27, 2002, from http://www.professional.asha .org/resources/legislative/ih_index.cfm

Apgar, V. (1953). A proposal for a new method of evaluation of the newborn infant. *Anesthesia and Analgesia, 32,* 260.

Bergman, I., Hirsch, R. P., Fria, T. J., Shapiro, S. M., Holzman, I., & Painter, M. J. U. (1985). Cause of hearing loss in the high-risk-premature infant. *Journal of Pediatrics, 106,* 95–101.

Bergstrom, L. (1984). Congenital hearing loss. In J. L. Northern (Ed.), *Hearing disorders* (2nd ed.). Boston: Little, Brown.

Bess, F. H., & Tharpe, A. M. (1986, January/February). Case history data on unilaterally hearing-impaired children (pp. 14–19). In F. H. Bess et al. (Eds.), Children with unilateral hearing loss. *Ear and Hearing Monograph.*

Bluestone, C. D., & Klein, J. O. (1996). Otitis media, atelectasis, and eustachian tube disfunction. In C. D. Bluestone, S. E. Stool, & M. A. Kenna (Eds.), *Pediatric otolaryngology* (3rd ed., Vol. I, pp. 388–582). Philadelphia: Saunders.

Brookhouser, P. E., Worthington, D. W., & Kelly, W. J. (1993). Middle ear disease in young children with sensorineural hearing loss. *Laryngoscope, 103*(4), 371–378.

Church, M. W., & Gerkin, K. P. (1988). Hearing disorders in children with fetal alcohol syndrome: Findings from case reports. *Pediatrics, 82*(2), 147–154.

Clarren, S. K., & Smith, D. W. (1978). The fetal alcohol syndrome. *New England Journal of Medicine, 198,* 1063–1067.

Cohn, E., & Kelley, P. (1999). Clinical phenotype and mutations in connexin 26 (DFNB1/GJB2), the most common cause of childhood hearing loss. *American Journal of Medical Genetics, 89,* 130–136.

Davis, A., Wood, S., Healy, R., Webb, H., & Rowe, S. (1995). Risk factors for hearing disorders: Epidemiologic evidence of change over time in the United Kingdom. *Journal of the American Academy of Audiology, 6*(5), 365–370.

deVries, L. S., Lary, S., & Dubowitz, L. M. S. (1985). Relationship of serum bilirubin level to ototoxicity and deafness in high-risk low-birth-weight infants. *Pediatrics, 76,* 351–354.

Fria, T. J., Cantekin, E. I., & Eichler, J. A. (1985). Hearing acuity of children with otitis media with effusion. *Archives of Otolaryngology, 111,* 10–16.

Healthy People 2000. (1990). U.S. Department of Health and Human Services, Public Health Service, DHHS Publication No. (PHS) 91-50213. Washington, DC: U.S. Government Printing Office.

Hendricks-Munoz, K. D., & Walton, J. P. (1988). Hearing loss in infants with persistent fetal circulation. *Pediatrics, 81,* 650–656.

Joint Committee on Infant Hearing. (2000). Year 2000 position statement: Principles and guidelines for early hearing detection and intervention programs. *American Journal of Audiology, 9,* 9–29.

Kallio, M. J. T., Kilpi, T., Anttila, M., & Peltola, H. (1994). The effect of a recent previous visit to a physician on outcome after childhood bacterial meningitis. *Journal of the American Medical Association, 272*(10), 787–791.

Klein, J. O. (1992). Epidemiology and natural history of otitis media. In F. H. Bess & J. W. Hall, III (Eds.), *Screening children for auditory function.* Nashville, TN: Bill Wilkerson Center Press.

Klein, J. O. (1994). Antimicrobial therapy and prevention of meningitis. *Pediatric Annals, 23*(2), 76–81.

Kleinman, L. C., Kosecoff, J., DuBois, R. W., & Brook, R. H. (1994). The medical appropriateness of tympanostomy tubes proposed for children younger than 16 years in the United States. *Journal of the American Medical Association, 271*(16), 1250–1255.

Krishnamoorthy, K. S., Shannon, D. C., DeLong, G. R., Todres, I. D., & Davis, K. R. (1979). Neurologic sequelae in the survivors of neonatal intraventricular hemorrhage. *Pediatrics, 64*(2), 233–237.

Leavitt, A. M., Watchko, J. F., Bennett, F. C., & Folsom, R. C. (1987). Neurodevelopmental outcome following persistent pulmonary hypertension of the neonate. *Journal of Perinatology, 7*(4), 288–291.

Leon, P. E., Raventos, H., Lynch, E., Morrow, J., King, M. C. (1992). The gene for an inherited form of deafness maps to chromosome 5q31. *Proceedings of the National Academy of Sciences, 89*(11), 5181–5184.

Lloyd, L. L., Spradlin, J. E., & Reid, M. J. (1968). An operant audiometric procedure for difficult-to-test patients. *Journal of Speech and Hearing Disorders, 33*, 236–245.

Moore, J. M., & Wilson, W. R. (1978). Visual reinforcement audiometry (VRA) with infants. In S. E. Gerber & G. T. Mencher (Eds.), *Early diagnosis of hearing loss.* New York: Grune & Stratton.

Morton, N. (1991). Genetic epidemiology of hearing impairment. *Annals of the New York Academy of Sciences, 630*, 16–31.

Naulty, C. M., Weiss, I. P., & Herer, G. (1986). Progressive sensorineural hearing loss in survivors of persistent fetal circulation. *Ear and Hearing, 7*, 74–77.

National Institutes of Health (NIH). (1993). *Early identification of hearing impairment in infants and young children.* NIH Consensus Statement online. March 1–3, *11*, 1–24.

Northern, J. L., & Downs, M. P. (1991). *Hearing in children*, Baltimore: Williams & Wilkins.

Oyler, R. F., Oyler, A. L., & Matkin, N. D. (1988). Unilateral hearing loss: Demographics and educational impact. *Language, Speech, and Hearing Services in Schools, 19*, 201–210.

Parving, A. (1993). Congenital hearing disability: Epidemiology and identification; A comparison between two health authority districts. *International Journal of Pediatric Otolaryngology, 27*, (etc.) 29–46.

Pediatric Working Group. (1996). Amplification for infants and children with hearing loss. *American Journal of Audiology, 5*(1), 53–68.

Pukander, J. (1982). Acute otitis media among rural children in Finland. *International Journal of Pediatric Otorhinolaryngology, 4*, 325–332.

Sabo, D. L., Brown, D. R., & Watchko, J. F. (1992). Sensorineural hearing loss in high-risk infants. In F. H. Bess & J. W. Hall (Eds.), *Screening children for auditory function.* Nashville, TN: Bill Wilkerson Center Press.

Salamy, A., Eldredge, L., & Tooley, W. J. (1989). Neonatal status and hearing loss in high-risk infants. *Journal of Pediatrics, 114*, 847–852.

Sell, E., Gaines, J., Gluckman, C., & Williams, E. (1985). Persistent fetal circulation. *Archives of the Journal of Disorders of Children, 139*, 25–28.

Shaver, K. (1988). Genetics and deafness. In F. H. Bess (Ed.), *Hearing impairment in children* (pp. 15–32). Parkton, MD: York Press.

Simmons, F. B. (1980). Patterns of deafness in newborns. *Laryngoscope, 90*, 448.

Sipila, M., Karma, P., Pukander, J., Timonen, M., & Kataja, M. (1988). The Bayesian approach to the evaluation of risk factors in acute and recurrent acute otitis media. *Acta Otolaryngology, 106*, 94–101.

Stahlberg, M. R., Ruuskanen, O., & Virolainen, E. (1986). Risk factors for recurrent otitis media. *Pediatric Infectious Disease Journal, 5*, 30–32.

Steel, K. P., & Bussoli, T. J. (1999). Deafness genes: Expressions of surprise. *Trends in Genetics, 15*, 207–211.

Stein, L. K., & Boyer, K. M. (1994). Progress in the prevention of hearing loss in infants. *Ear and Hearing, 15*(2), 116–125.

Streissguth, A. P., Clarren, S. K., & Jones, K. L. (1985). Natural history of the fetal alcohol syndrome: A 10-year follow-up of eleven patients. *Lancet, 2,* 85–91.

Streissguth, A. P., Landesman-Dwyer, S., Martin, J. C., & Smith, D. W. (1980). Teratogenic effects of alcohol in humans and laboratory animals. *Science, 209,* 353–361.

Sundstrom, R., Van Laer, L., Van Camp, G., & Smith, R. (1999). Autosomal recessive nonsyndromic hearing loss. *American Journal of Human Genetics, 89,* 123–129.

Tharpe, A. M., & Bess, F. H. (1991). Identification and management of children with minimal hearing loss. *International Journal of Pediatric Otolaryngology, 21,* 41–50.

Thompson, G., & Weber, B. A. (1974). Responses of infants and young children to behavior observation audiometry (BOA). *Journal of Speech and Hearing Disorders, 2,* (etc.) 140–147.

Vuori, M., Lahikainen, E. A., & Peltonen, T. (1962). Perceptive deafness in connection with mumps. *Acta Otolaryngologica, 55,* 231–236.

Walton, J. P., & Hendricks-Munoz, K. (1991). Profile and stability of sensorineural hearing loss in persistent pulmonary hypertension of the newborn. *Journal of Speech and Hearing Research, 34,* 1362–1370.

Watkin, P., Baldwin, M., & McEnery, G. (1991). Neonatal at risk screening and the identification of deafness. *Archives of Diseases in Children, 66,* 1130–1135.

Wilson-Costello, D., Friedman, H., Minich, N., Fanaroff, A. A., & Hack, M. (2005). Improved survival rates with increased neurodevelopmental disability for extremely low birth weight infants in the 1990s. *Pediatrics, 115*(4), 997–1003.

## READINGS FROM THE POPULAR LITERATURE

Bowers, T. (1999). *Alandra's lilacs.* Washington, DC: Gallaudet University Press. (hearing parents, deaf child)

Cohen, L. H. (1994). *Train go sorry: Inside a deaf world.* New York: Vintage Books. (deafness)

Greenburg, J. (1071). *In this sign.* New York: Henry Holt. (novel about a deaf family)

Keller, H. (1961). *The story of my life: The autobiography of Helen Keller.* New York: Dell. (deaf-blind)

Kisor, H. (1990). *What's that pig outdoors: A memoir of deafness.* New York: Hill and Wang. (deafness)

Sidransky, R. (1990). *In silence: Growing up hearing in a deaf world.* New York: St. Martin's Press. (hearing child, deaf parents)

Walker, L. A. (1986). *A loss for words: The story of deafness in a family.* New York: Harper & Row. (hearing child, deaf parents)

# CHAPTER TWELVE

# DISORDERS OF HEARING IN ADULTS

LINDA NORRIX
FRANCES P. HARRIS

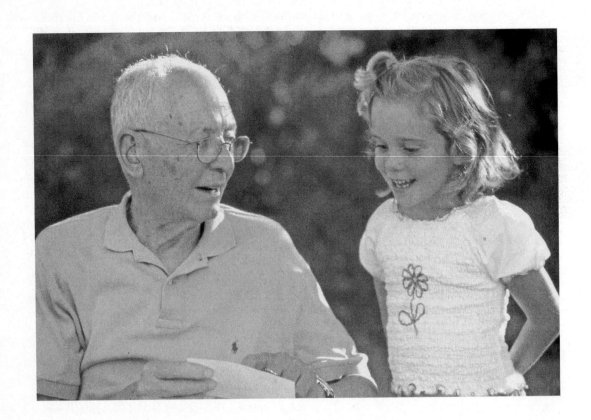

## PREVIEW

About 29 million Americans report difficulty with their hearing. Common causes of hearing loss in adults include prolonged exposure to noise, specific medical conditions, and simply the effects of aging. Regardless of the cause, hearing loss can affect communication, and in turn disrupt family relationships, social interactions, work performance, and overall well being. After documenting the degree of hearing loss and its impact on the individual's life, the audiologist can offer a variety of means to improve hearing performance, including amplification, assistive and alerting devices, and may offer strategies to maximize communication.

Approximately 29 million Americans, most of whom are adults, report difficulty hearing (Kochkin, 2001). Most individuals with hearing impairments develop these difficulties in adulthood, and our focus in this chapter will be on this group. It is important to understand the terminology associated with hearing problems and the effects of those problems on individuals and society (ASHA, 1995). *Hearing impairment* is defined as a loss or abnormality in the structure or function of the auditory system. Impairments can be measured using laboratory techniques (Stephens & Hetu, 1991). Hearing-impaired individuals may exhibit reduced sensitivity for detection of sound, poor understanding of speech, or both. Although Giolas (1994) recommended that the term **hearing loss** be used to quantify the degree of the impairment (e.g., Frank has a 50 dB hearing loss), it is often used interchangeably with the term *hearing impairment*. **Hearing disability** refers to the restrictions in daily activities that a person may experience as a result of a hearing impairment; therefore, one's social environment must be considered in determining disability (Stephens & Hetu, 1991). A hearing impairment may or may not result in a disability. For example, an individual who is socially active and who has a high-frequency hearing impairment is likely to report difficulties understanding speech in noisy environments. In contrast, a person with the same impairment who has few social contacts may not report such problems.

**Handicapping** situations are sometimes experienced by individuals with hearing disabilities (ASHA, 1995). In addition to the hearing impairment, individuals may also experience social isolation, reduced economic resources, and difficulty maintaining independence. Audiologists working with adults need to understand not only the degree of hearing impairment but also the disability and handicapping situations that can be associated with the impairment. The World Health Organization (WHO) has adopted the terms *activity limitations* and *participation restrictions* to describe the effects of impairment on peoples lives. Physical, social, and attitudinal factors are also considered in the classification system (WHO, 2001). The newer terms and classification system emphasize how individuals live with their health conditions, specify what an individual can and cannot do, and eliminate some of the negative connotations associated with older terms once used. The audiologist's goal of management is to optimize the client's ability to live a full life in both the workplace and society. By considering the hearing impaired individual's abilities, restrictions, and limitations in the context of his or her personal situation, an appropriate rehabilitation plan may be developed.

## CONDUCTIVE HEARING LOSS

Although conductive hearing loss is relatively frequent in childhood, it is less frequent in adults. A conductive hearing loss occurs when the sound cannot get to the inner ear efficiently; consequently, there is less stimulation of sensory receptors in the inner ear (see Chapter 10). The audiogram for a conductive loss will exhibit elevated thresholds by air conduction and normal thresholds by bone conduction, so that an air-bone gap will be present (see Chapter 11). The person with hearing impairments typically has good word recognition, provided that speech is loud enough to be heard. Causes of conductive impairments include excess *cerumen*, or ear wax, blocking the ear canal, fluid behind the eardrum within the middle ear space (see Chapter 11 for a discussion of middle ear fluid in children), a perforated eardrum, or damage to the ossicles within the middle ear. **Otosclerosis** is an example of a disorder that occurs in adulthood and causes a progressive conductive hearing impairment. In otosclerosis, bony tissue is replaced by spongy or fibrous bone growth. The most common place for this abnormal bone growth to occur is in the area of the oval window, resulting in reduced motion of the stapes and a conductive hearing loss. Otosclerosis is commonly found in both ears rather than in just one. It is more common in women than in men, and in Caucasians than in Asian or African Americans. Genetics seem to play a role, and a family history is often reported (Balloh, 1998).

> *Ms. Garrett*, age 35, reported that within the last several years she has had difficulties understanding speech in background noise, localizing sounds, hearing people talk when they are positioned to her left, and using the telephone with her left ear. Figure 12.1 illustrates Ms. Garrett's audiogram and word recognition ability. She has otosclerosis in the left ear. Notice that when tested in the left ear at a normal conversational level (45 dB HL), she repeated only 44 percent of the single-syllable words correctly. This was because the speech signal was not entirely audible to her.

To appreciate the effect of hearing loss on the ability to understand speech, it is helpful to examine the relative contribution of the different frequency and intensity combinations for speech audibility, as shown in Figure 12.2. One hundred dots are displayed on the graph. The denser the distribution of dots, the greater the amount of speech energy that falls within that frequency band. An **articulation** or **audibility index** is calculated by assigning 0.01 (one percent) to each dot that is within a person's audibility range. Ms. Garrett's left ear air conduction thresholds are superimposed on the graph.

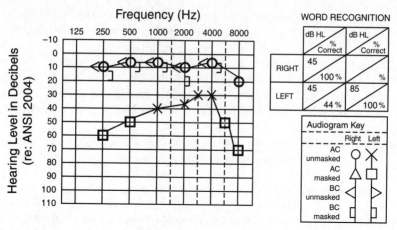

**FIGURE 12.1  Audiogram illustrating a conductive hearing loss in the left ear due to otosclerosis.**

**FIGURE 12.2  The left ear thresholds of an individual with unilateral otosclerosis superimposed on the Count-the-Dot audiogram for calculation of the articulation index. The shaded portion of the graph indicates the frequency range and hearing levels that are audible when speech is presented at a normal conversational level. Note that it was necessary to use masking at levels of 50 dB and above to prevent crossover of sounds to the opposite ear. Masked thresholds are represented by squares on the audiogram.**

Adapted from Mueller & Killion (1990).

Ms. Garrett's audiogram reveals approximately 36 dots that fall below her audiometric curve (between her thresholds and 110 dB HL), which results in an audibility index of 0.36. The audibility index can then be used in a formula to estimate syllable, word, or sentence intelligibility (Mueller & Killion, 1990). In Ms. Garrett's case, a left ear intelligibility score of approximately 56 percent would be predicted based on her audibility index of 0.36. This is close to the 44 percent that was measured directly during testing. When words were presented at a higher level (85 dB HL), Ms. Garrett's word recognition ability was excellent (100% correct).

Ms. Garrett's profile indicates that she is an excellent candidate for wearing a hearing aid because her hearing loss is primarily conductive, which results in little or no sound distortion. With appropriate amplification, the client with a conductive hearing impairment will have few if any limitations or restrictions in their daily life. Depending on the cause of the conductive hearing loss, surgery or medical treatment may improve or even restore hearing. Surgeries, however, are not risk free, as we will see when we continue to follow Ms. Garrett's history.

Ms. Garrett had surgery in an attempt to eliminate the conductive hearing loss due to otosclerosis. The surgery, performed by an ear, nose, and throat (ENT) specialist, is known as a **stapedectomy** and often reduces or nearly eliminates the conductive component of a hearing impairment. During her surgery, the footplate of the stapes was removed and replaced with a wire prosthesis. Although initial results indicated almost complete elimination of the conductive hearing impairment, one month after the surgery she returned to the clinic because she was hearing a loud roaring noise in the left ear. Figure 12.3 illustrates the audiogram obtained from this visit. Her left ear thresholds had deteriorated and her audiogram revealed a sensorineural hearing loss (note that the air and bone conduction thresholds are now in the same place) with very poor word recognition ability (20% correct) even when words were presented well above her thresholds for tones (95 dB HL). Because of the poor word recognition ability, she was no longer a candidate for amplification in this ear.[1] Amplification would make sounds audible but not very clear, possibly interfering with speech understanding in the good ear.

## SENSORINEURAL HEARING LOSS

The majority of hearing impairments in adulthood are sensorineural. A sensorineural hearing impairment occurs when there is damage to the inner ear, the nerve leading to the brainstem, or both (see Chapter 10). Prior to the now widespread use of imaging and electrophysiological techniques, cochlear damage was not easily differentiated from damage within the auditory nervous system. Therefore, all hearing impairments in which the audiogram does not exhibit an air-bone gap, signalling a conductive loss, are generally described as sensorineural (Northern & Downs, 2002). A sensorineural hearing loss usually means cochlear damage. The three most common conditions in adulthood that are associated with sensorineural hearing impairments due to cochlear processes are aging, noise exposure, and Ménière's disease. A less common cause is cochlear insult due to toxic influences (e.g., drug exposure). Additional problems may include tumors on the auditory nerve and diseases of the central nervous system. Pathology within the auditory nervous system, beyond the cochlea, is known as retrocochlear. Retro-

---

[1]Only 1 to 3 percent of stapedectomies result in sensorineural hearing loss.

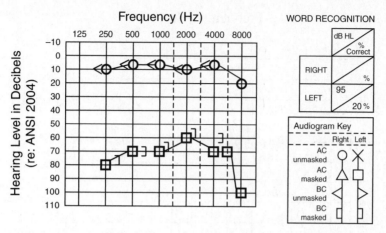

FIGURE 12.3   **Audiometric results after an unsuccessful stapedectomy that resulted in a moderate-to-severe sensorineural hearing loss in the left ear. Word recognition was also very poor.**

cochlear pathology generally does not affect pure-tone thresholds, unless the cause of the hearing loss also affects the cochlea. Individuals with damage to the central auditory nervous system find it difficult to understand speech, especially in difficult listening environments.

## Aging Process

The proportion of people with hearing loss increases with age. It is estimated that 43 percent of those with hearing loss are age 65 years or older (National Academy on an Aging Society, 1999). A decrease in hearing associated with the aging process is known as **presbycusis**. A lifetime of environmental noise exposure, disease processes, drug effects, and genetic predisposition to hearing impairment contribute to presbycusis. Although changes to the cochlea probably begin earlier in life, it is generally not until middle age that people begin to have difficulties understanding speech. Initial changes occur in the basal end of the cochlea, which is responsible for detecting high-frequency sounds (see Chapter 10). Because low-frequency hearing is relatively normal, individuals with early presbycusis typically report that they can hear people talk, but that they cannot understand what is being said. This is because consonants, which are composed of high-frequency, low-intensity sounds, are inaudible. These are most important for understanding spoken words. Figure 12.4 depicts the general frequency and intensity characteristics of four classes of speech sounds: nasals, vowels, stops, and fricatives (Olsen, Hawkings, & Van Tasell, 1987). Notice that stops and fricatives are high in frequency compared to nasals and vowels. Stops and fricatives, therefore, are easily missed by the person with a high-frequency hearing loss. Distinguishing place of articulation (e.g., distinguishing /b/ from /d/ from /g/) is also dependent on

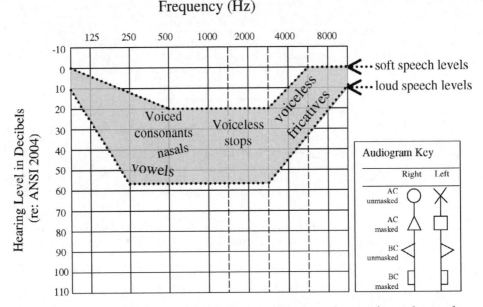

**FIGURE 12.4    The frequency and decibel levels of various classes of speech sounds.**

From Olsen, W., Hawkins, D., & Van Tasell, D. [1987]. Representations of the long term spectra of speech. *Ear and Hearing, 8(5)* 1000. Reprinted with permission of Lippincott Williams & Wilkins.

high-frequency cues. Without using speechreading or contextual cues, a person with a high-frequency hearing loss might report hearing "ben" for "den" or "gay" for "day" or "bay." Another common complaint of individuals with high-frequency hearing loss is the inability to understand speech in the presence of background noise, because it masks the weaker components of the speech signal (e.g., the high-frequency consonants and place-of-articulation cues). Rooms with reverberation (echoes) are also difficult listening environments for those with hearing impairment.

Typical thresholds for individuals of various ages are illustrated in Figure 12.5. Notice that hearing at high frequencies shows the most marked changes with age. However, in the oldest individuals, low-frequency sounds also become more difficult to detect. It is also the case that hearing thresholds decline at an earlier age and more quickly in men than women (Pearson et al., 1995). With advanced presbycusis, a loss of neurons in the central nervous system may accompany the changes within the cochlea, resulting in central presbycusis or a **central auditory processing disorder**. A sign of central presbycusis is **phonemic regression**. This refers to word recognition that is very poor and cannot be explained based on the amount of hearing loss for pure tones. A common report of individuals with central presbycusis is "I can hear fine but everyone mumbles."

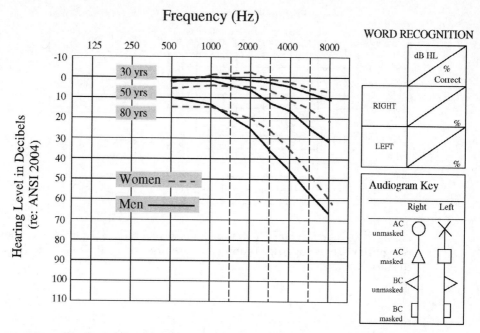

**FIGURE 12.5    Hearing thresholds at three ages. Note that thresholds at the higher frequencies show the most change with age. Adapted from Pearson et al., 1995.**

Central auditory processing disorders associated with the aging process may be difficult to distinguish from the cochlear damage that almost always accompanies aging.

> *Mr. Robinson*, age 70, came to the clinic to have his hearing evaluated. He was accompanied by his two daughters, who reported that their father was answering questions inappropriately and saying "huh" constantly. Although Mr. Robinson admitted that he had some difficulty hearing, he commented that his hearing "was not all that bad" and that he would be able to hear better if people "would speak more clearly." Figure 12.6 illustrates Mr. Robinson's audiogram. He has central presbycusis. He shows signs of a central auditory processing disorder along with the cochlear impairment. This is evident because his ability to understand words is poorer than expected based on his pure-tone audiogram. His word recognition ability was 28 percent in his left ear and 32 percent in his right ear when words were presented at a level well above his thresholds.

By way of comparison Mr. Robinson's ability to recognize words is much worse than that of a 44-year-old man with the same degree of hearing loss. This younger man, who was tested at the same clinic, had 80 percent word recognition ability. Stach, Spretnjak, and Jerger (1990) estimated that over 50 percent of those

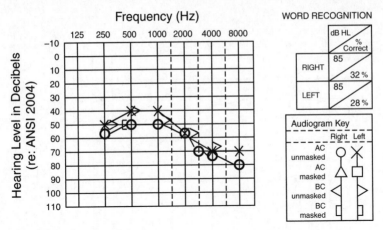

**FIGURE 12.6** **Audiogram illustrating a sensorineural hearing loss. The poor word recognition scores suggest a central auditory processing disorder in addition to cochlear damage.**

over 65 years of age will have a central auditory processing disorder. This population has more difficulty extracting speech from noise, understanding speech when reverberation is present, and benefitting from amplification devices than those with hearing impairment who do not have central auditory processing disorders.

The increased prevalence of central auditory processing disorders with increasing age is important to consider when working with the people over 65. As the baby boomer generation ages, there will be more elderly people living in retirement and nursing home facilities. It is estimated that, by the year 2030, the nursing home population will reach 3 million residents (Sahyoun, Pratt, Lentzner, Dey, & Robinson, 2001). Of these, nearly half are estimated to have a hearing impairment that interferes with communication (Schow & Nerbonne, 1980). Retirement and nursing homes impose particular demands on hearing. For elderly individuals with hearing loss, communication difficulties are likely to occur in areas such as meeting rooms, dining areas, and recreational rooms. In addition, communication impairments may adversely affect patient–staff relationships. Hearing-impaired residents may be labeled withdrawn, uncommunicative, or confused.

Hearing impairment can also be associated with poor performance on cognitive tests, especially if they are administered verbally. For example, Weinstein and Amsel (1986) gave a test of mental function to hearing-impaired patients. Patients were tested both with and without their hearing aids. Results indicated that, when amplification was used, 33 percent of patients were classified as less severely demented than they had been when tested without hearing aids.

Although some nursing home residents may have personal hearing aids, many aids are likely to be malfunctioning (Erber & Heine, 1996; Thibodeau &

Schmitt, 1988). In addition, few health care providers have received formal training in the management of patients with communication disorders. Because of the high prevalence of hearing loss in the elderly population, an audiologist might be employed to provide audiologic evaluation, fit hearing aids, and train staff members how to use strategies to enhance communication as well as how to troubleshoot hearing aids. These services are important to prevent social isolation due to hearing loss, which can dramatically decrease quality of life for those in nursing home facilities.

Many factors contribute to hearing impairment among the elderly. Each person's hearing capabilities and communicative contexts are unique, and therapies must be tailored to individual needs. Hearing rehabilitation for the elderly presents an exciting challenge for the audiologist.

## Noise Exposure

Many Americans are exposed to potentially hazardous noise levels in the workplace, at home, and during recreational activities. The National Institute on Deafness and Other Communication Disorders (1999) estimated that 30 million Americans are exposed to dangerously high sound levels on a regular basis. They also estimated that noise exposure contributed to about one-third of all hearing impairments reported. Noise exposure can cause a "threshold shift" initially observed around 4000 Hz. That is, hearing a tone in the 4000 Hz frequency region will be more difficult after noise exposure than before.

> *Mr. McGee*, age 52, has been employed in a manufacturing plant for twenty-five years. He also enjoys carpentry work and snowmobiling as recreational activities. He reported that he hears ringing in his ears (**tinnitus**) and that speech sounds are muffled. The audiologist employed by his company evaluated his hearing (see Figure 12.7) and compared the results to previous evaluations. She noted a threshold shift—that is, his hearing for the frequencies 3000, 4000, and 6000 Hz had become poorer since his previous tests.

Thresholds that are poor around 4000 Hz (4k Hz) and improve at 8000 Hz are known as the "4k notch" because of the dip that appears on the audiogram (see Figure 12.7). This threshold shift is due to damaged sensory cells in the cochlea, resulting in sensorineural hearing loss. Initially, the threshold shift may be temporary. After removing oneself from the high noise levels, thresholds may return to normal. This is known as a *temporary threshold shift*, or TTS. However, it is likely that some damage to the sensory cells has been done. Furthermore, with repeated exposures, or after exposure for a longer period of time, or with personal susceptibility to noise damage, recovery may not be complete. The result can be a *permanent threshold shift*, or PTS. Like those with presbycusis, individuals with noise-induced hearing loss have difficulty understanding speech in noisy environments and in rooms with high levels of reverberation.

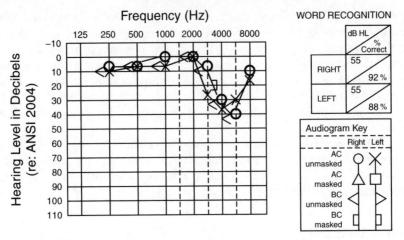

**FIGURE 12.7** **Audiogram illustrating a sensorineural hearing loss centered around the 4000 Hz region as a result of excessive noise exposure.**

Mr. McGee received a complete audiometric evaluation and was counseled about the harm that noise exposure causes, as well as the effects of his high-frequency hearing loss on communication ability. He was shown how to wear ear plugs appropriately, and instructed to limit his exposure to noise and wear hearing protectors at work as well as during recreational activities that involve high noise levels.

## Ménière's Disease

*Mrs. Hill*, age 55, experiences episodic attacks of vertigo, nausea, tinnitus, and a sensorineural hearing loss in the right ear that is more severe in the low frequencies than in the high frequencies. A feeling of pressure in her right ear often precedes the attacks. The most distressing symptom for her is the vertigo that comes on suddenly with little warning. Because of the unpredictability of these attacks and the embarrassment she feels, Mrs. Hill is no longer employed and has stopped socializing with friends. She was diagnosed with **Ménière's disease** ten years ago. The hearing loss has become slightly worse over the last five years. Figure 12.8 displays her audiogram.

Between 3 and 5 million people in the United States suffer from Ménière's disease (National Institute on Deafness and Other Communication Disorders, 1998). Although the exact cause of Ménière's disease is unknown, it is thought to be due to an excess buildup of inner ear fluid called *endolymph*. Ménière's disease fluctuates and is often unilateral. One-third of those with the disease will develop it in both ears. It is common for the first episode to occur from early to mid-adulthood. As the disease progresses, the low-frequency hearing loss becomes more severe and permanent. The role of the audiologist with this population is to provide information about the disease and the available audiologic rehabilitation methods. Amplification may be necessary depending on the nature and degree of

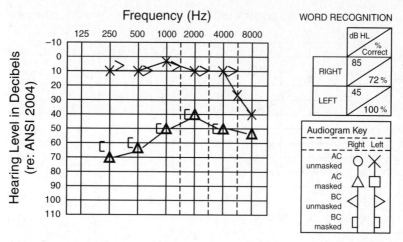

**FIGURE 12.8    Audiogram illustrating a right sensorineural hearing loss due to Ménière's disease.**

hearing impairment. Noise maskers may also be necessary to help the patient with Ménière's disease become less aware of the tinnitus.

Sensorineural hearing impairments associated with the aging process, noise exposure, and Ménière's disease are the most prevalent causes of hearing impairments in the adult population. There are a variety of other less frequent causes as well. The audiologist must know how to differentiate among these causes of hearing loss. Some examples follow.

## Ototoxicity

**Ototoxicity** results when certain drugs damage the inner ear, resulting in sensorineural hearing loss. The damage is usually in the high frequencies and can be reversible or permanent. Ototoxic drugs are often used for treatment of life-threatening medical conditions. The audiologist's role is to obtain periodic audiograms prior to, during, and after drug therapy. For those individuals who develop hearing loss, the audiologist provides rehabilitation services that may consist of providing amplification, support, and encouragement. Education about hearing conservation is also important, because individuals on drug therapies may be more susceptible to noise damage than those not receiving such therapies.

## Acoustic Neuroma

*Ms. Parker*, age 56, came to the ENT clinic because she was having pain on the left side of her face, tinnitus in the left ear, and dizziness. Her audiogram (Figure 12.9) revealed a sloping, mild-to-moderate sensorineural hearing loss in the left ear and mild high-frequency sensorineural hearing loss in the right ear. Her word recognition was excellent in the right ear when words were presented at normal and loud

**FIGURE 12.9** **Audiogram illustrating a left sensorineural hearing loss associated with an acoustic neuroma. Note that the word recognition score for the left ear (seen at upper right) decreased when words were presented at 90 dB HL compared to 70 dB HL (rollover).**

conversational levels (50 and 90 dB HL, respectively). Left ear results revealed good word recognition at 70 dB HL but poor recognition when words were presented at 90 dB HL.

This dramatic decrease in word recognition as the presentation level of the words is increased is known as **rollover** and is often associated with pathology in the auditory nervous system.

The audiologist evaluated Ms. Parker using the auditory brainstem response (ABR) test (see Chapter 11). Four electrodes were placed on the surface of her scalp, and clicking sounds were presented to each ear. The electrodes detected the brain's electrical activity that occurred in response to the clicks. Samples of the electrical activity that occurred after each click were recorded and processed with a computer.

An ABR typically includes, several positive peaks of electrical activity that normally occur within milliseconds following each click. Delayed electrical peaks, in the absence of a conductive hearing loss, or delayed intervals between peaks are a strong indication that the pathology is located in the neural pathways of the auditory system (see Chapter 10).

Ms. Parker's ABR results are shown in Figure 12.10. The peaks for waves III and V for the left ear were at 5.16 ms and 7.44 ms, respectively. These were much longer than the latencies for waves III and V for the right ear (4.64 ms and 6.72 ms, respectively). Ms. Parker subsequently had an MRI of the internal auditory canal (the bony canal that extends from each cochlear nucleus to its corresponding cochlea), and an **acoustic neuroma** (tumor) on the auditory nerve was confirmed. The tumor was surgically removed, but the surgery, unfortunately, left Ms. Parker with no measurable hearing in the left ear. Ms. Parker, being active in her vocation and community, found that the unilateral hearing loss restricted her participation in everyday activities. As is common with unilateral hearing loss, she had difficulties localizing sounds, understanding speakers positioned on the side of the poorer ear, and understanding speech in noise. The audiologist fit her with a hearing aid that placed a microphone at the unusable left ear and a receiver on the good right ear. The microphone picked up the signal reaching the impaired ear and sent it to the good ear to allow sound detection.

A hearing aid arrangement in which a microphone placed behind an unaidable ear sends the signal to the good ear is known as *contralateral routing of signals*, or a CROS hearing aid. Wearing a CROS hearing aid makes it easier for the individual with a unilateral hearing impairment to hear sounds directed to the impaired ear. It also restores a sense of sound balance and an improvement in the signal-to-noise ratio when the signal is on the side of the poorer ear.

| | Latencies | | |
|---|---|---|---|
| I | 2.60 | I | 2.56 |
| III | 5.16 | III | 4.64 |
| V | 7.44 | V | 6.72 |
| I-III | 2.56 | I-III | 2.08 |
| III-V | 2.28 | III-V | 2.08 |
| I-V | 4.84 | I-V | 4.16 |

**FIGURE 12.10** The auditory brainstem response of a patient with a left acoustic neuroma. When clicks were presented to the left ear, waves III and V were abnormally delayed compared to the waves associated with right ear click stimulation.

Although acoustic neuromas only affect 1 out of 100,000 people, if undetected this condition can result in death due to pressure on brainstem structures from tumor growth. If detected early and surgically removed, hearing may be preserved. Therefore, patients experiencing unilateral hearing loss or unilateral tinnitus should be tested to determine if an acoustic neuroma is the cause of their symptoms.

### Diseases of the Central Auditory System

Audiologists may also evaluate and participate in the rehabilitation of patients who have lesions to the brain or brainstem that affect hearing (see Chapter 10 for a discussion of the central auditory pathways). Such disorders include multiple sclerosis, strokes, and cortical and brainstem tumors. A lesion of the brain can disturb the blood supply to the cochlea, resulting in damage to the hair cells and a reduced ability to hear pure tones. However, most often a central auditory disorder will cause difficulties with speech processing without affecting pure-tone hearing sensitivity. Individuals with central auditory lesions report difficulties listening in background noise, with reverberation, if visual cues are not available, and when speech is spoken at a rapid rate. An elderly person with a central auditory lesion will likely have some difficulty hearing pure tones due to the effects of aging on the cochlea.

## MIXED HEARING LOSS

Finally, a hearing loss that has both conductive and sensorineural components is known as a *mixed hearing loss*.

> *Mrs. Leon*, age 84, reported a sudden decrease in her hearing. Her family, who accompanied her to the evaluation, reported that for many years she had some difficulties understanding speech and had to turn the television to higher-than-normal loudness levels in order to hear most programs. Recently, her neighbors had complained about the loud noise coming from her apartment. Mrs. Leon reported a sudden hearing loss coincident with a cold that she developed approximately two months prior. She expressed much concern about her deteriorating hearing ability, as it was a sign of "getting old" and "one more thing going wrong."
>
> Mrs. Leon's audiometric results are displayed in Figure 12.11. The audiogram showed that she had a mixed hearing loss. Notice the 30 to 40 dB air-bone gap, which reflects a mild-to-moderate 30 to 50 dB sensorineural hearing loss (thresholds for bone conduction range from 30 to 50 dB HL) with an added conductive component. The conductive component of her hearing impairment was due to bilateral middle ear infection (otitis media, see Chapter 11). The sensorineural component was diagnosed as presbycusis. Pressure equalization tubes were placed in her ears by an ENT specialist. After medical intervention, the audiologist recommended hearing aids and assisted her in the rehabilitation process. Mrs. Leon adapted quite well to her new hearing aids and showed a renewed interest in communicating with her family and friends. Comforted by the knowledge that she was not rapidly going deaf, and assisted with amplification, she was better able to participate in community functions and religious services.

**FIGURE 12.11** **Audiogram illustrating a mixed hearing loss due to otitis media (which caused the conductive component) and presbycusis (which caused the sensorineural component).**

## PSYCHOSOCIAL IMPACT OF HEARING LOSS

Ramsdell (1960) distinguished three psychological levels of hearing: primitive level or the auditory background of daily living, signal/warning level, and symbolic or social level. Any or all of these levels can be affected by a hearing impairment. For example, an individual with a sudden and total hearing loss will have difficulties at all three levels. In contrast, a person with a mild hearing loss still feels connected to the world (still hears background noises) and is able to hear warning signals. However, the social level of hearing may be affected by a mild hearing loss if it impacts communication. When this happens, emotional difficulties can also arise.

> *Mr. Cohen*, a 42-year-old salesman, experienced a sudden, severe, and bilateral sensorineural hearing loss. Mr. Cohen had provided the sole financial support for his family that included three children. Because of the severity of the loss and the communication demands that his job required, he had to quit his job. His wife became employed, and Mr. Cohen became more responsible for daily activities in the home. He often declined social invitations because he tired easily when trying to participate in the conversations. He relied on his wife to interpret for him and often pretended to understand what people were saying.

A hearing impairment also impacts the family and significant others. Often a hearing-impaired individual is seen in the clinic at the urging of a spouse or partner. Family members may become frustrated at continually repeating and interpreting for the individual with a hearing loss. The extra effort required to include the hearing-impaired individual in conversations and spectator activities such as plays, movies, and lectures can put stress on family relationships and result in exclusion of the hearing-impaired person. It is not uncommon to hear an elderly person with hearing loss say, "If I don't do something about my hearing, my spouse will leave me." Even said in jest, the statement reflects the seriousness of communication breakdown and its impact on relationships. Likewise, hearing impairment can interfere with activities of daily living. Communicating on the telephone and asking a passerby for directions are just two examples of the many activities that may become more difficult with hearing impairment.

The audiologist must be knowledgeable and competent in assessing the effects of hearing loss on functional communication, including how it influences the psychosocial, educational, and occupational well-being of the client (ASHA, 2002). Training the hearing-impaired individual and significant others to use effective communication strategies and offering counseling for those adjusting to hearing loss are two very important services that an audiologist provides.

## AUDIOLOGICAL EVALUATION

### Hearing Screenings

The audiologist may screen for hearing loss or oversee such a screening program. The purpose of screening is to identify individuals who have a high probability of having a hearing loss (those who fail the screening) so that they can be referred for appropriate diagnostic testing (ASHA, 1995). ASHA recommends that adults be screened at least every ten years through age 50 and then at three-year intervals after that. Common settings for screenings include health fairs and medical facilities. High-noise industries are particularly important sites for screening because noise damage to the cochlea can be prevented. Nursing homes are also important screening sites because of the high prevalence of hearing impairments in the elderly population. In these high-risk environments, screenings are needed on a regular basis (see Figure 12.12).

Hearing screenings consist of presenting pure tones at a predetermined level. The American Speech-Language-Hearing Association (1997) recommends that, if an individual responds to pure-tone air conducted stimuli at 25 dB HL at 1000, 2000, and 4000 Hz in both ears, then he or she passes the screening. If no response is obtained at one or more frequencies in *either* ear, then the individual fails the screening. The 25 dB HL level was recommended because even mild hearing loss can negatively influence a person's health and well-being.

In addition to pure-tone screening, a hearing disability index should be used to identify individuals who perceive themselves as having a disability (ASHA, 1997). Self-assessment measures gauge the client's perceptions by asking them to rate the degree to which their hearing loss interferes with their daily activities or social interactions. Use of a measure that asks clients to report on activities that involve hearing (e.g., Ventry & Weinstein, 1982) can help identify those individuals who believe that they have a disability. These individuals will be most motivated to attempt rehabilitation and actively utilize strategies for improved communication. Individuals who fail the pure-tone screening and report problems with hear-

**FIGURE 12.12** **The hearing of an adult is screened using a portable audiometer.**

ing in their daily lives should be counseled regarding hearing impairment and the need for a referral for a complete hearing assessment.

## Hearing Assessment

A second task of the audiologist is to assess a client's hearing status. A complete audiologic evaluation will determine the need for medical referral, additional audiologic follow-up, or both. The test results will assist the physician in diagnosing and treating the patient. A complete evaluation also provides the basis for a rehabilitation plan.

The audiologic evaluation begins with a case history. The audiologist obtains information about the hearing difficulties that the person is experiencing, family history of hearing loss, medical history, and previous experience with hearing aids. Next, the audiologist examines the patient's external ears with a handheld **otoscope** or **video otoscopy**. With video otoscopy, enlarged images of the tympanic membrane and ear canal can be projected on a video monitor (see Figure 12.13). A photoprint of these structures can be made to document pathology and medical treatment outcomes. If excessive *cerumen* (wax) is observed in the ear canal, it must be removed prior to testing. Cerumen removal can be performed by an audiologist with specialized training or by appropriate medical personnel. Audiologic testing is performed to determine if a hearing impairment exists, the type of impairment (conductive, sensorineural, or mixed), and the severity of the impairment for various frequencies and for speech. We can examine the stages of the audiologic evaluation by following the case of Mr. Peterson.

**FIGURE 12.13    An audiologist uses visual otoscopy to examine the ear canal and tympanic membrane.**

*Mr. Peterson* came to the clinic because he was having difficulties hearing his coworkers. He reported more difficulty hearing from his right ear than his left ear. After a case history was obtained and an otoscopic examination revealed the ear canals to be free of cerumen, immittance measures were obtained (see Chapter 11 for a discussion of immittance). Next, Mr. Peterson was seated inside a sound-treated booth, and miniature earphones were inserted in his ear canals. The audiologist tested the hearing of each ear individually using an audiometer. The test began with the audiologist saying two-syllable words (such as "cowboy" and "arm-chair") to Mr. Peterson, who was not allowed to "lip read" by watching the audiologist's face. The lowest level at which Mr. Peterson was able to repeat the two-syllable words 50 percent of the time was recorded for each ear. These were his speech reception thresholds (SRTs). Next, the pure-tone air conduction and bone conduction thresholds were obtained. Finally, word recognition ability was assessed. Single-syllable words were presented at normal and loud conversational levels, and the audiologist recorded the percent of words Mr. Peterson repeated correctly.

Audiologists also test adults who are not able to respond verbally to the test stimuli, such as adults with developmental disabilities, severe head injury, or stroke. Written or picture-pointing responses can be used during word recognition testing. *Otoacoustic emissions* (see Chapter 10) also can be used to screen for hearing loss in difficult-to-test adults, because such tests do not require a volitional response. If a person fails the screening, then an auditory brainstem response threshold search can be obtained.

### Assessing Participation Restrictions

For those hearing impairments that are not medically correctable, the audiologist has the task of developing and implementing a rehabilitation plan in conjunction with the patient. Results from the audiologic evaluation are combined with information about the individual's daily life in order to formulate an appropriate plan. Some individuals may be homebound, with few visitors; others are involved actively with work or social activities. There are a variety of potential communicative needs, and the difficulties each person may perceive may be greater or less than what the audiogram might suggest (Matthews, Lee, Mills, & Schum, 1990; Weinstein & Ventry, 1983). For that reason, self-assessment tools have been used to gauge functional communication.

The audiologist must understand the individual's hearing abilities as they relate to communication demands. An understanding of each patient's hearing and his or her communication needs will assist the audiologist in jointly developing rehabilitation goals with the patient and the patient's family.

## MANAGEMENT STRATEGIES

According to ASHA (2002), "Audiologic/aural rehabilitation (AR) is an ecological, interactive process that facilitates one's ability to minimize or prevent the limitations and restrictions that auditory dysfunctions can impose on well-being and communication, including interpersonal, psychosocial, educational, and vocational functioning" (p. 90). The audiologist achieves these goals with a variety of methods. One of the most important goals of rehabilitation is to facilitate accurate understanding of speech. This may involve the use of hearing aids.

### Hearing Aids

Hearing aids are electronic devices that amplify sound. To provide maximum benefit to an individual client, they must be selected and fit appropriately. ASHA (1998) defined several stages in the hearing aid selection and fitting process, including *assessment, selection and fitting, verification, orientation,* and *validation.* By completing each of these stages carefully, the audiologist increases the likelihood that clients will not only receive amplification that is appropriate for them but also will use it successfully. Hearing aids come in various styles (Figure 12.14). The ear-

**FIGURE 12.14  Types of hearing aids. From left to right, top to bottom: body (A), behind-the-ear (B), in-the-ear (C), in-the-canal (D), and completely-in-the-canal (E).**

level hearing aids are the most commonly dispensed devices and include the behind-the-ear, in-the-ear, in-the-canal, and completely-in-the-canal styles. Special fittings, such as the CROS aid described earlier for Ms. Parker, are also available.

All hearing aids, no matter the style, have the same basic components: a microphone for sound input and conversion to an electrical signal, an amplifier to increase the level of sound, a receiver to convert the electrical signal to an acoustic signal, and a battery to power the device. The circuitry of a hearing aid, or how it processes the electrical signal, may vary across instruments. Many hearing aids in today's market are digital rather than analog. This means that the hearing aid uses a computer chip and special mathematical algorithms to manipulate the incoming signal after it is converted to a series of digits. The digital signal is tailored to the individual's audiometric configuration. For example, if a client has a hearing loss in the high frequencies only, then the hearing aid would produce more amplification in the high-frequency range and little if any amplification in the lower frequencies.

Decisions concerning the circuitry of the hearing aid are determined primarily by *assessment* of the degree of the hearing loss. Hearing aid *selection* depends on both the nature of the hearing impairment and the client's preferences and lifestyle. For example, the behind-the-ear hearing aid has the most flexibility for fitting any magnitude of hearing loss, but may not be accepted by a client as readily as a smaller style such as a completely-in-the-canal aid. However, this smaller hearing aid cannot compensate for more severe hearing losses and is difficult for many elderly clients to insert and remove. For clients with binaural hearing loss, the use of two hearing aids (binaural amplification) is generally recommended because of the advantages for localizing sound and for understanding speech in background noise. Guidance and counseling are important to help each client to understand the advantages and disadvantages of each style so that an appropriate selection may be made. The advanced technology now available in hearing aids makes them more flexible; however, many of the limitations of using amplification for an individual with a sensorineural hearing loss remain. Two of these limitations include distortion of the signal and intolerance for loud sounds. Having realistic expectations improves satisfaction with a hearing aid.

Hearing aids are custom-fitted to the client's ear. After *fitting* the hearing aid, the audiologist must *verify* the fitting to assure that it is correct and appropriate for the client. One way is to insert a small probe microphone in the ear canal, near the tympanic membrane. The microphone measures the characteristics of sounds near the plane of the eardrum. These recordings are referred to as *real ear* or *probe microphone measurements*. Sounds of various frequencies are presented through a loudspeaker while the probe microphone measures the sound pressure level with the hearing aid in the ear and turned on (aided condition) and without the hearing aid in the ear (unaided condition). The difference in sound pressure level between the aided and unaided conditions tells the audiologist how much gain the hearing aid provides at different frequencies. Because probe microphone measurements require no response from the patient, they are reliable and can be used to verify hearing aid fittings even with a difficult-to-test patient. Although this is the preferred verification method, other means of verification are available if real ear measurements cannot be made.

During the *orientation* stage, the patient is instructed in the use and care of the hearing aids. Following the orientation, the patient is usually given a trial period with the devices during which time any problems with the fitting may be resolved. Let us examine this aspect of the rehabilitation process by following Mrs. Leon, the woman who received pressure equalization tubes to correct the conductive component of a mixed hearing impairment (see Figure 12.11 for a review of Mrs. Leon's audiogram).

> Written and oral instructions were provided to Mrs. Leon and her family regarding her hearing aids. A gradual listening program was recommended. Mrs. Leon was instructed to wear the hearing aids initially in quiet environments such as when watching television or having a conversation with one or two people. After she became comfortable using the hearing aids in quiet, she was instructed to wear them in noisier environments. Listening activities were also recommended. Mrs. Leon was instructed to make a list of common, everyday background sounds in her environment (e.g., water running, the refrigerator humming) and to listen to these sounds while wearing the hearing aids. She was informed that these exercises

would assist her in relearning how to tune out or ignore the background noises that she may not have heard for quite some time due to her hearing loss.

A needs assessment tool was administered to her both before and after a trial use period with her hearing aids. She indicated that she wanted to hear the minister in her church during the Sunday sermon. The needs assessment revealed that the hearing aids had achieved this goal for her, thus validating one aspect of the fitting.

Although hearing aids are the most common form of treatment for sensorineural hearing impairment, only 6.35 million people own them, while 22.3 million individuals with hearing impairments do not (Kochkin, 2001). The low percentage of hearing aid users is likely due to denial, embarrassment, or a belief that a hearing aid will not help. The statistics are unfortunate given the research that shows hearing aid use to be associated with improvements in social, emotional, psychological, and physical well-being (National Council on the Aging, 1999). These improvements in the quality of life are found not only for those with severe hearing loss but for those with mild loss as well.

Technological advances as well as skillful counseling are likely to increase the number of adults who become successful hearing aid users. Two of the strongest predictors of hearing aid success are a patient's motivation and his or her perception of handicap. An individual who purchases a hearing aid because he or she is missing out on conversations during social interactions is much more likely to make a successful adjustment than is a person who has stopped socializing and purchases a hearing aid because of family pressure. Presbycusic listeners with severe central auditory processing disorders are also less likely to benefit from wearing hearing aids.

## Assistive Listening and Alerting Devices

An **assistive listening device** is any device, excluding hearing aids, designed to improve a hearing-impaired individual's ability to communicate and therefore function more independently than without the device. Closed captioning of television broadcasts is one example of an assistive device that can be used in the home. A **closed caption decoder** displays the television dialogue in written form at the bottom of the television screen. Many public venues, such as theaters and meeting halls, are equipped with frequency-modulated or **FM systems**. These systems use radio waves to send signals such as a speaker's voice or a movie sound track to a listener equipped with a receiver and earphones or a hearing aid with an FM connection. Because an FM system is wireless, the hearing-impaired individual and the talker are able to move around freely within the listening environment. Other types of assistive listening devices are designed for one-on-one communication. For example, a simple amplified handset is often sufficient to allow the hearing-impaired individual to communicate over the telephone. For more profound hearing losses, the telephone message can be typed by a relay operator and transmitted to a special **telecommunication device for the deaf (TDD)** for the hearing-impaired individual to read.

In addition to assistive listening devices, **alerting devices** are also available for the hearing-impaired individual. These include devices that provide a visual signal for common environmental sounds (e.g., the ringing of a phone or a doorbell). Vibrotactile devices, such as an alarm clock that vibrates the pillow, are also available. Alerting devices can be used to indicate dangerous situations (e.g., the sounding of a smoke alarm). Finally, hearing-ear dogs are also trained to help alert their owners to auditory signals.

Not all hearing-impaired persons come to the audiologist's office with the intent to purchase hearing aids or assistive listening and alerting devices. Mrs. Lough is an example of a client who continued to deny that she had a hearing problem and had no intention of trying amplification.

> *Mrs. Lough* came in for testing urged by her husband, who was having difficulty communicating with her. He reported that when she does not hear him (which is most of the time), he raises his voice, and then Mrs. Lough gets angry because she feels like he is yelling at her. Mrs. Lough's first comment to the audiologist was "I hope you're not going to fit me with hearing aids because I don't want them." She had tried hearing aids twice previously at other clinics and was very dissatisfied with them. The hearing evaluation was performed, and as Figure 12.15 indicates, Mrs. Lough had a moderate sensorineural hearing loss in both ears. Her word recognition ability was fair at a high presentation level. Once the testing was completed, the audiologist used a handheld amplifier to describe the hearing impairment and its implications for understanding speech. Oral and written information was provided to Mrs. Lough and her husband about hearing aids (what hearing aids could and could not do) and strategies that could facilitate the communication process. Assistive listening devices (ALDs) were also discussed as an alternative to hearing aids. Mrs. Lough was resistant to purchasing any type of amplification including ALDs.

**FIGURE 12.15** **Audiogram of a moderate sensorineural hearing loss with fair word recognition ability. Although amplification would make more speech sounds audible to this client, she refused to try it.**

Unfortunately, sometimes counseling cannot undo the negative impact of bad experiences with prior amplification or poor motivation to communicate more effectively. To benefit from amplification, a patient must accept the hearing loss and be ready to work with the audiologist to improve his or her communication abilities.

## Cochlear Implants

For those with severe to profound hearing loss who do not benefit substantially from amplification, cochlear implants might be recommended. To date, the cochlear implant has been more successful in adults with acquired hearing loss than with adults who have been deaf since childhood. As we saw in Chapter 11, the implant consists of multiple electrodes surgically placed within the cochlea. The electrodes conduct electrical current that directly stimulates auditory nerve fibers to produce hearing sensations. Audiologists play an important role in education and counseling of potential candidates for cochlear implants. Although inserted into the cochlea by a surgeon, the audiologist activates and maps the implant approximately four weeks after surgery. Mapping involves determining the appropriate levels of electrical stimulation for each electrode. The audiologist also participates in the follow-up and long-term rehabilitation plan that involves teaching the client to use available auditory cues in conjunction with speechreading.

## Auditory Training and Speechreading

Historically, **auditory training** and speechreading were used to teach children who were deafened before or shortly after birth to understand speech. However, these techniques may be useful for adults who use amplification but still have difficulty understanding speech. Auditory training involves teaching the individual to optimize use of available sound cues. Several approaches to auditory training exist. These range from drill on sound sequences (e.g., /ba/ vs. /da/) to teaching strategies that capitalize on knowledge of the topic of conversation to assist speech comprehension.

The short- and long-term effects of auditory training on speech perception in those with acquired hearing loss are not known. However, there is indirect evidence that auditory training in individuals learning a second language can facilitate speech discrimination (Logan, Lively, & Pisoni, 1991) and even effect changes in the central auditory nervous system (Kraus, McGee, Carrell, King, & Tremblay, 1995; Tremblay, Kraus, Carrell, & McGee, 1997).

Adding visual information to auditory speech signals improves identification relative to auditory input alone (Hardison, 1998). **Speechreading** is a technique that capitalizes on this improvement. In face-to-face communication, listeners can improve their ability to understand speech considerably by watching the speaker's mouth as words are formed (Sumby & Pollack, 1954). Attending to the speaker's face provides information about the place of articulation (see Chapter 3). This provides a significant benefit because the acoustic cues are most severely affected by background noise and high-frequency hearing loss.

The ability to speechread varies widely across individuals. However, there are some factors that can increase the likelihood of success (see also Montgomery, 1993, for suggestions to maximize speechreading in combination with amplification). Training in speechreading might include strategies such as making sure that a speaker's face is visible and well lit so that mouth movements can be seen. A client also learns to focus on understanding phrases and ideas, rather than phonemes and words.

## Counseling and Communication Strategies

The audiologist provides critical information to the client and significant others. Individuals must understand the nature of their hearing impairment and its implications for day-to-day life. Furthermore, it is important for hearing-impaired individuals and their significant others to understand the limits of available technologies and rehabilitative methods. For example, the client should understand that hearing aids will not restore normal hearing. Strategies to improve the communication process are also discussed with the patient and family members. Kaplan (1988) listed several strategies that can be used by both the hearing-impaired person and the person speaking. For example, the client with a hearing loss may be advised to ask a speaker to repeat or rephrase a statement that was not understood. Hearing-impaired individuals are also counseled to read reviews prior to seeing a movie to better follow the plot. Significant others might be advised to face the client when speaking and not to talk to the client from other rooms.

In addition to informational counseling, the audiologist must be sensitive to how an individual reacts to his or her hearing impairment and to any psychosocial adjustment problems related to the impairment. Tanner (1980) provided an excellent article about loss related to communication disorders and Kübler-Ross's (1969) five stages of the grieving process (i.e., denial, anger, bargaining, depression, acceptance). It is important to keep in mind that an individual may not only be grieving the loss of hearing but also the loss of independence, vocation, and group or self-identity. Hard-of-hearing support groups offer an excellent opportunity for those with hearing impairments to share their experiences and feelings with others experiencing similar problems.

## Support Groups

Members of national and local support groups work together to improve communication and teach self-management skills. Information about hearing impairment is often provided at support group meetings, as are discussions about communication problems and solutions. The meetings provide an opportunity for the hearing-impaired individual to practice assertive communication strategies in a nonthreatening environment. The groups also offer opportunities for members to be proactive in political issues related to the civil rights of those with a hearing loss. For example, members of Self-Help for the Hard of Hearing (SHHH) were actively involved in developing regulations for section 255 of the Telecommunications Act of 1996. This section requires telecommunication products and services to be accessible to people with disabilities. The group was also instrumental in developing regulations for the Americans with Disabilities Act (ADA) of 1990. The ADA was designed to ensure that those with disabilities (including hearing loss) are not discriminated against in employment, public accommodations, transportation, state and local government services, and telecommunications.

## CLINICAL PROBLEM SOLVING

Mr. Westrich, age 76, reported that he has difficulty understanding his wife and grandchildren when they talk. He also has difficulty understanding speakers on television. He suggested that "all newscasters must go to the same school of mumbling." At family gatherings, he relies on his wife to repeat what people have said and often gets left out of conversations. He was a pilot in the military for thirty years and enjoyed hunting before he retired. Figure 12.16 displays his audiogram and word-recognition ability.

1. What type of hearing loss does Mr. Westrich have?
2. What factors are likely to have contributed to Mr. Westrich's hearing loss?

**FIGURE 12.16   Audiogram of a client who came to the clinic because of difficulties communicating with his family.**

3. What class(es) of speech sounds will Mr. Westrich have most difficulty hearing?
4. Is Mr. Westrich a candidate for amplification? Why or why not?
5. What types of communication strategies might Mr. Westrich use when communicating? What might the speaker do to facilitate Mr. Westrich's speech understanding?

## REFERENCES

American National Standards Institute. (2004). *Specifications for audiometers* (ANSI S3.6-R2004). New York: Author.

American Speech-Language-Hearing Association (ASHA). (1995, February). Report on audiological screening. *American Journal of Audiology, 4.* 24–40.

American Speech-Language-Hearing Association (ASHA). (1997). *Guidelines for audiologic screening* (pp. 49–59). Rockville, MD: Author.

American Speech-Language-Hearing Association (ASHA 1998). Guidelines for hearing aid fitting for adults. *American Journal of Audiology, 7,* 5–13.

American Speech-Language-Hearing Association (ASHA). (2002). *Knowledge and skills required for the practice of audiologic/aural rehabilitation.* Rockville, MD: Author.

Americans With Disabilities Act of 1990, Pub. L. No. 101–336, §2, 104 Stat. 328 (1991).

Balloh, R. W. (1998). *Dizziness, hearing loss, and tinnitus.* Philadelphia: FA Davis.

Erber, N. P., & Heine, C. (1996). Screening receptive communication of older adults in residential care. *American Journal of Audiology, 5,* 38–46.

Giolas, T. G. (1994). Aural rehabilitation of adults with hearing impairment. In J. Katz (Ed.), *Handbook of clinical audiology* (pp. 776–789). Baltimore: Williams & Wilkins.

Hardison, D. M. (1998). Acquisition of second-language speech: Effects of visual cues, context and talker variability (Doctoral dissertation, Indiana University, 1998). *Dissertation Abstracts International, 59*(5-A), Z5053.

Kaplan, H. (1988). Communication problems of the hearing-impaired elderly: What can be done? *Pride Institute Journal of Long Term Home Health Care, 7,* 10–22.

Kochkin, S. (2001). The VA and direct mail sales spark growth in hearing aid market. *The Hearing Review, 8,* 16–24.

Kraus, N., McGee, T., Carrell, T. D., King, C., & Tremblay, K. (1995). Central auditory system plasticity associated with speech discrimination training. *Journal of Cognitive Neuroscience, 7,* 25–32.

Kübler-Ross, E. (1969). *On death and dying.* New York: Macmillan.

Logan, J. S., Lively, S. E., & Pisoni, D. B. (1991). Training Japanese listeners to identify /r/ and /l/: A first report. *Journal of the Acoustical Society of America, 89,* 874–886.

Matthews, L. J., Lee, F., Mills, J. H., & Schum, D. J. (1990). Audiometric and subjective assessment of hearing handicap. *Archives of Otolaryngology—Head and Neck Surgery, 116,* 1325–1330.

Montgomery, A. A. (1993). Management of the hearing-impaired adult, In J. Alpiner & P. McCarthy (Eds.), *Rehabilitative audiology: Children and adults* (pp. 311–330). Baltimore: Williams & Wilkins.

Mueller, H., & Killion, M. (1990). An easy method for calculating the articulation index. *Hearing Journal, 3,* 14–17.

National Academy on an Aging Society. (1999). Hearing loss: A growing problem that affects quality of life. Retrieved 3/23/07 from http://www.agingsociety.org/profiles.htm

National Council on the Aging. (1999). *The consequences of untreated hearing loss in older persons*. Conducted by the Seniors Research Group. Retrieved 3/23/07 from http://www.ncoa.org/ news/hearing/01_intro.htm

National Institute on Deafness and Other Communication Disorders. (1998, July). *Because you asked about Ménière's disease*. Retrieved 3/23/07 from http://www.nidcd.nih.gov/health/pubs_ hb/meniere.htm.

National Institute on Deafness and Other Communication Disorders. (1999, April). *Noise-induced hearing loss* (NIH Pub. No. 97-4233). Retrieved 3/23/07 from http://www.nidcd.nih.gov/health/pubs_hb/noise.htm#who

Northern, J. L., & Downs, M. P. (2002). *Hearing in children* (5th ed.). Baltimore: Lippincott Williams & Wilkins.

Olsen, W., Hawkins, D., & Van Tasell, D. (1987). Representations of the long-term spectra of speech. *Ear and Hearing, 8*(5), 1003–1085.

Pearson, J. D., Morrell, C. H., Gordon-Salant, S., Brant, L. J., Metter, E. J., Klein, L. L., & Fozard, J. L. (1995). Gender differences in a longitudinal study of age-associated hearing loss. *Journal of the Acoustical Society of America, 97*, 1196–1205.

Ramsdell, D. (1960). The psychology of the hard of hearing and deafened adult. In H. Davis & S. Silverman (Eds.), *Hearing and deafness*. New York: Holt, Rinehart & Winston.

Sahyoun, N. R., Pratt, L. A., Lentzner, H., Dey, A., & Robinson, K. N. (2001). *The changing profile of nursing home residents: 1985–1997*. Aging Trends, No. 4. Hyattsville, MD: National Center for Health Statistics. Retrieved 3/23/07 from http://www.cdc.gov/nchs/data/agingtrends/04nursin.pdf

Schow, R., & Nerbonne, M. (1980). Hearing level in nursing home residents. *Journal of Speech and Hearing Disorders, 45*, 124–132.

Stach, B. A., Spretnjak, M. L., & Jerger, J. (1990). The prevalence of central presbycusis in a clinical population. *Journal of the American Academy of Audiology, 1*, 109–115.

Sumby, W. G., & Pollack, I. (1954). Visual contributions to speech intelligibility in noise. *Journal of the Acoustical Society of America, 26*, 212–215.

Tanner, D. (1980). Loss and grief: Implications for the speech-language pathologist and audiologist. *Asha, 22*, 916–928.

Thibodeau, L. M., & Schmitt, J. (1988). A report on condition of hearing aids in nursing homes and retirement centers. *Journal of the American Academy of Audiology, 21*, 99–112.

Tremblay, K., Kraus, N., Carrell, T. D., & McGee, T. (1997). Central auditory system plasticity: Generalization to novel stimuli following listening training. *Journal of the Acoustical Society of America, 102*, 3762–3773.

Ventry, I., & Weinstein, B. (1982). Identification of elderly people with hearing problems. *Ear and Hearing, 3*, 128–134.

Weinstein, B. E., & Amsel, L. (1986). Hearing loss and senile dementia in the institutionalized elderly. *Clinical Gerontology, 4*, 3–15.

Weinstein, B. E., & Ventry, I. M. (1983). Audiometric correlates of hearing handicapped inventory for the elderly. *Journal of Speech and Hearing Disorders, 48*, 379–384.

World Health Organization (WHO). (2001, November). WHO publishes new guidelines to measure health. Retrieved 3/23/07 from http://www.who.int/inf-pr-2001/en/pr2001-48.html

## READINGS FROM THE POPULAR LITERATURE

Biderman, B. (1998). *Wired for sound: A journey into hearing*. Toronto: Trifolium Books. (cochlear implant to restore hearing)

Lane, H. (2000). *The mask of benevolence: Disabling the deaf community*. San Diego: Dawn Sign Press. (deafness)

Lane, H., Bahan, B., & Hoffmeister, R. (1996). *A journey into the deaf world*. San Diego: Dawn Sign Press. (Deaf culture)

Merker, H. (1999). *Listening*. Dallas: Southern Methodist University Press. (sudden adult-onset hearing loss)

Nieminen, R. (1990). *Voyage to the island*. Washington, DC: Gallaudet University Press. (deaf woman, teaching deaf children)

Niesser, A. (1990). *The other side of silence*. Washington, DC: Gallaudet Press. (deafness)

Padden, C., & Humphries, T. (1990). *Deaf in America: Voices from a culture*. Cambridge, MA: Harvard University Press. (Deaf culture)

Romoff, A. (1999). *Hear again: Back to life with a cochlear implant*. New York: League for the Hard of Hearing Publications. (adult restoration of hearing via implant)

Sacks, O. (1989). *Seeing voices: A journey into the world of the deaf*. New York: Harper Perennial. (deafness and Deaf culture)

Schaller, S. (1995). *A man without words*. Berkeley: University of California Press. (adult learning to talk)

# CHAPTER THIRTEEN

# PROFESSIONAL ISSUES

# PREVIEW

In this book, we have reviewed normal communication processes and disorders of communication that require the professional services of speech-language pathologists and audiologists. Along the way, we have introduced various aspects of clinical practice. In this final chapter, we will provide an overview of professional work settings, discuss interdisciplinary interactions, and address some professional issues such as standards, ethics, and certification requirements. Future advances in the understanding of communication processes and disorders will influence approaches to evaluation and treatment. In addition, professional practice patterns are likely to undergo change in response to social, political, and economic influences. We will touch on some foreseeable future trends.

Speech-language pathologists and audiologists work in a variety of settings. Each work environment is shaped by the clinical caseload, professional colleagues, administrative and support personnel, and the physical and procedural characteristics of the work site. A change in clinical setting can mean a drastic change in the characteristics of one's employment. Some professionals enjoy the opportunity to shift the nature of their work by changing clinical environments over the course of their career. Even those who remain in one type of setting are likely to experience considerable variety in their professional activities from day to day and year to year.

# CLINICAL SETTINGS

## School Settings

Public and private schools employ 55 percent of all speech-language pathologists and 9 percent of all audiologists, making them the most common work settings for ASHA members (ASHA, 2005). The start of school-based speech and hearing programs dates back to 1910 in the Chicago public school system (Paden, 1970). Programs developed because educators recognized that speech and hearing problems affected performance in the classroom, and they deemed it appropriate to provide services on-site. The scope of public school services has expanded over the years to include any child who has a communication disorder that negatively affects his or her education. Services for "educationally handicapped children" became nationwide in 1975 with the passage of Public Law 94-142, the Education for All Handicapped Children Act. Subsequent public laws were passed that govern services for children within the schools. Public Law 95-561 expanded remedial services by providing federal support to improve children's basic educational skills, including listening and speaking. With the passage of Public Law 99-457, preschool children who appear to have a speech, language, or hearing problem became eligible for assessment and remediation services through their local school system. Refinements in the laws governing service delivery to infants, preschoolers, and school-age children continue with the most recent legislation, the No Child Left Behind Act of 2001 and the Individuals with Disabilities Education Improvement Act (IDEA) of 2004. The public schools also conduct periodic hearing screening programs that may involve the direct or indirect participation of the audiologist.

Speech-language pathologists in the public schools may work with children individually, in small groups, or in an entire classroom. The caseload can vary from multiply handicapped children to those with specific speech or language difficulties. Some professionals serve children in only one school, whereas others are itinerant, traveling to several schools. Audiologists provide a range of services to public school children, including screening, diagnostic, and aural habilitation programs. They also assist students with the wide variety of personal and classroom amplification systems. One notable feature of work in the public school setting is the nine- to ten-month academic calendar, with a long summer break or extended breaks throughout the year. This schedule holds appeal for some professionals, particularly if their own children are of school age.

## Medical Settings

Medical settings are the second most common employment sites for speech, language, and hearing professionals. In 2005, 72 percent of audiologists and 36 percent of speech-language pathologists worked in medical settings (ASHA, 2005b). These work sites include a broad spectrum of health care delivery environments, including hospital-based acute care and rehabilitation units, inpatient and outpatient rehabilitation facilities, residential health care facilities, private practice offices, and medical clinics. Even within one hospital, speech-language pathologists and audiologists may work in a variety of settings. In the 1970s and 1980s, it was common for audiology and speech-language pathology to comprise a single unified department, but that is no longer standard practice. In most hospitals, speech-language pathologists and audiologists are members of various medical teams or departments within the hospital. For example, audiologists may be associated with otolaryngology or physical medicine and rehabilitation. Speech-language pathologists are often members of multidisciplinary teams that focus on different stages of the rehabilitation process, from acute to subacute to outpatient rehabilitation. Similarly, some teams focus on specific disorders, such as dysphagia or cognitive assessment and rehabilitation. It is most common for speech-language pathologists to work within a rehabilitation department, but in some hospitals they may be allied with other medical specialties, such as neurology, neurosurgery, pediatrics, surgery, or physical and rehabilitation medicine. The particular demands of medical settings have been addressed in several excellent resources, including a practitioner's guide (Johnson & Jacobson, 2006) and the *Journal of Medical Speech-Language Pathology.*

Just as clinical practice in the public schools has been influenced by public laws, service delivery in medical settings is greatly influenced by forces such as health care legislation, managed care, and health insurance policies. Hospital stays have shortened considerably in recent years, and there has been an increase in service delivery in the home, provided through home health care agencies. Patients tend to receive therapy for shorter durations than in the past, and clinicians must clearly justify their patients' need for therapy and the benefits of their services. These changes have been accompanied by an emphasis on the functional outcomes of treatment, so that clinicians focus on very practical aspects of the patients' needs and how treatment will make a difference in their everyday lives.

## Academic and Clinical Training Programs

Clinical training in the evaluation and treatment of communication disorders is conducted in many colleges and universities. The departments that provide course-work and professional preparation in speech-language pathology and audiology have various names, such as Speech and Hearing Sciences, Audiology and Speech-Language Pathology, and Communication Disorders. Clinical training involves academic course work at the undergraduate and graduate levels and supervised clinical training. Most university programs include an on-campus clinic for student training opportunities and off-campus practicum training with cooperating clinical placement sites in the community. University clinics typically serve both children and adults who have hearing, language, articulation, voice, and fluency problems. The clinics may offer students the opportunity to observe evaluation and treatment procedures in communication disorders prior to beginning direct clinical work. They also provide supervised clinical training for graduate students. Many training programs confer bachelor's, master's, and doctoral degrees.

University programs also contribute to the knowledge base of the professions through the conduct of basic and applied research. The research endeavors within a particular department reflect the areas of interest of faculty members. Students may become involved in research in a variety of informal and formal ways through work-study programs, volunteering, independent study, and thesis options. Research doctoral degree programs (e.g., PhD, ScD) are research oriented and require completion of original research in the form of a dissertation. There are also doctoral programs that focus on the clinical aspects of the professions.

## Community Speech and Hearing Centers

Many of the first speech and hearing service programs in the United States were provided in community speech and hearing centers. Such clinics are often housed in freestanding buildings rather than within an educational or medical facility. Community clinics are not as common as they once were, but those that still exist often derive some of their financial support from supplemental sources. For example, they may be funded by agencies such as the United Way or county public health programs, philanthropic groups such as Scottish Rite, or national organizations such as the Easter Seal Society. The clientele may be specific to certain disorders, such as children with cerebral palsy, or may include a wide variety of disorders that affect individuals of all ages.

## Private Practice

Some audiologists and speech-language pathologists provide clinical services in private practice settings. In 2005, 17 percent of certified audiologists were in full-time private practice, and another 10 percent worked in part-time private practice. In speech-language pathology, about 6 percent of certified professionals were in full-time private practice, and another 11 percent worked part-time in private practice (ASHA, 2005b). These individuals may provide services in their own office, at patients' homes, or through contractual arrangements with other care providers (e.g., hospitals, schools, nursing facilities). Practitioners who work part-time in a private practice may spend the rest of the day in another clinical setting (such as a public school or hospital). Private practitioners treat a wide variety of disorders. Adults may seek a private practice speech-language pathologist to continue treatment for a chronic condition, such as aphasia or a motor speech disorder. Parents may contract a private practitioner to supplement the services their child receives through the schools or to treat conditions not otherwise covered in school-based programs (e.g., tongue thrust). Schools, hospitals, and other agencies may contract with private practitioners in order to relieve personnel shortages. In such cases, the private practitioner operates as an independent contractor to these businesses and organizations rather than as one of their employees. This autonomy often appeals to clinicians who choose to maintain a private practice.

## INTERDISCIPLINARY INTERACTIONS

Almost all speech-language pathologists and audiologists work in conjunction with other professionals to some degree. Some of the cases presented earlier in this text provide examples of interdisciplinary interactions in the treatment of communication disorders. We can find out more about the nature of these interactions by reading about the experiences of clinicians who work on interdisciplinary teams. We will also consider the professionals who comprise these teams and work with speech-language pathologists and audiologists in a variety of settings.

### Team Approach in Public Schools

We begin with professionals who work with children in a public school setting. These individuals are jointly involved at all levels of case management, from the initial referral through the day-to-day implementation of therapy goals.

Patty is a speech-language pathologist with ten years' experience in the public school setting. She currently works with Cheryl, an occupational therapist (OT), and Jean, a physical therapist (PT), along with psychologists and several preschool and special education teachers. "An obvious motor impairment or speech-language problem is usually the cause for referral at our center. But often, with years of experience, you can just watch a kid and know that this kid needs to be seen by other professionals," Cheryl reported. The initial screening team in this school consisted of the classroom teacher, speech-language pathologist, and psychologist, with additional professionals brought in as needed.

All team members participate in joint evaluation of the child. However, their participation fluctuates according to the relevance of each assessment task to their area of expertise. For example, Patty may do the formal language testing of a child, but she may also observe during the PT's assessment of gross motor activities, because she knows that children are likely to use the most spontaneous language during that time. Cheryl reported that the group has come to work smoothly by getting to know what each other does. "Initially, it was intimidating, not knowing when it was my turn to do something. Then [over time] it just kind of smoothed out." "We pretty much follow the child's lead," added Patty. "When I'm preparing my next set of materials, Cheryl is already in there doing her next activity. The nice thing is it really speeds up the evaluation, so the child doesn't get bored."

The group pointed out several factors that made their work as an evaluation team effective. "First, it really helped that we all had experience with this population. Then, it was a matter of picking up on each other's pace," reported Jean. Patty added, "It's also a matter of knowing which activities of the others are going to provide me with language information. Or when I'm presenting information, Cheryl might say, 'You want to hold that at an angle because you can tell he's got low vision,' which helps me get optimal performance." The group agreed that teams work well when there is a respect for other professions and some knowledge of what each can contribute. The members must understand that the domains represented by each profession really do affect each other. As Cheryl put it, "I think that if you go in thinking that your own profession is the only one that is going to make a difference for the child, you're missing out on an integrated picture of the whole child."

This group offered many examples of ways the goals of different therapists interrelate for a particular child. For example, the positioning guidelines from the physical therapist may also be used by the occupational therapist and speech-language pathologist to provide the stability the child needs for learning to occur. To maximize their efforts, they often develop methods that address multiple goals at the same time.

Patty related, "If I am working to increase requests by a child, I can have the child ask for materials during an art project. When the request is made, I hand the crayon or straw to the child. I can do that in a way that reinforces the reaching or grasping behaviors I know Cheryl is working on as well." Often, motor activities can serve as the reinforcement for training speech goals. One popular activity is an obstacle course that primarily serves OT and PT goals. Children are "allowed" to run the course after producing three correct articulation targets. Jean remarked that she often watches Patty to see the level at which she presents language to the child: "It doesn't do me any good if a child can't perform a movement because he didn't understand my directions." In return, Patty has "borrowed" techniques from both Cheryl and Jean because she has noticed their effectiveness in helping children maintain their attention during various activities.

In the example above, we have seen how some of these professionals may work together in public schools. Let us now take a closer look at the professional interactions of a speech-language pathologist in a pediatric clinic.

## Team Approach in a Pediatric Clinic

Lora is a speech-language pathologist who serves as the coordinator of her hospital's cleft palate team (see Chapter 4 for a discussion of this condition). This team consists of an audiologist, geneticist, nurse, otolaryngologist (ENT), pediatrician, plastic surgeon, dentist, orthodontist, prosthodontist, and social worker, all of whom interact as a full team or as individuals with the parents and child.

"We get notified [that a child has been born with a cleft palate] from the birthing clinic. If it's feasible, we try to do a hospital visit within that first 24 to 48 hours," Lora reports. This visit usually involves a speech-language pathologist, a social worker, and a nurse. These individuals provide the parents with initial information concerning their child's condition, what can be done, and what to expect as the child develops. Lora also provides important information about feeding the child. Lora commented, "We feel that this early visit provides a valuable service."

Soon after, the audiologist will see the child to evaluate hearing status and to counsel the parents about possible concerns with hearing health as their child develops. Other early appointments will be with the geneticist, ear-nose-throat doctor, and the plastic surgeon. "As the child grows," related Lora, "he or she will be seeing the ENT, plastic surgeon, and some of the other team members on a regular basis. Then our program requires that the child visit the entire team, which meets once a month, for certain procedures to be approved. They want [the treatment] to be a team consensus to be sure that it is the appropriate treatment for the child." Procedures that routinely involve team discussion include pharyngeal flap, bone grafts, and lip and nose revisions. The team may brainstorm ideas about the timing and course of treatment, taking into consideration the various aspects of the child's condition.

The team meeting starts with a preconference. "I type a summary of what surgeries have already been done, the diagnosis, presenting concerns and [histories of all other services] ahead of time," reported Lora. "One of the physicians will act as the presenting or attending physician, who will say what the main concerns are. If any questions come up right then, we will discuss them." Then the parents come into the meeting, and the team members have an opportunity to examine the child. This is also an opportunity for the parents to provide all the professionals with input on treatment decisions and to ask questions about possible future intervention. "We really try to encourage the parents to consider themselves a member of the team," said Lora, "and I know that it can sometimes be a bit intimidating for some of them."

The team meeting is an opportunity for the parents and professionals to see how all the components of intervention come together for the child. Through these meetings, Lora has learned from the other professionals about state-of-the-art techniques for the management of cleft palate. In addition, she has provided the team with valued contributions. She provides this example: "I've had to sell the team on the usefulness of videoendoscopy (see Chapter 6), and they've pretty much bought into it now. We've had a couple of cases where we discovered that the child didn't need surgery [based on the videoendoscopy results]. I feel really good about how that has developed." Lora concludes with this thought, "I know that I have grown tremendously in this role professionally. I used to be so intimidated. I would dread the conference and I would know inside 'Oh, it's three days away,' and now I've been doing it for six years. I've grown much more confident. Over time, I've earned the other team members' respect. And I had to earn it."

## Team Approach in a Medical Setting

Tom is a speech-language pathologist with twelve years of professional experience. Most of his work has been in medical settings with adults with acquired communication disorders, typically related to stroke or head injury. Tom currently works in a hospital-based skilled nursing unit that provides subacute care. The patients in the subacute program are medically stable, but in need of rehabilitation and nursing care. Many of them were transferred to the unit after a stay in the acute care unit of the hospital, where they were admitted following a medically significant event, such as a stroke. Other patients were admitted directly to the subacute unit for a period of diagnostic and rehabilitative care to improve their independent living skills. Although the facility where Tom works is in a hospital setting, many skilled nursing facilities are not located on a hospital campus.

Tom is part of a multidisciplinary rehabilitation team that includes a physical therapist, occupational therapist, dietician, nurse, and medical doctor. His workspace is part of a common rehabilitation area where the physical therapist and occupational therapist also work with patients. Interdisciplinary interaction is completely natural and occurs in both planned and spontaneous ways. For example, Tom had a patient who fatigued easily and had a limited amount of time when he was awake, alert, and able to participate in therapy. In order to maximize the patient's optimal treatment time, Tom conducted speech and language therapy at the same time that the PT was working with the patient on balance. The simultaneous attention to two tasks, balance and speech, offered an additional challenge to the patient that was more representative of real life than treating each in isolation. In other cases, therapy goals may be common across several disciplines and may be referred to as *conjoint treatment goals*. Tom told of a patient with a hip fracture who could not remember the precautions he was given by the physical therapist to protect his healing hip; therefore, part of the cognitive training that Tom implemented with this patient included strategies to assist him in learning the hip precautions. In this case, all of the therapies had common treatment goals that related to safety and achieving independent living.

Team interaction is a big part of what Tom enjoys about his current job. In fact, he selected his current work site because the team approach appealed to him. He said that "it is important to go beyond what you have been taught" to be successful in a given setting. Working side by side with other professionals is one important way to continually expand and integrate professional knowledge.

## THE PROFESSIONAL ASSOCIATION: THE AMERICAN SPEECH-LANGUAGE-HEARING ASSOCIATION

### History and Purpose

The professions of speech-language pathology and audiology emerged and grew over the course of the twentieth century. In the early 1900s the focus was on speech disorders, particularly articulation and stuttering. In 1925, a group of professionals devoted to the treatment of communication disorders started an association called the American Academy for Speech Correction (Paden, 1970). The profession of audiology developed after World War II, owing to the needs of many soldiers who returned home with acquired hearing loss (Cherry & Giolas, 1997). As the audiology profession was established, audiologists were included among the ranks of professionals dealing with communication disorders. In 1948, the professional organization became the American Speech and Hearing Association (ASHA). As clinical attention to language impairments increased, the profession changed the name again in 1978 to the American Speech-Language-Hearing Association, although the ASHA acronym was retained. In 2005, over 123,000 speech-language pathologists, audiologists, and speech, language, and hearing scientists held ASHA membership. Information about this organization can be found on the ASHA website at www.asha.org. Additional discussion concerning professional issues is found in Lubinski, Golper, and Frattali (2007).

Although there are other related professional organizations to which audiologists and speech-language pathologists belong, ASHA is the primary professional organization for speech, language, and hearing professionals. The mission of ASHA is to promote the interests of the professions and to advocate for people with communication disabilities. The purposes are reflected in the Association bylaws (ASHA, 2006), which are paraphrased here:

1. To encourage basic research and scientific study of human communication and its disorders.
2. To promote appropriate academic and clinical preparation for individuals preparing to enter the professions, and to promote continuing education within the profession.
3. To promote investigation and prevention of communication disorders.
4. To foster improvement of clinical procedures used in treating disorders of communication.

5. To stimulate exchange of information pertinent to communication and communication disorders.
6. To advocate for individuals with communication disorders.
7. To promote the interests of members of the Association.

ASHA is an organization that is intended to serve the interests of the membership. There are two bodies that govern and establish the policies of the Association: the Legislative Council and the Executive Board. The Legislative Council establishes the policies of the organization and is composed of elected representatives from every state; the Executive Board consists of officers elected by the ASHA membership, as well as the Executive Director of the Association. Many of the ASHA policies, such as defining the scope of practice of the professions, have significant impact on speech-language pathologists and audiologists, and therefore are of great interest to members of the Association. The executive board also manages the affairs of the Association, and board members often serve as official representatives of the Association. The committees, task forces, and boards that operate within the ASHA structure provide opportunities for the membership to significantly contribute to the professions.

## Certification and Accreditation

Most practitioners in speech-language pathology and audiology in the United States are members of ASHA and have received the Certificate of Clinical Competence (CCC) in either audiology, speech-language pathology, or both, from ASHA. To be eligible to obtain the CCC, ASHA requires the completion of graduate course work and graduate clinical practicum from a program certified by ASHA (ASHA, 2005a). Academic preparation includes basic sciences and professional course work that meets the ASHA standards. Clinical observation and supervised practicum must be completed across a range of ages and disorders as specified by ASHA (2005a). Following the completion of the graduate degree, the CCC applicant must spend a Clinical Fellowship Year (CFY) working in an approved clinical setting under the direct supervision of a clinically certified clinician. The applicant also must pass a certification examination. ASHA membership is not required for certification by the organization, but the number of nonmembers holding certification is small. Most states require a license to practice, although those requirements are often consistent with the standards set forth by ASHA for the CCC. Evidence of continuing education also may be required for periodic state licensure renewal.

## Continuing Education

ASHA is devoted to continuing education and advancement of scientific clinical knowledge in the professions. The Association publishes several scholarly journals that are available to members and are carried in many libraries: *American Journal of*

*Audiology; American Journal of Speech-Language Pathology; Journal of Speech, Language, and Hearing Research; and Language, Speech, and Hearing Services in Schools.* These journals contain research articles that have been reviewed by experts in the professions (a process called peer review) and have been deemed worthy of publication. A monthly newspaper called *ASHA Leader* helps keep members abreast of current events of interest to the profession. Another continuing education opportunity is provided by the annual ASHA Convention. This convention often draws more than 10,000 participants, who have the opportunity to listen to professional presentations, view new books and clinical materials, and meet for a variety of formal and informal gatherings. Although the ASHA Convention is the largest educational event each year, there are many other learning activities available throughout the year that are sponsored by ASHA, state and local organizations, academic programs, and private groups. The opportunities include workshops, telephone seminars, videoconferences, and electronic learning activities, such as web-based workshops.

## Ethical Conduct

A primary concern of ASHA is for certified speech-language pathologists and audiologists to practice their professions ethically. Consequently, all certified audiologists or speech-language pathologists (regardless of ASHA membership) must adhere to the Association's Code of Ethics (ASHA, 2003). The Code of Ethics provides guidelines for professional practice and is a helpful resource when ethical questions arise (Figure 13.1). A timely example of the value of the Code of Ethics pertains to the discussion of clinical cases via electronic mail and listserv discussion groups. There are many opportunities for clinicians to solicit the opinions and advice of other professionals regarding the diagnosis or treatment of a particularly difficult or unusual case by Internet and email interactions. When seeking information, common sense would suggest that it would be inappropriate for a clinician to reveal the name or other identifying information about a specific patient in the context of a listserv discussion (Principle I). However, it might not be so obvious that it is unethical to conduct evaluation or treatment solely by correspondence, as indicated by Principle I-I (see Figure 13.1). That principle should caution clinicians who seek and offer advice about practice via email, because there are potential problems when diagnostic treatment suggestions are given by someone who has not seen the actual patient. Therefore, advice proffered by mail (electronic or otherwise) should be taken as suggestions rather than prescriptions for treatment. The Code of Ethics can help clarify these issues for the clinician.

## Student Membership

There is a student organization, the National Student Speech Language Hearing Association (NSSLHA), that undergraduate and graduate students may join as they pursue preprofessional education in speech-language pathology, audiology,

Ethics    2003 / I - 185

AMERICAN
SPEECH-LANGUAGE-
HEARING
ASSOCIATION

# Code of Ethics

*Last Revised January 1, 2003*

## Preamble

The preservation of the highest standards of integrity and ethical principles is vital to the responsible discharge of obligations by speech-language pathologists, audiologists, and speech, language, and hearing scientists. This Code of Ethics sets forth the fundamental principles and rules considered essential to this purpose.

Every individual who is (a) a member of the American Speech-Language-Hearing Association, whether certified or not, (b) a nonmember holding the Certificate of Clinical Competence from the Association, (c) an applicant for membership or certification, or (d) a Clinical Fellow seeking to fulfill standards for certification shall abide by this Code of Ethics.

Any violation of the spirit and purpose of this Code shall be considered unethical. Failure to specify any particular responsibility or practice in this Code of Ethics shall not be construed as denial of the existence of such responsibilities or practices.

The fundamentals of ethical conduct are described by Principles of Ethics and by Rules of Ethics as they relate to the conduct of research and scholarly activities and responsibility to persons served, the public, and speech-language pathologists, audiologists, and speech, language, and hearing scientists.

Principles of Ethics, aspirational and inspirational in nature, form the underlying moral basis for the Code of Ethics. Individuals shall observe these principles as affirmative obligations under all conditions of professional activity.

Reference this material as: American Speech-Language-Hearing Association. Code of ethics (revised). *ASHA Supplement*, 23, pp. 13–15.

Index terms: ASHA reference products, ethics (professional practice issues), ethics and related papers

Document type: Ethics and related documents

Rules of Ethics are specific statements of minimally acceptable professional conduct or of prohibitions and are applicable to all individuals.

## Principle of Ethics I

Individuals shall honor their responsibility to hold paramount the welfare of persons they serve professionally or participants in research and scholarly activities and shall treat animals involved in research in a humane manner.

### Rules of Ethics

A. Individuals shall provide all services competently.

B. Individuals shall use every resource, including referral when appropriate, to ensure that high-quality service is provided.

C. Individuals shall not discriminate in the delivery of professional services or the conduct of research and scholarly activities on the basis of race or ethnicity, gender, age, religion, national origin, sexual orientation, or disability.

D. Individuals shall not misrepresent the credentials of assistants, technicians, or support personnel and shall inform those they serve professionally of the name and professional credentials of persons providing services.

E. Individuals who hold the Certificates of Clinical Competence shall not delegate tasks that require the unique skills, knowledge, and judgment that are within the scope of their profession to assistants, technicians, support personnel, students, or any nonprofessionals over whom they have supervisory responsibility. An individual may delegate support services to assistants, technicians, support personnel, students, or any other persons only if those services are adequately supervised by an individual who holds the appropriate Certificate of Clinical Competence.

**FIGURE 13.1   ASHA Code of Ethics.**

Used with permission of the American Speech-Language-Hearing Association.

*ASHA Desk Reference 2002 Volume 1 • Cardinal Documents of the Association*

F. Individuals shall fully inform the persons they serve of the nature and possible effects of services rendered and products dispensed, and they shall inform participants in research about the possible effects of their participation in research conducted.

G. Individuals shall evaluate the effectiveness of services rendered and of products dispensed and shall provide services or dispense products only when benefit can reasonably be expected.

H. Individuals shall not guarantee the results of any treatment or procedure, directly or by implication; however, they may make a reasonable statement of prognosis.

I. Individuals shall not provide clinical services solely by correspondence.

J. Individuals may practice by telecommunication (for example, telehealth/e-health), where not prohibited by law.

K. Individuals shall adequately maintain and appropriately secure records of professional services rendered, research and scholarly activities conducted, and products dispensed and shall allow access to these records only when authorized or when required by law.

L. Individuals shall not reveal, without authorization, any professional or personal information about identified persons served professionally or identified participants involved in research and scholarly activities unless required by law to do so, or unless doing so is necessary to protect the welfare of the person or of the community or otherwise required by law.

M. Individuals shall not charge for services not rendered, nor shall they misrepresent services rendered, products dispensed, or research and scholarly activities conducted.

N. Individuals shall use persons in research or as subjects of teaching demonstrations only with their informed consent.

O. Individuals whose professional services are adversely affected by substance abuse or other health-related conditions shall seek professional assistance and, where appropriate, withdraw from the affected areas of practice.

## Principle of Ethics II

Individuals shall honor their responsibility to achieve and maintain the highest level of professional competence.

### Rules of Ethics

A. Individuals shall engage in the provision of clinical services only when they hold the appropriate Certificate of Clinical Competence or when they are in the certification process and are supervised by an individual who holds the appropriate Certificate of Clinical Competence.

B. Individuals shall engage in only those aspects of the professions that are within the scope of their competence, considering their level of education, training, and experience.

C. Individuals shall continue their professional development throughout their careers.

D. Individuals shall delegate the provision of clinical services only to: (1) persons who hold the appropriate Certificate of Clinical Competence; (2) persons in the education or certification process who are appropriately supervised by an individual who holds the appropriate Certificate of Clinical Competence; or (3) assistants, technicians, or support personnel who are adequately supervised by an individual who holds the appropriate Certificate of Clinical Competence.

E. Individuals shall not require or permit their professional staff to provide services or conduct research activities that exceed the staff members competence, level of education, training, and experience.

F. Individuals shall ensure that all equipment used in the provision of services or to conduct research and scholarly activities is in proper working order and is properly calibrated.

## Principle of Ethics III

Individuals shall honor their responsibility to the public by promoting public understanding of the professions, by supporting the development of services designed to fulfill the unmet needs of the public, and by providing accurate information in all communications involving any aspect of the professions, including dissemination of research findings and scholarly activities.

### Rules of Ethics

A. Individuals shall not misrepresent their credentials, competence, education, training, experience, or scholarly or research contributions.

B. Individuals shall not participate in professional activities that constitute a conflict of interest.

C. Individuals shall refer those served professionally solely on the basis of the interest of those

**FIGURE 13.1   (continued)**

being referred and not on any personal financial interest.

D. Individuals shall not misrepresent diagnostic information, research, services rendered, or products dispensed; neither shall they engage in any scheme to defraud in connection with obtaining payment or reimbursement for such services or products.

E. Individuals' statements to the public shall provide accurate information about the nature and management of communication disorders, about the professions, about professional services, and about research and scholarly activities.

F. Individuals' statements to the public—advertising, announcing, and marketing their professional services, reporting research results, and promoting products—shall adhere to prevailing professional standards and shall not contain misrepresentations.

## Principle of Ethics IV

Individuals shall honor their responsibilities to the professions and their relationships with colleagues, students, and members of allied professions. Individuals shall uphold the dignity and autonomy of the professions, maintain harmonious interprofessional and intraprofessional relationships, and accept the professions' self-imposed standards.

### Rules of Ethics

A. Individuals shall prohibit anyone under their supervision from engaging in any practice that violates the Code of Ethics.

B. Individuals shall not engage in dishonesty, fraud, deceit, misrepresentation, sexual harrassment, or any other form of conduct that adversely reflects on the professions or on the individual's fitness to serve persons professionally.

C. Individuals shall not engage in sexual activities with clients or students over whom they exercise professional authority.

D. Individuals shall assign credit only to those who have contributed to a publication, presentation, or product. Credit shall be assigned in proportion to the contribution and only with the contributor's consent.

E. Individuals shall reference the source when using other persons' ideas, research, presentations, or products in written, oral, or any other media presentation or summary.

F. Individuals' statements to colleagues about professional services, research results, and products shall adhere to prevailing professional standards and shall contain no misrepresentations.

G. Individuals shall not provide professional services without exercising independent professional judgment, regardless of referral source or prescription.

H. Individuals shall not discriminate in their relationships with colleagues, students, and members of allied professions on the basis of race or ethnicity, gender, age, religion, national origin, sexual orientation, or disability.

I. Individuals who have reason to believe that the Code of Ethics has been violated shall inform the Board of Ethics.

J. Individuals shall comply fully with the policies of the Board of Ethics in its consideration and adjudication of complaints of violations of the Code of Ethics.

**FIGURE 13.1   (continued)**

and the associated sciences. Many colleges and universities have NSSLHA chapters. NSSLHA membership offers students the opportunity to receive professional journals, participate in educational activities, and even become involved in association governance activities. NSSLHA also has its own journal: *Contemporary Issues in Communication Science and Disorders.*

## Special Interest Divisions

Although members of ASHA are generally trained to manage a broad array of communication disorders, many members have special interests in particular disorders or aspects of the profession. In 1988, special interest divisions were established to allow ASHA members with common interests to identify themselves and affiliate with one another. The divisions have different objectives, but their common purposes are to advance the education of their affiliates and represent their special interests within ASHA. There are sixteen special interest divisions, which are listed in Table 13.1. In addition to ASHA members and international affiliates, members of NSSLHA may choose to affiliate with one or more of the divisions, which may provide them with insight into current issues in prospective areas of interest. Affiliation with special interest divisions is optional; affiliate dues may be paid at the same time that ASHA or NSSLHA dues are paid.

**TABLE 13.1   Special Interest Divisions of the American Speech-Language-Hearing Association**

| | |
|---|---|
| Division 1: | Language Learning and Education |
| Division 2: | Neurophysiology and Neurogenic Speech and Language Disorders |
| Division 3: | Voice and Voice Disorders |
| Division 4: | Fluency and Fluency Disorders |
| Division 5: | Speech Science and Orofacial Disorders |
| Division 6: | Hearing and Hearing Disorders: Research and Diagnostics |
| Division 7: | Aural Rehabilitation and Its Instrumentation |
| Division 8: | Hearing Conservation and Occupational Audiology |
| Division 9: | Hearing and Hearing Disorders in Childhood |
| Division 10: | Issues in Higher Education |
| Division 11: | Administration and Supervision |
| Division 12: | Augmentative and Alternative Communication |
| Division 13: | Swallowing and Swallowing Disorders (Dysphagia) |
| Division 14: | Communication Disorders and Sciences in Culturally and Linguistically Diverse Populations |
| Division 15: | Gerontology |
| Division 16: | School-Based Issues |

# TRENDS IN THE PROFESSION

## Specialty Recognition

Professional preparation in speech-language pathology and audiology is relatively broad based, and there are many clinical populations and settings from which to choose. However, many professionals find over time that they tend to specialize in a particular area (or areas) of clinical practice. In 1994, the Legislative Council of ASHA approved a program for specialty recognition within the professions of speech-language pathology and audiology. This voluntary program allows practitioners within a given specialty to petition for the establishment of specialty recognition in their area of expertise. The Clinical Specialty Board established by ASHA oversees the application process, but it does not initiate the establishment of specialty recognition; the initiative comes from a group of practitioners in a given specialty. So, in effect, speech-language pathologists and audiologists who have become specialists in a particular area take the responsibility to establish the criteria for such specialization. In some cases, the Special Interest Division may choose to petition for specialty recognition, in other cases, the petitioner may be a related professional organization. The specialty recognition process is in its infancy. Students and new professionals in speech, language, and hearing may be interested in researching the status of specialty recognition as they prepare to enter their profession.

## Use of Support Personnel

The use of support personnel is an emerging trend within the professions. There are different levels of support personnel, including speech-language pathology assistants, or aides, audiometric technicians, or audiology assistants. These individuals work in a variety of settings under the supervision of an ASHA-certified speech-language pathologist or audiologist. Unlike the requirements for clinical certification of master's-level clinicians, there is no widely accepted training standard for support personnel. However, ASHA has provided guidelines for the training, credentialing, use, and supervision of these individuals in clinical and educational settings (ASHA, 2004). In addition, the ASHA Code of Ethics provides principles related to work performed by support personnel. The use of support personnel is intended to occur as an adjunct to and under the supervision of clinically certified personnel. When managed properly, a program that includes both certified personnel and support personnel can be effective. Let's take a look at one such team.

> *Kendall,* an ASHA-certified speech-language pathologist, "inherited" a speech aide when she took a part-time job at a state residential facility for adults with severe developmental disorders. Her aide, Julie, had been working at this center for twenty

years, the last six as a speech aide. Julie has a high school education and received on-the-job training for her current position. Kendall and Julie have been working together for three years.

Kendall is responsible for initial assessments of the center's residents. She interviews the center staff concerning the residents' level of functioning and develops programs designed to increase their functional communication. She discusses a new program with Julie to get her insights on how it might be integrated into the daily activities at the center. Julie is at the center on a daily basis and she oversees the implementation of those programs. She works with the center staff to explain the communication goals and provides them with materials for training those communication behaviors during the day. She also collects and compiles data on the frequency with which goals were addressed by the staff and the effectiveness of the program for a resident.

Julie's duties are fairly typical of support personnel. They include clerical work, making materials for intervention programs, and implementing the programs planned by the certified clinician. Julie's contribution on a daily basis increases frequency of services to the residents beyond what Kendall could provide on her own. Effective use of support personnel may mean that the certified clinician has to rethink the components of his or her job and how to best carry them out.

"One of the things that has been very important for me in working with my aide was learning to prioritize," said Kendall. "I had to decide which tasks were critical for me to complete, and let Julie do the rest."

As Kendall's experience shows, support personnel can make a positive contribution to the professions. However, the use of support personnel in clinical settings is not without controversy. Some clinicians are concerned that bureaucratic decisions will be made that increase the duties of support personnel beyond their training and abilities, eroding the quality of services. Professionals who have had experience working with support personnel have offered guidance for others who might also have the opportunity (Kimbarow, 1997). Their advice includes the following:

- Establish clear guidelines for use of support personnel.
- Establish minimum competencies for the work setting.
- Learn how to supervise and train support personnel.
- Allow for a training period for developing competencies before working with patients.
- Explain the rationale behind therapy procedures so that they are implemented correctly.
- Do not assign support personnel to work with new clients or with certain types of complex disorders.
- Establish a plan of supervision and feedback.

## Employment Outlook

Speech-language pathology and audiology are relatively young professions that continue to grow. The U.S. Bureau of Labor Statistics (2006–2007) estimates that employment of speech-language pathologists and audiologists will increase by about 9 to 17 percent by 2014. Among the job settings that will see the biggest demand are colleges and universities seeking teaching and research-oriented faculty in communication sciences and disorders. Data from the Council on Graduate Programs (2002) suggest that job openings for those with research doctorates will exceed the number of doctoral graduates for much of this decade.

The outlook is good for the professions, given factors such as increased awareness of communication disorders; early detection of hearing, speech, and language disorders in children; the aging of the population and associated increased prevalence of age-related communication impairments; and increased concern over occupation-related hearing disorders (ASHA, 1998). These trends suggest continued growth of the professions well into the future. Although work settings and models of service delivery are likely to change over time, the professions will remain devoted to increased understanding of the nature and treatment of communication disorders.

## REFERENCES

American Speech-Language-Hearing Association (ASHA). (2004). *Guidelines for the training, use, and supervision of speech-language pathology assistants.* Available at http://www.asha.org/members/deskref-journals/deskref/default

American Speech-Language-Hearing Association (ASHA). (1998, Spring). Position statement and guidelines for support personnel in audiology. *Asha, 40* (Suppl. 18), 19–21.

American Speech-Language-Hearing Association (ASHA). (2003). Code of ethics. *ASHA Supplement, 23,* 13–15. Retrieved November 12, 2006, from ASHA website http://www.asha.org/NR/rdonlyres/F51E46C5-3D87-44AF-BFDA-346D32F85C60/0/v1CodeOfEthics.pdf

American Speech-Language-Hearing Association (ASHA; 2005a). *Membership and certification handbook of the American-Speech-Language-Hearing Association.* Rockville, MD: Author.

American Speech-Language-Hearing Association (ASHA). (2005b). *Highlights and trends: ASHA member counts.* Retrieved November 12, 2006, from http://www.asha.org/about/membership-certification/member-counts.htm

American Speech-Language-Hearing Association (ASHA). (2006). *Bylaws and policies associated with the bylaws of the American Speech-Language-Hearing Association.* ASHA Desk Reference. Rockville, MD: Author.

Cherry, R., & Giolas, T. G. (1997). Preface to aural rehabilitation with adults. *Seminars in hearing, 18,* 75.

Council on Academic Accreditation in Audiology and Speech-Language Pathology (2004). *Standards for accreditation of graduate programs in audiology and speech-language pathology.* Available at http://www.asha.org/members/deskref-journals/deskref/default.

Council on Graduate Programs in Communication Sciences and Disorders. (2002). *Demographic survey of undergraduate and graduate programs in communication sciences and disorders.* Minneapolis, MN: Author.

Johnson, A. F., & Jacobson, B. H. (2006). *Medical speech-language pathology: A practitioner's guide* (2nd ed.). New York: Thieme.

Kimbarow, M. L. (1997). Ahead of the curve: Improving services with speech-language pathology assistants. *Asha, 39,* 41–44.

Lubinski, R., Golper, L.C. & Frattali, C. (2007). *Professional issues in speech-language pathology and audiology: A textbook.* Florence, KY: Thomson Delmar Learning.

Paden, E. (1970). *A history of the American Speech and Hearing Association, 1925–1958.* Bethesda, MD: American Speech and Hearing Association.

U.S. Bureau of Labor Statistics, U.S. Department of Labor. (2006-2007). *Occupational outlook handbook, 2006-07 edition.* Retrieved November 12, 2006 from http://www.bis.gov/oco/ocos099.htm

**acoustic neuroma**   A nonmalignant tumor that involves the myelin sheath of the VIIIth nerve.

**addition error**   A type of speech articulation error characterized by adding a sound to the target phoneme or word; for example, for the word, *blue,* a child pronounces it *bolu.*

**affricate**   A consonant that begins with a plosive phoneme and ends with a fricative, such as *ch,* written phonetically as /ʧ/.

**agraphia**   An acquired impairment of writing caused by brain damage.

**air conduction audiometry**   Testing hearing by introducing the tone into the ear canal, with the sound waves then traveling to the ear drum at the end of the canal (as opposed to bone conduction).

**alerting devices**   Devices to warn a hearing-impaired person to sounds in the environment (e.g., a telephone ringing, a doorbell, a baby's cry, or an emergency alarm) through vibration, a light signal, or a combination.

**alexia with agraphia**   An acquired impairment of reading and writing due to brain damage.

**alexia without agraphia**   An acquired impairment of reading that is not accompanied by a writing impairment; also called pure alexia.

**alexia**   An acquired impairment of reading caused by brain damage.

**allophone**   One of the variant forms of a phoneme that is recognized by the listener as the target phoneme.

**alveolar ridge**   The ridge of bone just behind the upper front teeth.

**Alzheimer's disease**   The most common form of dementing illness; a chronic, progressive disease that results in intellectual decline affecting language, memory, and cognition.

**anarthria**   A severe impairment of motor control for speech resulting in complete lack of articulate speech.

**anomia**   A reduced ability to name objects or retrieve desired words.

**anomic aphasia**   A fluent aphasia that is characterized by relatively good verbal expression and auditory comprehension but notable difficulty coming up with the names of things.

**APGAR**   A five-point evaluation system for identifying the status of newborns.

**aphasia**   An acquired impairment of language due to damage to the language-dominant hemisphere, typically the left.

**aphonia**   Attempts to produce a voice that results in a whisperlike sound. This usually occurs with voice disorders that prevent the vocal folds from vibrating to produce sound.

**apraxia of speech**   An impairment of motor planning for the movements for speech so that voluntary control for speech is disrupted.

**arcuate fasciculus**   A bundle of nerve fibers (white matter) that originate in cell bodies in the superior temporal gyrus and project anteriorly to the frontal lobe.

**articulation**   Production of speech sounds.

**arytenoid cartilage**   The paired, pyramid-shaped cartilages that sit on the posterior portion of the cricoid cartilage and aid in abduction and adduction of vocal folds.

**aspiration**   Inhalation of fluids or other matter into the airway.

**assistive listening device (ALD)**   Any device designed to reduce the effects of distance, background noise, and reverberation on the perception of speech.

**ataxia**   A motor disorder characterized by marked loss of coordination, often associated with cerebellar disease.

**athetosis**   A form of cerebral palsy characterized by twisting and flailing of the extremities, neck, and trunk.

**audibility index**   An estimation of what percent of acoustic energy from speech will be audible to a particular person.

**audiogram**   A graphic representation of the results of a hearing test with axes for hearing level and frequency.

**audiologist**   A professional who is concerned with the prevention, evaluation, and rehabilitation of auditory, balance, and related disorders.

**audiology**   The study of normal and disordered hearing.

**audiometer**   An electronic instrument used to evaluate the auditory system.

**auditory brainstem response**   An electrophysiological response to sounds that results in five to seven peaks that appear within 10 ms after the presentation of a signal (usually a click).

**auditory training**   The training of a hearing-impaired individual to make use of residual hearing abilities.

**auricle**   The external ear, also known as pinna.

**basal ganglia**   A collection of subcortical gray matter structures, including the putamen, globus pallidus, and caudate, that contribute to control of motor behavior.

**basilar membrane**   A thin tissue layer found within the cochlea on which the organ of Corti rests.

**bolus**   Refers to a cohesive mass of some substance such as food.

**bone conduction audiometry**   In hearing testing, introducing the sound waves directly into the cochlea via the bones of the skull.

**brainstem**   The brain structures at the base of the brain excluding the hemispheres above, the cerebellum, and the spinal cord below.

**Broca's aphasia**   A nonfluent aphasia with relatively preserved auditory comprehension, associated with damage to the inferior portions of the left frontal lobe.

**canonical babbling**   Consonant-vowel or consonant-vowel-consonant-vowel combinations produced by babies.

**carcinoma**   A cancer or malignancy.

**central auditory processing disorder**   Difficulties understanding speech as a result of structural changes in the central auditory nervous system. The difficulties are most pronounced in background noise and other difficult listening situations (e.g., reverberation).

**central nervous system**   The brain and spinal cord, exclusive of the cranial and peripheral nerves.

**cerebellum**   A brain structure that sits below the cerebral hemispheres and above the pons, playing an important role in muscular coordination.

**cerebral localization**   A theory of brain function that associates particular functions and behaviors to particular sites of the brain.

**cerebral palsy**   A developmental motor disorder related to brain injury; the most common forms are spasticity, athetosis, and ataxia.

**cerebrovascular accident**   *See* stroke.

**cerebrum**   The largest division of the brain, containing the cerebral hemispheres and corpus callosum.

**cerumen**   A waxy substance produced by glands that lie within the skin of the ear canal.

**chromosome**   A structure containing genes that transmit genetic information.

**cilia**   Hairlike structures that extend from the surface of a cell.

**circumlocution**   Talking with an excess number of words; or talking around the topic rather than being direct because of a failure to retrieve desired words, as in anomia.

**closed caption decoder**   An electronic device that decodes the captioned signals that are often broadcast with television programs. It enables captions to appear on the television screen and helps hearing-impaired individuals to understand the dialogue of television programs and movies.

**cluttering**   A disorder of fluency characterized by rapid speech, breaks in fluency, and faulty articulation.

**coarticulation**   The simultaneous production of two or more consonants or vowels in normal speech production of a word, such as the word *tram*—the first three phones (/t/ /r/ /æ/) might overlap in production.

**cochlea**   The snail-shaped part of the inner ear containing the sensory organs of hearing.

**cochlear implant**   A coil and electrodes surgically placed in the inner ear and connected to an external transmitter/signal processor. It is intended to produce sensations of sound for those with profound hearing impairments.

**code switching**   Shifting by speakers among one or more dialects or languages to accommodate social rules or situational demands.

**cognate**   A pair of sounds, such as /p/ and /b/, produced similarly except that one (/p/) is unvoiced and one (/b/) voiced.

**communication**   An interaction or exchange of one's feelings, ideas, thoughts, and wants among two or more people by such modes as speech, writing, facial expression, gesture, or touch.

**conduction aphasia**   A fluent aphasia characterized by relatively good auditory comprehension and poor verbal repetition.

**conductive hearing loss**   A loss of hearing related to obstruction or disease in the outer or middle ear in which sound transmission fails to reach the cochlea in the inner ear.

**congenital**   Present at birth.

**content**   The elements of language that carry meaning; also called semantics.

**continuant**   A speech sound that can be continued or prolonged, such as /m/ or /s/.

**corpus callosum**   A large band of fibers that joins the two hemispheres of the brain.

**cortex**   The surface layer of the brain that contains the bodies of neurons.

**cranial nerves**   Twelve paired peripheral nerves that derive from or come into the cranial cavity, such as cranial nerve I, olfactory, or II, optic.

**cricoid cartilage**   The ring of cartilage that forms the base of the larynx.

**criterion-referenced test**   A type of measure that is used to compare a child's performance against a standard, or criterion, for behavior.

**decibel (dB)**   A logarithmic unit of measurement of sound intensity.

**delayed auditory feedback**   An event produced when a device presents the listener's own speech or voice after a time delay. One effect of delayed auditory feedback is fluency enhancement in individuals who stutter.

**dementia**   A behavioral syndrome of generalized intellectual deficit that results from a number of diseases.

**denasality**   Insufficient nasal resonance; hyponasality.

**developmental language disorder**   A condition involving poor language skills that appears during childhood.

**diadochokinesis**   The rapid, alternating movements of a body part, such as in the lips and tongue rapidly saying puh-tuh-kuh repeatedly.

**diagnosogenic theory of stuttering**   Theory that posits stuttering begins when normal disfluencies are labeled as stuttering.

**diaphragm**   The muscular-tendonous partition that separates the thorax from the abdomen, serving as the primary muscle of respiration.

**diphthong**   A blending together of two vowels in the same syllable, such as heard as /aI/ in the word *right*.

**diplophonia**   This describes a voice that has two pitches occurring at the same time.

**distortion error**   The production of a target phoneme utilizing a sound that is not in the language, such as in a lateral lisp.

**dyslexia**   An impairment of reading due to developmental or acquired brain damage.

**dysphagia**   An impairment of the ability to swallow.

**dysphonia**   A disorder of voice, such as hoarseness, breathiness, or harshness.

**effusion**   Fluid that has exuded into the middle ear space.

**electrolarynx**   An electronic device that creates sound that can be used as a substitute for the voice (usually because the larynx has been surgically removed).

**endogenous**   Caused by genetic factors.

**epiglottis**   An oblong cartilage that sits at the top of the larynx and covers its opening during swallowing.

**Eustachian tube**   The air tube that connects the middle ear with the nasopharynx.

**exogenous**   Acquired or caused by factors outside the genes.

**external ear canal**   The external opening into the ear.

**fluent aphasia**   An aphasia profile that is characterized by spoken output of relatively normal utterance length, ease of production, and prosodic variation.

**FM system**   A device that uses a transmitter to send the desired signal to a receiver using a radio wave. The receiver is coupled to the listener via earphones or a hearing aid.

**form**   The phonological, syntactic, and morphological elements of language.

**four kilohertz (4 kHz) notch**   An increase in hearing impairment in the 3000 to 6000 Hz region with recovery of hearing at 8000 Hz. This pattern is associated with noise-induced hearing impairment.

**frequency**   The number of cycles per second of a sound wave; perceived as pitch.

**frontal lobe**   The anterior part of each cerebral hemisphere, from the Rolandic fissure forward.

**global aphasia**   A nonfluent aphasia characterized by marked impairment of verbal expression and auditory comprehension, typically caused by large lesions to the perisylvian region of the left hemisphere.

**glossectomy**   The surgical removal of the tongue.

**glottis**   The opening between the vocal folds.

**habituate**   Exhibit gradual decrease in responsiveness following repeated exposure to a stimulus.

**handicap**   A disadvantage resulting from an impairment or disability that limits the fulfillment of a role that is normal for an individual.

**hearing**   The perception of sound.

**hearing disability**   The restrictions in daily activities that result from a hearing impairment.

**hearing impairment**   Any loss or abnormality of structure or function of the auditory system.

**hearing loss**   The degree of hearing impairment.

**hemiparesis**   Weakness of one side of the body.

**hemisphere**   Literally, half circle. In reference to brain anatomy, hemisphere indicates the half of the cerebrum or cerebellum to each side of midline.

**Hertz (Hz)**   Unit of measure that reflects cycles per second.

**hyperlexia**   A reading disorder characterized by strong phonological decoding despite poor or very poor reading comprehension.

**hypernasality**   Excessive nasal resonance.

**immittance audiometry**   Air-pressure and air-volume differences measured in the external and middle ear as a method of detecting conductive hearing loss.

**incidence**   The number of new cases that appear in a population over a set period of time.

**incus**   An anvil-shaped bone found in the middle ear.

**intensity**   A measure of the magnitude or pressure of a sound wave; perceived as loudness.

**involuntary repetitions**   A form of stuttering characterized by unexpected syllable or word repetitions.

**jargon aphasia**   An acquired impairment of language characterized by meaningless utterances.

**language**   The coding of meaning into a system of arbitrary symbols that are recognized by members of the community. Language may be spoken, written, or manual (signed).

**learning disability**   Educational difficulties in reading, writing, listening, speaking, or arithmetic, believed to be related to some kind of central brain dysfunction.

**left neglect**   Reduced awareness or responsiveness to sensory input from the left side of the body (intrapersonal space) or left half of the environment (extrapersonal space) that cannot be attributed to sensory or motor defects.

**lesion**   Damage to the nervous system.

**malleus**   A hammer-shaped bone attached to the tympanic membrane within the middle ear.

**mandible**   The lower jaw.

**Ménière's disease**   A disease of the inner ear thought to be associated with an overproduction of endolymph. Symptoms include tinnitus, vertigo, and hearing loss.

**mental retardation**   Reduced cognitive abilities, confirmed by measured intelligence quotients of 70 or below and poor adaptive abilities.

**middle ear**   The air-filled space located in the temporal bone containing the three small middle-ear bones, incus, malleus, and stapes.

**misarticulations**   Speech articulation errors of omission, addition, substitution, or distortion.

**mixed hearing loss**   A hearing loss caused by both conductive and sensorineural problems.

**morpheme**   Words or the smallest unit of a word that has meaning. For example, the word *cat* is one morpheme; in the plural form *cats,* the *s* is an added morpheme.

**morphology**   The study of words and word forms; the study of morphemes.

**multi-infarct dementia**   A form of dementia related to many small strokes (or infarcts).

**myofunctional therapy**   Muscle training of the tongue to reduce tongue pressures on dentition, that is, therapy for reverse swallow and tongue thrust.

**nasoendoscope**   A scope used during a videoendoscopy examination of the larynx. This scope is shaped like a long, thin tube that is flexible. It is placed through the nose to view the soft palate and can also be positioned in the pharynx to view the larynx.

**neologism**   A nonword, or literally "new word," produced by an individual with aphasia.

**neuron**   Cell within the brain that supports activity through the conduction of chemical-electrical signals.

**nonfluent aphasia**   An aphasia profile that is characterized by effortful speech production, reduced grammatical complexity, and short utterance length.

**normative sample**   A representative sample of individuals whose performance on a test or measure serves as a reference against which a single individual's performance can be compared.

**norm-referenced test**   Test designed to allow comparisons between an individual's performance and a group of individuals of similar age.

**occipital lobe**   The posterior part of each cerebral hemisphere.

**omission error**   One of the four types of articulatory errors, in which the sound is totally omitted.

**oral-peripheral examination**   An examination of the structure and function of the face, mouth, and oral cavity, intended to assess the integrity of the articulatory mechanisms of speech.

**organ of Corti**   Area within the cochlea containing the tectorial membrane and hair cells.

**ossicles**   The three small bones (incus, malleus, stapes) that form the ossicular chain in the middle ear.

**otitis media**   Inflammation of the middle ear.

**otoacoustic emissions**   Sounds produced by the inner ear.

**otosclerosis**   A disorder of the ear that is characterized by increased vascularity and bone resorption of the stapes. It results in a progressive, conductive hearing loss when it interferes with the movement of the stapes.

**otoscope**   A lighted device with a speculum on the end used to visualize the tympanic membrane and ear canals.

**ototoxicity**    Sensory damage to the cochlear or vestibular systems from exposure to a chemical.

**oval window**    A membrane-covered opening of the vestibule of the cochlea that is attached to the footplate of the stapes. Vibration of the stapes footplate sets the oval window in vibration.

**palate**    The roof of the mouth. Anteriorly, the hard palate is bone, covered with a membrane; posteriorly, the soft palate (velum) is muscle covered with a membrane. The palate separates the oral and nasal cavities.

**paraphasia**    An erroneous word or a nonword that reflects disorders of word choice (e.g., *man* for *woman*) or sound substitution errors (e.g., *tike* for *bike*).

**parietal lobe**    One of the four lobes of the cerebral hemisphere, extending posteriorly from the Rolandic fissure to the occipital lobe.

**perinatal**    The period surrounding birth; between the twenty-ninth week of gestation to one to four weeks after birth.

**peripheral nervous system**    The nervous system that extends beyond the brain and the spinal cord, including peripheral sensory nerves that send impulses to the central nervous system and motor nerves that carry effector impulses to peripheral structures.

**peristaltic contractions**    In the esophagus, this term describes how the muscles squeeze together starting at the top and moving downward. Each neighboring segment squeezes together to push food toward the stomach.

**perisylvian region**    The region of the brain that surrounds the Sylvian fissure, which is the primary horizontal fissure for each cerebral hemisphere.

**perseveration**    Involuntary repetition of a word, phrase, sentence, or idea.

**pharynx**    The tube-shaped cavity at the back of the mouth that extends from the posterior nasal cavity to just above the larynx and trachea.

**phone**    A speech sound.

**phoneme**    The smallest sound unit of speech represented by a symbol of the International Phonetic Alphabet.

**phonemic regression**    Poor auditory comprehension often associated with advanced age.

**phonological process**    The systematic simplification by children of the production of adult-modeled articulation, such as deleting the final consonant of words or deleting a syllable within a word.

**phonology**    The study of the sounds of spoken language, including the rules of phoneme use, phonemes, phonetic production, and voicing characteristics.

**Pick's disease**    A dementing disease that is associated with atrophy of the frontal and temporal lobes.

**pinna**    The visible outer ear, also known as the auricle.

**pitch**    The perceptual correlate of the frequency of a sound as heard by the ear.

**plosive**    A speech sound produced by impounding air behind an articulator and suddenly releasing it, as in /p/ or /b/.

**postnatal**    Occurring after birth.

**prelingual**    Before the development of speech.

**prenatal**    Preceding birth.

**presbycusis**    Hearing impairment associated with the aging process.

**prevalence**    The total number of cases present in a population in a given period of time.

**primary progressive aphasia**    An acquired impairment of language that follows a slowly progressive, rather than abrupt, onset and is not associated with dementia.

**prosody**    The melody, flow, and rhythm of a spoken language; melodic changes in syllable stress, pitch, loudness, and duration.

**protoword**    Early form of an actual word that usually contains some of the sounds of the target word.

**pure tone**    A periodic sound wave of a particular frequency that is generated in the audiometric testing of hearing.

**recessive**   A term to describe genetic conditions that are only expressed when two copies of the gene causing the condition are present.

**reflux**   Refers to backward movement of food during swallowing. Often, reflux refers to acid from the stomach spilling upward into the throat, causing irritation to the tissues.

**reliability**   Quality of providing consistent information.

**Rolandic fissure**   The central fissue that divides the posterior frontal lobe from the anterior parietal lobe.

**rollover**   A phenomenon in which word recognition scores decrease as the presentation level of the stimuli increases.

**round window**   An opening in the vestibule of the cochlea beneath the oval window on the cochlea, permitting the displacement or movement of fluid within the cochlea.

**seizures**   The convulsions of an epileptic attack; epilepsy.

**semantics**   The study of the history and meaning of words.

**sensorineural hearing loss**   A hearing loss caused by disease of the inner ear or eighth cranial nerve.

**sound–symbol correspondence**   The ability to associate individual sounds with printed letters.

**spasticity**   A paralysis characterized by extreme tension and hypercontraction of muscles with hyperactive tendon reflexes.

**specific language impairment**   A diagnosis of a child who demonstrates impairment in understanding spoken language, speaking, reading, and writing with no other demonstrable impairment.

**spectrogram**   A visual display of the sound frequencies of a spoken utterance.

**speech-language pathologist**   A professional who specializes in the diagnosis and treatment of communication and swallowing disorders.

**speech-language pathology**   A profession that specializes in the diagnosis and treatment of communication disorders related to problems of hearing, articulation, language, voice, fluency, and swallowing.

**speech**   Sound production via changes in the vocal mechanism and oral structures to form words and sentences in auditory-oral communication.

**speechreading**   The use of visual cues from a talker's face to identify this or her speech.

**spinal cord**   The lower portion of the central nervous system, originating at the medulla and extending down within the spinal vertebra.

**spinal nerves**   Thirty-one pairs of nerves that enter or exit the spinal cord.

**spondaic words**   Two-syllable words pronounced with equal stress on each syllable.

**stapedectomy**   An operation in which the stapes is removed and replaced with a prosthesis in an attempt to improve a hearing impairment that was caused by otosclerosis.

**stapes**   A stirrup-shaped bone within the middle ear that attaches to the round window of the inner ear.

**stimulability testing**   In testing articulation, a determination of how well the client can produce the target sound when the sound has been repeatedly presented (visually and auditorially).

**STORCH**   Acronym for syphillis, toxoplasmosis, other, rubella, cytomegalovirus, and herpes simplex infections.

**stroke**   Sudden onset of disturbed neurological functioning caused by disruption of blood flow. Also called a cerebrovascular accident (CVA), usually one of three types: thrombosis, embolus, or hemorrhage.

**stuttering**   The involuntary repetition, interruption, and prolongation of speech sounds and syllables, which the individual struggles to end.

**subglottal air pressure**   The air pressure within the airway below the vocal folds; outgoing air moves between the vocal folds when pressure below the folds is greater than air pressure above them.

**substitution error**   A type of articulation error characterized by an incorrect phoneme used in place of a target phoneme, such as /w/ said for /r/.

**Sylvian fissure**   The horizontal fissure that divides the inferior border of the frontal and parietal lobes from the superior temporal lobe.

**syndrome**   A collection of physical features that co-occur and characterize a disorder or condition.

**syntax**   The grammatical structure and word order of a language.

**telecommunication device for the deaf (TDD)**   A keyboard that attaches to a telephone to allow typewritten communication with other TDDs. It enables individuals with hearing difficulties to communicate using the telephone.

**telegraphic speech**   Spoken communication that consists primarily of content words and is lacking functor words, such as pronouns, auxilary verbs, and articles.

**temporal lobe**   One of the four lobes of a cerebral hemisphere, lying below the Sylvian fissure.

**thalamus**   A large gray mass of sensory nuclei deep within the hemisphere, bordering the third ventricle.

**thyroid cartilage**   The shield-shaped outer cartilage protecting the larynx; popularly called the Adam's apple.

**tinnitus**   Noises in the ear(s) usually described as ringing, hissing, or roaring.

**tongue thrust**   Abnormal tongue positioning, particularly during swallowing, that may have an adverse effect on the anterior dental bite.

**tracheostoma**   A permanent opening in the neck that is surgically created. This is usually done because the larynx has been surgically removed or is not able to open enough to allow breathing, such as with bilateral vocal fold paralysis or injury to the larynx.

**transformer**   A device or mechanism that changes the nature or properties of a signal or substance.

**traumatic laryngitis**   A dysphonia related to excessive use of harmful voicing behaviors such as yelling and screaming.

**tympanic membrane**   The round membrane between the ear canal and middle ear, also known as the eardrum.

**use**   The rules for communicative interactions, including the social-interactive aspects of language, sometimes called pragmatics.

**validity**   The quality of providing accurate or true information.

**velum**   The soft palate.

**videoendoscopy**   This procedure uses special fiberoptic equipment to obtain views of the internal structure of the larynx.

**videofluoroscopy**   The process whereby X-ray images of motion are recorded on videotape for the purpose of examination of function, such as in the study of swallowing.

**video otoscopy**   A system that provides enlarged images that can be viewed on a monitor, stored on disk, or printed. Applications include visualization of the outer ear, tympanic membrane, and middle ear and counseling regarding hearing instrument insertion, operation, and hygiene.

**vocal nodules**   Benign growths on the vocal folds, usually bilateral, which are typically the result of laryngeal abuse and voice misuse.

**vocal polyps**   Benign growths on the vocal folds that usually occur unilaterally and are soft and compliant fluid-filled bags. These occur as a result of excessive use of harmful vocal habits such as yelling and screaming.

**vocalization**   Voicing or phonation.

**voice**   The production of sound by vibration of the vocal folds.

**waveform**   The graph of the oscillations corresponding to the frequency of a sound.

**Wernicke's aphasia**   A fluent aphasia characterized by poor auditory comprehension and paraphasic utterances.

# AUTHOR INDEX

# SUBJECT INDEX